Deus in Machina

Deus in Machina

Religion, Technology, and the Things in Between

Edited by

Jeremy Stolow

FORDHAM UNIVERSITY PRESS

New York 2013

Copyright © 2013 Fordham University Press

All rights reserved. No part of this publication may be reproduced, stored in a retrieval system, or transmitted in any form or by any means—electronic, mechanical, photocopy, recording, or any other—except for brief quotations in printed reviews, without the prior permission of the publisher.

Fordham University Press has no responsibility for the persistence or accuracy of URLs for external or third-party Internet websites referred to in this publication and does not guarantee that any content on such websites is, or will remain, accurate or appropriate.

Fordham University Press also publishes its books in a variety of electronic formats. Some content that appears in print may not be available in electronic books.

Library of Congress Cataloging-in-Publication Data

Deus in machina : religion, technology, and the things in between / edited by Jeremy Stolow. — 1st ed.
  p. cm.
 Includes bibliographical references.
 ISBN 978-0-8232-4980-0 (cloth) — ISBN 978-0-8232-4981-7 (pbk.)
 1. Technology—Religious aspects. 2. Medicine—Religious aspects. 3. Religion and science. I. Stolow, Jeremy, 1965–
 BL265.T4.D48 2013
 201'.66—dc23

2012028202

15 14 13 5 4 3 2 1
First edition

CONTENTS

List of Illustrations   vii
Acknowledgments   ix

Introduction: Religion, Technology, and the Things in Between
    JEREMY STOLOW   1

EQUIPMENT

Calendar, Clock, Tower
    JOHN DURHAM PETERS   25

Ticking Clock, Vibrating String: How Time Sense Oscillates Between Religion and Machine
    WOLFGANG ERNST   43

The Electric Touch Machine Miracle Scam: Body, Technology, and the (Dis)authentication of the Pentecostal Supernatural
    MARLEEN DE WITTE   61

The Spiritual Nervous System: Reflections on a Magnetic Cord Designed for Spirit Communication
    JEREMY STOLOW   83

BIO-POWER

An Empowered World: Buddhist Medicine and the Potency of Prayer in Japan
    JASON ĀNANDA JOSEPHSON   117

Does Submission to God's Will Preclude Biotechnological Intervention? Lessons from Muslim Dialysis Patients in Contemporary Egypt
    SHERINE F. HAMDY   143

The Canary in the Gemeinschaft? Disability, Film,
and the Jewish Question
  FAYE GINSBURG   159

(RE)LOCATING RELIGION IN A TECHNOLOGICAL AGE
Thinking about Melville, Religion, and Machines That Think
  JOHN LARDAS MODERN   183
Amazing Stories: How Science Fiction Sacralizes the Secular
  PETER PELS   213
Virtual Vodou, Actual Practice: Transfiguring the Technological
  ALEXANDRA BOUTROS   239
TV St. Claire
  MARIA JOSÉ A. DE ABREU   261

Notes   281
List of Contributors   353

ILLUSTRATIONS

1	Anchor Escapement Mechanism in a Clockwork	49
2	Advertisement for the Electric Touch Magic Trick	62
3	Stage Backdrop to the International Central Gospel Church	70
4	Book cover, *Catch the Anointing*, by Dag Heward-Mills	75
5	"The Magic Rope"	85
6	"Clairvoyance and Spirit Impression"	94
7	Austrian participants holding photos of child victims of the Holocaust	166
8	"Robot-Worship"	206
9	"God" (1917)	207

ACKNOWLEDGMENTS

This book was first conceived during conversations that took place while I was a visiting fellow at the Center for Religion and Media at New York University in 2003–2004. My thanks to all the members of the Center during that time, especially Faye Ginsburg, Angela Zito, Elizabeth Castelli, and Mazyar Lotfalian. In January 2007 I convened a colloquium at the Art Gallery of Hamilton (Hamilton, Ontario, Canada) entitled "Deus in Machina," which led to the present volume. I wish to acknowledge the following financial supporters, without whom this colloquium would not have happened: the Social Sciences and Humanities Research Council of Canada; the Office of the Dean of Social Science, McMaster University; the Office of the Vice President (Research), McMaster University; the Office of the Provost, McMaster University; and the Office of the Dean of Humanities, McMaster University. Acknowledgement must also be given to the participants in that colloquium who greatly sharpened our collective understanding of religion and technology, especially, but not only: James Benn, Ellen Badone, Thomas A. Carlson, Yasser Haddarah, Stephen Hughes, Barbara Kirshenblatt-Gimblett, Travis Kroeker, Mazyar Lotfalian, Carly Machado, Valentina Napolitano, Celia Rothenberg, Mark Rowe, and Dorien Zandbergen. A special word of thanks goes to Benjamin Fleming for his tremendous help as the colloquium's administrative assistant.

At Fordham University Press, I wish to thank above all Helen Tartar, whose vision, exacting standards, and scholarly passion are unparalleled in academic publishing. It has been a sheer pleasure to work with her, alongside the other diligent staff members of the press—not least, Thomas Lay—who helped bring this book to its successful conclusion.

For his contribution to this book, John Durham Peters wishes to thank Routledge for permission to adapt and revise the previously published entries "Calendar" and "Clock" in *The Encyclopedia of Religion, Communication, and Media*, ed. Daniel A. Stout (New York: Routledge, 2006), 57–59, 77–79. Sherine Hamdy wishes to thank the journal *Anthropology Quarterly* for allowing her to reprint several passages from her article "Islam, Fatalism, and Medical Intervention: Lessons from Egypt on the Cultivation of Forbearance (Sabr) and Reliance on God (Tawakkul)," 82, no. 1 (2009): 97–120. John Lardas Modern wishes to thank the journal *Method and Theory in the Study of Religion* for granting him permission to revise his previously published article "Deus in Machina Movet: Religion in the Age of Technological Reproducibility," 18, no.1 (2006): 1–36. Jeremy Stolow wishes to thank Routledge for permission to reprint a few lines from his earlier publication of "Technology" in *Key Words in Religion, Media and Culture*, ed. David Morgan (New York: Routledge, 2008), 187–97.

As the editor, I wish to thank all the contributors of this volume for their ongoing commitment to this project, as well as my many friends, colleagues, mentors, and students who offered valuable insight, lively debate, and encouragement on the long road that edited books so often must travel (there are too many of you to be listed by name; let me hope you know you are being addressed here). On behalf of all the book's contributing authors, I also wish to acknowledge the anonymous reviewers who provided helpful comments on earlier drafts of the book. For their help in preparing the manuscript for submission to the press, I thank my editorial assistants, Erin Despard and Brian Fauteux. The final word of thanks, as always, goes to my family, Danielle and Malka, for all their support and love; they are the deities who animate my machine.

Deus in Machina

Introduction

Religion, Technology, and the Things in Between

Jeremy Stolow

In ancient Greek tragedy it was not uncommon to resolve a particular dramatic crisis with the sudden intervention of a god, a strategy with which the playwright Euripides had a particular affinity. At the appointed moment during the play performers would utilize a trapdoor in the floor of the stage or employ a *mēchanê*, a sort of crane with a pulley attached to it, to lower, raise, or exhibit motionless in midair a statue or an actor dressed as a deity, often the god Zeus. Such a miraculous apparition would interrupt the dramatic events taking place on stage, typically for the purpose of rescuing characters from an impending doom.[1] But this dramaturgical convention, *apò mēchanês theós* ("the god out of the machine"), was denigrated by a long line of critics, starting with Aristotle, who lamented playwrights' overreliance on such a cheap and "merely mechanical" resolution of dramatic tensions.[2] In this tradition the convention of *apò mēchanês theós* and its Latin calque, *deus ex machina*, came to refer to any formulaic use of a plot device in which a conveniently perfect solution emerges for an otherwise inextricable problem in the story through the insertion of an entirely unexpected character, object, or event. Underlying the critics' longstanding disdain for the employment of *deus ex machina*, perhaps we might note an even deeper disdain for mechanical manipulation. Apparently, authentic divine presence, if it is to remain authentic, is not supposed to manifest itself as an instrument in the service of the human hand. Wherever we think we see gods sprouting out of our tools and machines we are merely bearing witness to the fruits of our own human labor, and only a poor poet (or a gullible spectator) would suppose otherwise. There is in fact a long history of association of the word *machina* with abject notions of trickery and deceit, as evident in the Latin verb *māchinārī*, "to invent, contrive, or devise," a reference still preserved in the English noun *machination*: a crafty scheme designed to accomplish a sinister end.[3] Here, perhaps, is one archaic trace preserved in the modern conception of religion as an ideological mechanism brought to bear upon superstitious populations by an impudent and cunning priesthood, as proposed by David Hume in his *Natural History of Religion* (1757), Ludwig Feuerbach in his *Lectures on the Essence of Religion* (1851), and Emile Durkheim in his *Elementary Forms of Religious Life* (1912), to name but three figures within a crowded lineage of scholars dedicated to exposing the machine hiding behind our ghostly illusions.[4]

The title of this book, *Deus in Machina*, purposefully inverts the presumed relationship between divine entities and the mechanisms that render them present. Rather than foreclosing discussion about whether and how one must choose between human-built machines and the authentic presence of gods, spirits, and other transcendent forces and things, this book seeks to revisit and revise the very supposition that religion and technology exist as two ontologically distinct arenas of experience, knowledge, and action. In common parlance, the word *religion* typically refers to the intangible realms of ritual expression, ethical reasoning, affect, and belief, whereas the word *technology* points to the material appurtenances, mechanical operations, and expert knowledge that enable humans to act upon, and in concert with, the very tangible domains of nature and society. The locution *religion and technology* thus operates alongside a series of analogous binaries, including *faith and reason, fantasy and reality, enchantment and disenchantment, magic and science,* and *fabrication and fact*. To talk about religion and technology, therefore, would appear to be a relatively straightforward matter of properly deploying the "and" that conjoins the two terms. Religiously derived emotions, beliefs, ethical motivations, and performative repertoires can be added to—or subtracted from—the otherwise independent operations of technologies that do their work "in the real world," producing their effects in accordance with established laws of physics. Religious actors can embrace, avoid, reject, or repurpose technologies; they can tell stories about the sources of inspiration that led to their creation; they can develop their own vocabularies to describe how and why they work; and they can even come to regard the things they or their fellow humans built with their own hands as idols, fetishes, talismans, or transubstantiations of ordinary matter into sacred matter. But *technology* refers to an order of things existing outside of and independent from all such dispositions, uses, and frameworks of meaning, and there is not supposed to be anything allegorical about the work technologies perform or the things they can or cannot do.

However, as Bruno Latour reminds us, it is not so easy, nor is it so desirable, to distinguish between reality and its construction. Facts about the natural world have always only come to us through the work of fabrication: through controlled modes of experimentation and observation and through the social allocation of credibility and expertise. And yet, once constructed, these facts manage to erase their own origins in order to present themselves, quite magically, as things that have been merely discovered, not made. For Latour it is this process of construction and denial of constructedness that brings the "real" world of technoscience into curiously close alignment with the "illusory" universe of idol-worship, fetishism, and other acts of bearing witness to transcendent powers of miracle, magic, and fate. One of the aims of this book is to take seriously Latour's attempt to shake us free from the ingrained wisdom that presumes there is a clear and unproblematic divide between reality and construction—or, as Latour provocatively suggests, between fact and fetish—in order to immerse ourselves in a labile, category-confusing universe of "autonomous creations," including such things as "lactic acid ferments, divinities, black holes, tangled genes, apparitions of the Virgin, and so on. What do we have to lose? What are we afraid of?"[5] In a similar vein this book asks: Is it still useful—is it still even possible—to imagine that religion and technology can be parceled out as two discrete dimensions of the cosmos? What is at stake in the provocation of this book's title to locate "god *in* the machine?" Who has the authority to weigh those stakes? What might be gained or lost once religious and technological things are allowed to mingle promiscuously with one another?

The chapters that follow suggest various answers to such questions. They do so by experimenting with different vocabularies, analytical approaches, and exemplary stories in order to revisit long-cherished assumptions about the overlaps and the differences among humans, techniques, tools, machines, spirits, gods, and other natural and supernatural entities and forces. The ensuing conversation (a term I choose intentionally to signal that readers should not expect to find a seamless unity of opinion among the contributors to this volume) brings together scholars from several disciplinary locations, including those of the anthropology and history of religion, media history, and media archaeology. This interdisciplinary dialogue was first staged at a conference on religion and technology held in Hamilton, Canada, in 2007 (although some of the contributors to this book joined the conversation later on), the aim of which was to take stock of the appearance in different disciplines of strikingly comparable research questions and thematic concerns with regard to the technologization of religion and the religiosity of technology, even if these overlaps have not always been properly acknowledged.

In particular *Deus in Machina* is premised on two scholarly discussions that have blazed significant trails for thinking in new ways about religion and technology. The first one comprises what has recently been dubbed the "media turn" in the study of religion.[6] Over the past decade or so, a remarkable body of historical and ethnographic work has pushed the study of religion beyond its customary modes of engagement with sacred texts, rituals, structures of belief, abstract principles of ethical conduct, and institutional definitions of identity and belonging.[7] This literature has called new attention to the many ways religious practice and imagination are inextricably bound up with the materialities of media and the labor of mediation—not just textual or iconographic systems of representation, but also a much broader terrain of sensorial techniques, tools, material artifacts, and systems of coordinated action. Some scholars have focused on the proliferation of technological platforms, institutional arrangements, and representational strategies gathered under the term *new media*, exploring how the functional logics of digital and mobile media bear elective affinities with the expanding public presence of transnational religious movements or, more broadly, with the restructuring of practices, discourses, patterns of adherence, and systems of exchange that has been visited upon religious communities in virtually every region of the world today, even (perhaps especially) at the frontiers of so-called secular society. Others have been busy reexamining and reassessing older modes of religious mediation, such as music, book publishing, sacred architecture, and markets for the circulation of magical goods and services, in each case attending to the ways both private and public arenas of religious power and experience have been shaped—historically and in the present—by technologies that reorganize social time and space or offer new means of storing, retrieving, and distributing knowledge. What unites all this work is a common commitment to (at least some version of) the claim that media provide

Introduction

the deep conditions of possibility for religious adherents to proclaim their faith, mark their affiliation, receive spiritual gifts, or participate in any of the countless local idioms for making the sacred present to mind and body.[8] Technology—in the enlarged sense of materials, techniques, instruments, and expertise—forms the gridwork of orientations, operations, and embedded and embodied knowledges and powers without which religious ideas, experiences, and actions could not exist, even if such mediations are denigrated or repressed in the name of transcendent immediacy (or an unmediated transcendent).[9]

At the very same time that anthropologists and historians of religion have been busy assessing the technological materialities of religious experience and expression, a parallel discussion has been unfolding among students of science, technology, and media aimed at revising received assumptions about the construction and functioning of modern technologies and their interface with human experience. In particular, historians as well as observers of the contemporary period have distanced themselves from the venerable "conflict thesis" of religion and science in order to attend more closely to the modes of wonder-making that shape public science and the systems of faith that undergird technoscientific knowledge and practice: not just the science and technology produced in laboratories, but also those produced at conferences and in schools, at factories and in offices, at public demonstrations and in museums, among other scenes for the construction, popularization, and domestic consumption of technoscientific instruments, practices, and bodies of knowledge.[10]

Having dismissed innocent accounts of technology as the instrument of human intention and the handmaiden of social progress, a growing chorus of scholars has placed a new premium on technology's sacral and/or magical dimensions. Because of their imponderable complexities, their autonomous, networked agency, and their capacities to compress time, erase distance, and reproduce sameness, modern technologies have thus come to be understood as possessing transcendent or uncanny features, the encounter with which is phenomenologically comparable with the performative techniques of prayer, ritual action, or magic, or with the "religious" experiences of ecstasy and awe—as famously argued by Jacques Derrida in his account of what he describes as the return of a repressed, "primitive" animism within modern tele-technoscience.[11] From the pixilated color screens that dazzle our eyes to the surveillance systems that track every moment of daily life to industrial megaprojects that threaten the planetary ecosystem, the advancement and diffusion of new technologies increasingly seem to play on longstanding religious themes of (in)finitude, salvation, and fate. In the rapidly evolving domains of robotics, bioengineering, and digitally mediated communications, observers have documented a steady erosion of once-confident distinctions between humans and other bodies, as the authority of Linnaean taxonomy appears to be giving way to a new cosmology of virtual projections, "cybergnostic" modes of dispersed intelligence, and the generation of all manner of half-human, half-machine hybrid "monsters."[12] More broadly still, one might say that myths, monsters, ghosts, angels, karmic forces, and enchanted objects seem everywhere to be on the rise: in the generation of visual phantasmagoria and cinematic illusions (and other mediated spectacles based on the logic of "special effects"); in the transnational circulation of Pokémon video games and trading cards; or in the vertiginous experience of the Internet as global society's collective "digital sublime"; among other instances where (as Peter Pels words it, in his contribution to this volume) "religious" modes of knowledge, practice, and experience are making their appearance in "nonreligious" contexts.[13]

Deus in Machina builds upon these discussions, seeking to bridge hitherto disconnected disciplinary perspectives on religion, technology, and the things in between. It does so by pursuing paths of inquiry that rub against the grain of common wisdom and that challenge the established scholarly consensus about where and how to divide religion and technology from one another. Having invoked the figure of "established scholarship," I ought to add a few words about the general shape of the existing literature. Of course it would be a daunting, if not tedious, task to enumerate and describe all the works that have some bearing on the topic of religion and technology.[14] One would have to consider not only the more recent discussions I have just enumerated, but also a much larger and older body of scholarship. Indeed, since at least the late nineteenth century, there has been a steady outpouring of books, conference proceedings, newspaper editorials, and special issues of journals penned by social scientists, theologians, philosophers, medical ethicists, engineers, ecologists, and others concerned with the ethical assessment of particular technological procedures or, more generally, with the conditions of social life, both historically and in our present "technological age." One strand of scholarship focuses on the contributions made by ancient and medieval theologians, monastic orders, magi, and other "religious folk" in the development of numerous technical arts, including medicine, pharmacology, architecture, astronomy, navigation, timekeeping, lenscrafting, and metal casting.[15] David Noble's widely read account of the origins of modern Western conceptions of technological mastery and popular forms of faith in technological progress highlights the eschatological context of medieval European Christianity and the role played by theological categories of redemption, the millennium, and Armageddon.[16] Other studies hone in on the Renaissance and early modern Europe in order to trace the contributions of mystical vision, natural magic, millenarian motivations, and ecclesiastical allegiances to the generation of modern scientific credibility.[17] Another body of literature documents the religious biographies of natural philosophers, doctors, inventors, and engineers—Abu Rayhan al-Biruni, the Muslim scientific polymath; Robert Boyle, the Puritan; Isaac Newton, the alchemist; and John Wesley, the Methodist electrotherapist—alongside history's countless autodidacts, self-styled inventors, witches, medicine men, and other non-elites whose technological engagements have been lost under the general sign *magic*.[18] Yet another body of work explores the ambiguously magical status of instruments within histories of scientific experiment and natural philosophy and their relationship with an expanding public culture of scientific exhibition and display.[19] Even further afield, the study of religion and technology has also been shaped by contributions of numerous engineers and scientists, from Norbert Wiener's colorful attempt (in 1964) to apply a version of the Turing Test to demonstrate the affinity between God and computers to Dean Hamer's more recent summary of ongoing neuroscientific efforts to locate "the god gene" or the "religion" function within the human brain.[20]

Deus in Machina thus finds itself at the crossroads of a dizzying number of pathways for the study of religion and technology. What can yet another book hope to accomplish? The contributors to this volume proceed on the assumption that critical engagement with religion and technology remains an incomplete task and that there is in fact plenty of room for further documentation, comparison, and, above all, reflection. As individual chapters and also as parts of a collective enterprise, the studies undertaken here intervene into the existing literature on several fronts. In the remainder of this introduction, I shall attempt to highlight what I take to be this book's key contributions.

Beyond Instrumentalism

The first contribution of *Deus in Machina* is its attempt to revisit and reconsider the dominant instrumentalist conceptions of technology that issue directly from ongoing efforts to keep religion and technology separate from one another. At the risk of caricaturing the literature referenced earlier, and despite its enormous variances in historical and cultural context, let us take note of a strikingly recurring analytical strategy. One begins by trying to identify the practices and beliefs of particular historical actors, who for their part are distinguished by their religious commitments, affinities, and habits, and *then* traces the decisions of these actors to use, refuse, or repurpose particular technologies in the service of religious goals such as spiritual purification, missionary conquest, salvation, and the expiation of sin. Sometimes this is an exercise of addition: religious actor plus technology equals religious outcome. The careers of British and American tract, Bible, and missionary societies provide a familiar illustration of this formula. Nineteenth-century Protestant intellectuals and activists are widely reported to have been enthusiastic champions of emerging technologies of communication and transportation (such as stereotypography, steam-powered transit, and electromagnetic telegraphy) and new methods of technical coordination of information (such as statistics and bookkeeping). These were greeted as signs of Providence and as tools perfectly designed to service of their mission to "spread good news" among mass populations on an unprecedented global scale.[21] At other times the exercise is one of subtraction: religious actor minus technology equals religious outcome. This formula structures many narratives about religious acts of resistance, censorship, or refusal in the face of technological change, whereby new instruments and practices are treated as threats to established hierocratic authority, as spiritual pollutants, or as violations of sacred law. In some of the more dramatic cases, new technologies herald the presence of the devil—an association emblematically conveyed in the declaration made by Pope Gregory XVI on the occasion of his decision (in 1836) to prohibit the construction of railways in the Papal States: *chemin de fer, chemin d'enfer* [the "iron road" is the road to hell].[22]

However, as each of the chapters of *Deus in Machina* shows, the calculus of addition and subtraction does not get us very far when it comes to trying to understand the exact role played by particular instruments and technical procedures for religious actors and within religious contexts of action. In the first instance technologies rarely (if ever) can be fully enclosed within the conceptual horizons and the operational intentions of their makers. Nor is it tenable to explain resistances to technology with recourse to some variant of the proposition that, because "lay people" tend to possess a limited understanding of the underlying principles and operational characteristics of technologies, their relationships are based on hearsay, superstition, or cognitive dissonance. What, then, helps instrumentalism retain its commonsense status?

Introduction 9

Hiding behind what I am here calling "instrumentalist" treatments of technology, it is perhaps possible to detect the half-buried presence of magic. Magic is the family of tools, techniques, and understandings of the world that, according to a long tradition of scholarship, is supposedly located within the province of "the primitive mind": as a parapractical mode of action and a prerational effort to explain causal forces in the universe. Magic is the ancestor (or illegitimate cousin) of what we moderns call technology. In the larger historical scheme of things, magic is something that was (or ought to have been) superseded by a more sober reliance upon techniques and instruments that "actually do their jobs" and by the advancement of scientific reasoning that "properly" frames knowledge about such work. The divide between religion and technology thus appears to be rooted in claims that are at once historical and epistemological, and to those extents the very divide is an outcome of a process Bruno Latour famously called "purification."[23] Magic—the third term that floats promiscuously in between the orders of knowledge and faith, action and fantasy, or the tangible and the merely ponderable—is that which must be systematically excluded for the sake of the integrity of religion, on the one hand, and technoscience, on the other.[24] In other words, it was precisely through the disavowal and repression of magic that both modern sciences and modern religions were born: religions and sciences that "know their place" by remaining safely segregated from each other's performative and epistemological prerogatives. This operation is necessary in order to lay the groundwork for further elaborations of technology as a "disenchanted" realm of tools, devices, techniques, and expert knowledges governed by its own internal logic: a realm that religious actors can only ever approach from the outside. And yet magic, the excluded middle, has never simply disappeared. As emphasized by a growing body of scholars (many of whom have already been cited), modernity is pervasively haunted by its very effort to disenchant the world.[25]

In the pages that follow, the reader will encounter a variety of instruments and technical processes—calendars, clocks, and towers (Peters), oscillating clocks (Ernst), feedback mechanisms (Modern), miraculous "touch machines" (de Witte), magnetized cables (Stolow), and kidney dialysis treatments (Hamdy), to name a few—the discussion of which greatly troubles instrumentalist presumptions about technological efficacy and about the chasm that supposedly divides scientific understanding from "religious" or "magical" modes of apprehending and working in the world. Some of the contributors to *Deus in Machina* explicitly align the objects of their study with magic in order to provoke a reconsideration of the terms on which technology is supposed to be divided from the supernatural, while others seek alternative means of calling instrumentalist presumptions into question. One theme running through several chapters has to do with the struggles among religious (and nonreligious) actors to recognize, authorize, and authenticate instances of technological efficacy. In his history of Buddhist therapeutic practices in Japan, Jason Josephson traces efforts to repress older conceptions of *kaji* (empowerment) through the systematic disempowerment of ritual healers and the domestication of Buddhist prayer as something merely supplementary (if not antithetical) to modern medical technique. Marleen de Witte explores how "miracle-working" Pentecostal pastors in contemporary Ghana produce extraordinary experiences of "God's touch" at the very same time that a broader public anxiety about the possibility of fraudulence and charlatanism has been reshaping the terms on which techniques for mediating the invisible realm of the Holy Spirit can be authenticated. Authenticity also emerges as a key theme in Alexandra Boutros's chapter, which documents the fraught terms on which Haitian Vodou is repackaged in the context of "cyberspace," a realm where diverse knowledge seekers and service providers encounter one another and where reliable access to "traditional" Vodou rituals and practices is routinely called into question by fiercely competing authority figures. In my own chapter on a nineteenth-century technology designed for spirit communication, I attend to the broader arena of popular science within which advocates as well as detractors of Spiritualism compete for the authority to define and operate instruments that purport to register the presence of "invisible" forces, variously described as electricity, nervous energy, sympathy, and spirit. Through these and other cases, *Deus in Machina* offers a far-reaching survey of things that are understood to serve as instruments of religious knowledge, power, imagination, and experience. In so doing, this book illuminates paths of inquiry that circumvent the instrumentalist cul-de-sac, allowing us to return with fresh eyes to the very question of what is a religious instrument.

Revis(it)ing Technology

Whereas instrumentalist accounts of religion and technology focus on the agency, motives, and strategic calculations of religious actors, other discussions turn on broader questions about the cosmological, ethical, and theological dimensions of technology itself: as a force of history-making and as a mode of being-in-the-world. One longstanding liberal tradition invokes technological change, and the rise of modern technology in particular, as the guarantor of convenience and abundance and of physiological and civic improvement, as voiced by a long line of techno-gurus from Thomas Edison to Bill Gates. When listening to such champions of technological progress, it is not difficult to hear echoes of the rhetoric and poetics of religious prophecy and the visualization of a salvific future free from toil, disease, isolation, forgetfulness, and other bodily catastrophes. Of course, that optimism is frequently countered by much darker assessments of our technological present and future: assessments that are no less indulgent in the language of cosmogony and prophecy, as epitomized by the work of Martin Heidegger, Jacques Ellul, Paul Tillich, and others who share an understanding of technology as a deep, systemic, and insidious mode of apprehending and dealing with the world.[26] In that tradition technology is positioned within a theology of creation and action that privileges the principle of efficiency over all other normative criteria, compelling us to regard the natural world as a legitimate object of mastery and control or, in Heidegger's terms, to reduce the world we encounter to *Gestell* ("standing reserve"). Heidegger's account of modern technological being-in-the-world has inspired successive generations of scholars to explore the internal logic that governs technology's steady colonization of our lived experience. As modern technologies develop, it is often noted, they incorporate larger and more complicated functions, their operational properties become increasingly difficult to discern, and they become increasingly unpredictable and unstable, having long freed themselves from the willful intentions of their original designers and users. Their apparent autonomy and self-determining functionality thus make modern technologies appear inexorable, sublime—even imperious. As Heidegger himself put it in a posthumously published interview, today we appear to have become so thoroughly subjugated to the imperatives of technological thinking that "only a God can save us."[27]

Heidegger was neither the first nor the last to comment on the growing discrepancy between "technical" and "cultural" systems of action and knowledge production, and the legacy of his meditations on technology are difficult to assess, not least because they have so readily been caricatured as a naïve form of technophobia.[28] At the risk of further perpetuating that caricature, I want to focus on one specific dimension of Heidegger's argument that seems most pertinent to the study of religion and technology and that helps to highlight the contributions offered by this book. My concern lies with the association of technology with the "merely machinic"—as opposed to the "poetic"—realm of thought and experience, which Heidegger and others seek to recuperate as that which make humans "authentically" human. In everyday language the word *technical* refers to a realm of dispassionate, disinterested, even "spiritless" activities. Technical operations are not supposed to "mean" anything; they just do their work (it is we humans who add the "poetic" meanings). In this sense technicality marks the zero-degree point of religious presence; neither positive nor negative, technical actions are thus understood to constitute the "dead letter" of the word or the "bare bones" of ritual performance. The spread of a technical mentality—governed by the cold laws of prosaics rather than the lyric laws of poetry—can thereby serve as the sign of a steady retreat from human authenticity, and by that token presumably as a retreat from authentic religiosity, as well. This argument borrows not only from (a version of) Heidegger's critique of technology, but also from Max Weber's account of the role of formal procedural rationality (*Zweckrationalität*) within a larger historical drive toward a world in which, as Weber put it, "one can, in principle, master all things by calculation. This means that the world is disenchanted. One need no longer have recourse to magical means in order to master or implore the spirits, as did the savage, for whom such mysterious powers existed. Technical means and calculations perform the service."[29] Weber's decision to counterpoise "magic" and "the technical" is part and parcel of a much broader effort to explain the force and direction of Western secularization or the supposed loss of aura in the mechanical age (as some readers of Benjamin would have it), and it has even made its appearance in interpretations of religious fundamentalism, which is often castigated for its "spiritless" textual literalism and its emphasis on the "machine-like" precision of ritual practice.[30]

Technology thus plays a leading role in some of the most prevalent accounts of modernity as the outcome of the disenchantment of nature and society: a historical process that has turned the world into an inert cosmos, subject to human powers of detached observation and calculated manipulation. But where does this conception of the "technical" (as opposed to the "magical") character of technology come from? As Heidegger himself was at pains to point out, modern technical rationality is rooted in a long history. In classical Greek philosophy, *techne*—a term that originally meant "to put together, to weave, or to connect things through art, artifice or craft"—was generally understood to furnish an inferior form of knowledge about the cosmos when compared to *episteme*, the systematic mode of contemplation that furnished universal and timeless truths.[31] It is only in the modern period that one begins to see an erosion of the classical division between the base "mechanical arts" and the lofty contemplative powers of

Introduction

natural philosophy. And it was only in the nineteenth century that people began referring to technology in the singular, an abstraction that was furthered over the course of the twentieth century with the rise of large-scale, increasingly bureaucratized networks of scientists, engineers, planners, and managers working in trade, industry, and government.[32]

A key development in the history of this shifting semantic terrain arguably begins with the collusion between post-Reformation Christianity and early modern natural philosophy, a marriage that had global consequences once interlaced with the history of European colonial conquest and the expansion of Western military and economic supremacy. The rise of modern science in the West has indeed often been interpreted as a radical break with medieval cosmologies and so-called primitive modes of magical thinking, a break coincident with the development of post-Reformation Christian accounts of the universe that were equally insistent on the need to separate knowledge of the natural world from higher forms of contemplation. One exemplary contribution to this effort was provided by Calvinist theology, which denied the intermediate power of bishops, kings, saints, angels, and even the Virgin Mary, and in so doing radically distanced both human subjects and the natural order from their absolute, unknowable, sovereign creator. For their part, figures such as Galileo, Descartes, Bacon, and Newton are said to have inaugurated modern science by having overturned once and forever the existing Thomist, neo-Platonic, and magical understandings of nature as a vast web of resemblances, sympathetic rapports, or final causes. As a new breed of "secular theologians," the fathers of modern science thus transformed nature into mere matter: a uniform entity, extended in space—and therefore amenable to precise measurement and controlled observation—and organized by universal principles of mechanical cause and effect, action and reaction.[33]

As a legatee of this process of desacralizing nature, the modern definition of technology thus posits a fundamental divide between human and nonhuman agents. This divide is precisely what makes technology potentially threatening for authentic human experience, including the modes of ethical living that are said to shape religious ways of being-in-the-world. But were technology and culture ever so neatly detached from one another? Is it really possible to recuperate forms of human existence "before" technology? Is the tradition of critique of technology's "inauthenticity" implicated in a deeper (unacknowledged?) set of assumptions about what it means to be human: assumptions that inform definitions of religion as a realm of experience, meaning, and authentic expression detached from and opposed to the instrumentality of technical things?

Over the course of the past half century a growing scholarly literature has called into question the ways humanity and technology are typically imagined to be distinct from one another precisely in order to find themselves in relationships of cooperation or conflict. For the paleoanthropologist André Leroi-Gourhan, technology was from the very beginning a partner in the evolution of humanity itself, forming a "curtain of objects" or an "artificial envelope" that mediates between the interior milieu of human subjectivity and the exterior milieu of geography, climate, flora, and fauna. The collaboration of humans and other living beings (prey, seeds, domestic animals), as well as nonliving matter (tools, shelter, clothing) form the very basis of life, action, and subjectivity stretching back to the darkest origins of the human species. Even the evolutionary transition to bipedality was implicated in a technogenetic process that freed hands for the activity of grasping objects and positioned the face for the development of complex techniques of gesture and speech. In this sense the emergence of the human species was inescapably tied to the history of technological invention and intervention in the form of memories and schemata of action exuded from human minds and bodies and inscribed onto tools: the hammer that multiplies our strength; the arrow that overcomes our slow-moving legs and weak teeth and nails; and the diagrams, tokens, and tallies (and later, more complex forms of numerical notation and writing) that store and retrieve information more effectively than our limited memories.[34]

Leroi-Gourhan's approach represents one eddy within a broader intellectual current addressing the relationship between technology and the human on terms that seek a way out of the conditions of war that supposedly rages between them. Drawing directly on Leroi-Gourhan (among other sources), Bernard Stiegler has coined the term *epiphylogenesis* to refer to the notion that humanity and technology have always been constitutive of one another in the form of Promethean "gifts" to compensate for what Stiegler calls "the fault of Epimetheus," referring to the Greek titan who, when charged to equip animals with the traits they needed for survival, overlooked humans and left them helpless.[35] Stiegler's orientation to technology merits comparison with other efforts to dissolve the distinction between human and nonhuman forms of agency, as in the case of actor-network theory, which also seeks to redistribute the epistemic privileges monopolized by human agents and to reevaluate the assumption that nonhuman agencies are mere supplements (or impediments) to human will.[36] The effort to displace the centrality of the human subject also forms a central plank of recent media theory, not least in the field of media archaeology, which has sought to challenge the hegemony of language-based models to describe technological operations and the human-machine interface, in order to rethink the relationship between technological operations and (human) conditions of perception and experience.[37]

In different ways each of these veins of critical thought has been concerned to transcend the distinction between (authentic) humans and (inauthentic) instruments and machines as presumed by (at least a version of) Heidegger and other critics of the technicity of technology. These divisions are breached in the name of a new appreciation of "the nonhuman," a category that not only includes such things as hydroelectric power plants, jet engines, staircases, ink, flowers, hair, animal blood, DVDs, and mobile telephones, but that also encompasses gods, angels, jinns, demons, bodhisattvas, saints, ethical principles, statements of fact, and many other "transcendent" creatures. These diverse entities define the horizons of human action at the same time that we humans define both ourselves and our "others." Taking the title of this book seriously thus requires that we place all the aforementioned creatures within a shared framework of traffic between and among humans and other actors and that we abandon ourselves, without predisposition, to the human/nonhuman hybrids that are generated in that traffic.

As part of a project to rethink the terms on which religion and technology can be related to one another, *Deus in Machina* thus casts its net widely in order to allow for the discovery of hybrids in both expected and unexpected places. In his chapter John Durham Peters introduces the category of "logistical media" in order to track how orientations to space and time (embodied in the technological forms of calendars, clocks, and towers) inform and enable religious meaning-making and religious practice, even if they are often imagined today as having been emancipated from this religious legacy as "merely secular" devices. Wolfgang Ernst also digs into the mechanics of timekeeping, but arrives at quite different conclusions from those of Peters. Whereas Peters is concerned with the traces of ancient religious purposes embedded in the history of timekeeping technologies—traces that continue to have an effect in the present—for Ernst what is paramount to consider is the *dis*-continuity between the history of religious timekeeping and the evolution of time-based media technologies. In other words, for Ernst, the challenge facing the study of religion and technology is not to bring them closer together, but to rethink the terms on which they must remain separate, an argument he pursues through his account of the history of the oscillating clock and its progressive detachment from its original locus in the monasteries of medieval Christian Europe. Questions about space, time, and technology also emerge in several other chapters—such as in de Abreu's meditation on Charismatic Catholic efforts to replenish modern technological "airspace," or in my own account of nineteenth-century Spiritualist conceptions of the cosmos as a vast "nervo-astronomy" of sympathetic linkages—but they also shape discussion of seemingly nonreligious modes of imagination and cultural practice, as Peter Pels demonstrates in his account of the development of the literary genre of science fiction over the course of the twentieth century and its various translations into science-fictionalized everyday life. Indeed, as Pels argues, images of spaceships and narratives about telepathic powers or time-traveling machines not only recuperate older religious discourses about space, time, and the transcendent, they also epitomize the ways religions are reinvented in order to fit the "secular" experiences of modern people.

Several chapters in this book offer new ways to think about religious subjectivity and community that also call into question settled assumptions about what divides human experience from techno-logic. In his chapter John Lardas Modern explores how the notion of "feedback loops" informs the tense relationship between American Protestant visions of a "purified" religious community and the haunting powers of technological modernity: tensions that productively informed diverse strands of the Melville revival of the 1920s, at a time of wrenching technological change. Maria José de Abreu offers a rereading of Walter Benjamin's famous theory of aura, now centered on the figure of the breathing body, which (for Catholic Charismatics in contemporary Brazil, among other actors who populate her narrative) invites a new conceptualization of the distinction between subject and object, or body and machine, through a reconsideration of the airspace that lies between and pervades them both. Sherine Hamdy challenges received notions of technological fatalism in the context of Muslims seeking (or avoiding) medical intervention in present-day Egypt, arguing that monolithic definitions of "fate" obscure the more nuanced strategies adopted by religious actors to make decisions about the risks, costs, and likely benefits associated with unpredictable (and for many, prohibitively expensive) medical procedures. In her chapter Faye Ginsburg also rubs against the grain of dominant notions of technological fate by exploring the work of disability activists, documentary filmmakers, and others concerned to overcome the marginalization of disabled persons within transnational Ashkenazi Jewish communities. As Ginsburg shows, the technoscientific data gathered under the sign of disability is never stable. It is always open to reappropriation and resignification for the sake of memorialization, restorative justice, political mobilization, and, in the specific case of Jewish disability, for the sake of new alignments of creed, kinship, bio-power, and belonging in the formation of Jewish religious community—as poignantly documented in Ginsburg's account of the efforts of disabled persons to construct new forms of "mediated kinship" and to imagine in a new register their own bodies as reflections of God's image. In these diverse studies the contributors to *Deus in Machina* make serious efforts to reevaluate the theological, cosmological, and ethical terms on which technology has been imagined as religion's "other" and to call attention to the multiple hybrids that begin to proliferate once that division has been superseded.

The Problem of Comparative Religions

If the discussion thus far has managed to cast doubt on the use of the word "technology," it is hardly the case that the word "religion" somehow deserves to escape from comparable scrutiny. In this respect a few words are also needed to clarify some of the ambitions, as well as the limits, of a study of religion and technology that adopts a comparative, historical, and cross-cultural perspective. The combination of chapters in this book does imply a purposeful eclecticism in which the reader is invited to traverse a wide range of time scales and geographic, cultural, and religious contexts, including engagements with: a site of Charismatic Catholic media production in Brazil (de Abreu); the public careers of Pentecostal pastors in Ghana (de Witte); the writings of a mid-nineteenth-century American Spiritualist (Stolow); the history of American Protestant readings of Herman Melville's epic novel *Moby-Dick* in the early twentieth century (Modern); local enactments of Islamic debates over organ transplantation in an Egyptian hospital (Hamdy); a history of the shifting doctrinal and legal discourses that defined the legitimacy and efficacy of Buddhist ritual healing practices in nineteenth-century Japan (Josephson); a transnationally dispersed community of Ashkenazi Jewish filmmakers and disability activists (Ginsburg); and the "virtual Vodou" cybercommunity (Boutros).

This is hardly an exhaustive list of religious frameworks for conceiving, engaging with, and assessing the ethical implications of technologies, both old and new. Readers can no doubt think of equally (if not more) compelling cases to consider within and across other religious traditions, including, for instance, Eastern Orthodox Christianity, Hinduism, Theravada Buddhism, Mormonism, and the innumerably diverse cosmologies and ritual practices of Fourth World peoples, none of which receives adequate attention in the following pages. But while the range of case studies explored here might seem limited, if not arbitrary, the decision to juxtapose them within a single book serves a larger purpose: to try to displace those reigning narratives of religion and technology that fail to reflect on their own parochial status as predominantly Christian and Western, or that are myopically focused on contemporary technoculture at the expense of a longer historical view. Prevailing accounts of scientific inquiry and technological invention have in fact been heavily biased toward the Euro-American context, and to that extent they are predicated on what should be acknowledged as parochial histories of economic patronage, ecclesiastical authority, public spectacle, and imperial imagination. It is regrettably commonplace, however, that commentators on religion and technology readily confuse particular narratives about the historical emergence of modern European and American science, biomedicine, industrial production, and military supremacy with a transcultural, normative account of technological change and modern fate. This slippage between the particular and the universal is especially clear in the way studies purporting to talk in general terms about "religion and technology" silently assume a model of post-Reformation Christianity: as a theological template; as a structure of belief; and as a mode of conduct distinct from the public domains of law and politics or, for that matter, of science, industry, and the capitalist market.

Of course, comparisons are always dangerous undertakings in that they encourage scholars either openly or unconsciously to reify the very terms on which discrete phenomena can be brought into alignment with one another. This problem has been commented upon with particular force in the field of religious studies, where it has been declared a nominalist error to presuppose the existence of a universally distributed, yet locally differentiated body of precepts, doctrines, affective dispositions, and modes of social affinity that all can be captured in the singular word "religion." As argued by Talal Asad, David Chidester, Tomoko Masuzawa, and Guy Stroumsa, among others, the very idea of religion as a transcultural category is rooted in a specifically Christian theological distinction between, on the one hand, the internal, timeless, private experience of faith and belief and, on the other hand, the external, temporal, public domains of politics, science, social habit, and cultural expression.[38] Hence the risk that every attempt to extend the scholarly gaze beyond the bounds of Western modernity carries with it a silent colonizing impulse to force different traditions of ethical and practical conduct and different modes of knowing the cosmos onto the Procrustean bed of post-Reformation Christianity.

Introduction

The assumed normativity—if not universality—of the Western Christian experience (if indeed such a monolithic entity has ever existed) thus represents a significant barrier for the integration of studies dealing with the conceptualization, reception, and use of technologies in non-Western and non-Christian religious contexts. Simply put, different religious regimes impose distinct constraints on the range of possible engagements with the pragmata of tools, devices, and machines, while at the same time through such appropriations enable quite different modes of embodied perception, action, and imagination. On the other hand, there is an equally great risk that a comparative study of religions and technologies scattered across different historical periods and regions of the world might proceed in a way that is innocent of the political and economic hegemony of the advanced Western industrial states in matters of technological development and in the global diffusion of modern technologies. In this respect, perhaps there still exist good reasons to relate questions of technology and modernity to specifically Christian powers of imagination and practice as proposed, for instance, by Jacques Derrida in his account of *mondialatinisation* [globalatinization].[39] The challenge facing any interdisciplinary comparative discussion of religion and technology is therefore this: How can one represent the legacy of Western Christian domination while at the same time provide room to explore the many ways the terms "religion" and "technology" might be applied to culturally varying, sometimes even incommensurable practices, techniques, symbolic repertoires, and sources of ethical judgment?

This is a challenge that *Deus in Machina* cannot possibly meet if both the words "religion" and "technology" are not first shorn of their nominalist trappings. Perhaps, therefore, the only safe way to make use of these terms is to place them in the category that rhetoricians call *catachresis*. A catachresis is a figure of speech that denotes a thing that otherwise cannot be named, because there is no proper referent, as in the popular example "the legs of a table."[40] By emptying out the words "religion" and "technology," and thereby drawing attention to the underlying disjuncture between these words and their (absent) referents, might not this serve to make new room for the many hybrids that lie beneath this semantic divide, each awaiting its own opportunity to be made visible as a god *in* the machine?

A Note on the Book's Structure

The foregoing discussion makes clear that there are multiple thematic threads tying the individual contributors of this book into larger conversations about religion and technology. Nevertheless, the ensuing eleven chapters have been grouped under three broad rubrics that are intended to highlight some particularly resonant questions and issues and to suggest some new lines of critical interrogation that might emerge from the juxtaposition of discrete case studies.

The first part, "Equipment," explores a range of instruments, tools, and devices that mediate between religious subjectivity and the cosmos in order to pose the question: What is religious—or *not* religious—about the equipment we humans use to organize space and time, to store and transmit knowledge, or to supplement our natural mnemonic, sensory, and perceptual faculties? Timekeeping devices receive prominent attention in the first two chapters, perhaps because they offer something like a litmus test for the study of religion and technology. Indeed, clocks, calendars, and related time-measuring technologies are long known to have originated in the context of religious institutions and to thus bear the mark of what were originally religious motivations and interests: to render the cosmos intelligible for the sacred imagination and to discipline and control populations for the sake of ritual order. But what significance, and what ongoing influence, ought we to attribute to the apparently religious origins of these and other technologies used to orient humans in time and space? What about the underlying metrics and logics of directionality, location, leverage, computation, or temporal progression that shape the way technologies are designed and the way the information they generate can be used? Do these always remain external to the domains of religious knowledge, sensibility, and practice? These questions are pushed further in the succeeding two chapters, each of which begins with the consideration of an instrument that defies credibility within the sanctions of modern scientific authority because it is presumed incapable of performing its advertised actions, and therefore needs to be located firmly in the province of superstition and religious fantasy. But how, precisely, are we supposed to draw the line between "proper" and "improper" uses of technological equipment, between accredited sources of knowledge and popular representations of technological efficacy, or between the reliability of professionally trained makers and operators of instruments and the deviousness of "religiously motivated" charlatans or the naïve credibility of ordinary users? By what standard is technological success to be measured, and by what authority are accounts of technological efficacy to be legitimated? How exactly can and should scholars disentangle the "merely instrumental" dimensions of instruments from other—dare one say transcendent?—powers that also seem to inhabit them and shape their representation and use?

The second part, "Bio-Power," further extends the first part's examination of the interface between culturally (or bodily) derived and mechanically derived perceptions and powers by turning to an arena that has long been central to religious imagination and practice: the assembly of concerns about health, fertility, desire, physical and mental suffering, and ethical governance that constitutes the biopolitics of individual as well as collective bodies and body projects. The chapters in this section explore how, especially (but not only) as a consequence of the development and global diffusion of the modern Western biomedical orthodoxy starting in the late nineteenth century, "religious" and "magical" epidemiological frameworks, diagnostic procedures, and modes of therapeutic intervention have been steadily displaced from their former position of dominance over the healing arts. At the same time, however, to the extent that human health remains an elusive end and the management of embodied differences (including, but not only, those differences marked by "disability") continues to be shaped by moral enigmas, the monopoly of modern medical authority is open to challenge in the form of alternative proposals for the governance of bodies and souls. It is in this context that Japanese Buddhist prayer (as a therapeutic technology), Islamic discourses about "fate" (as a mode of selective resistance to the application of advanced biotechnologies), and strategies to reconstitute Jewish genetic kinship in order to lift the stigma of disability (not least through the deployment of visual media technologies such as documentary cinema) all converge to suggest new ways of understanding the place of religious identity and practice within technologically mediated fields of bio-power and new ways of limning the religious imagination that lies buried in the contours of modern biopolitics.

The third and final part of this book, "(Re)Locating Religion in a Technological Age," returns once more to the figure of the machine in relation to religious perceptions and powers, but now with a sharpened focus on the definition of religion itself as a field of belonging, identity, knowledge, and performance folded into what Lewis Mumford once labeled our "neotechnic" modernity.[41] As John Lardas Modern poses the question in his chapter, "what separates histories of religion from histories of a secular haunted by the effects of mechanical reproduction?" Answers to that question are sought along various routes of investigation, including explorations of technology as a figure of literary as well as sacred imagination and representation (ranging from the epic modernism of Melville to the dark dystopianism of cyberpunk science fiction); a study of the reformulation of the longstanding Christian notion of "contemplation" within the contemporary techno-logic of televisual representation; or an instructive case study dealing with the modes of accumulation and consolidation of "authentic" religious knowledge via the Internet, a technological medium that upsets stable boundaries between religious insiders and outsiders through the unruly circulation of competing images and voices (as has been the case with the generation of online representations of Haitian Vodou).

Equipment

Calendar, Clock, Tower
John Durham Peters

"What is time?" asked Saint Augustine. He rightly considered this to be one of the great religious questions. His brilliant analysis did not quite solve the puzzle—but then, no one else has done better before or since. Whatever time is, clocks and calendars measure, control, and constitute it. Towers are related media—time-heralds that claim dominion over space via sight and sound. These media—so fundamental that they sometimes are not seen as media at all—negotiate heaven and earth, nature and culture, cosmic and social organization and define our basic orientation to time and space. As such, they are among the most profound technologies of political and religious power and control. Their analysis points to (1) the relevance of old media for understanding so-called new media and (2) the importance of the *logistical* or organizational role of religious technologies.

Calendar

Calendrical systems are abstract devices of cognitive, political, and religious organization. They are among the most basic of all human sense-making devices. Like the more elaborate institutions of science and religion, they render the cosmos intelligible for human use, only on a quotidian scale. Calendars are designed to coordinate periodic astronomical events (years, solstices, phases of the moon, days) with periodic human events (commemorations, anniversaries, holidays, Sabbaths). The double job of calendars—binding earthly history and celestial cycles—gives them their particular potency as media of communication. They are at once modes of representation and instruments of intervention: they constitute time in describing it. Calendars negotiate between the heavens and the state and orient us to time and eternity. Their basic unit is the year, as the basic unit of the clock is the day. Both devices mimic, with imperfect precision, the motions of the heavens and earth. As such they fulfill, even in a secular world, the classic religious function of providing a meaningful orientation to the universe.

Timekeeping is in some ways inherent to life itself. Life as we know it evolved on a planet having a daily rotation. The basic pulse of alternating day and night seems at some level to be built into all living beings. Oysters, potatoes, fruit flies, and bees—among many other creatures—can track the sun, locate themselves in geomagnetic fields, or consume oxygen in accordance with ancient daily rhythms.[1] These remarkable acts of geocosmic orientation take place at a precognitive level. Likewise the menstrual cycle among humans and the seasonal migrations of birds, fish, bats, and monarch butterflies are all achieved without the aid of conscious calendar-keeping. Though the internal time sense can be thrown off if organisms are deprived of environmental cues about time (so-called "zeitgebers"), there is no question that life itself is periodic, a nest of overlapping cycles.

The human avidity for timekeeping is likely coextensive with human culture as such. Hunting and gathering, pastoral nomadism, and agriculture all depend on close observation of natural cycles, and humans had surely accumulated a wealth of oral lore coordinating plants, animal migration, and seedtime and harvest with the cycles of the sun, moon, and zodiac long before literate and numerate calendar-keeping came into play.[2] More formal calendars require advanced knowledge of astronomy and are key ingredients of civilization, together with writing, mathematics, the division of labor, and centralized religious or state power. Two natural facts—the diurnal rotation of the earth and the annual orbit of the earth about the sun—shape all calendrical systems, and the monthly cycle of the moon is found in most. Other resources include solstices and equinoxes, even eclipses and comets. Much of the motivation of early calendar-making was the religious and political desire to synchronize everyday life with the motions of the celestial spheres: to do consciously what potatoes and oysters do instinctively.

Though all calendars have the day and the year, determining the precise boundaries of each of these units turns out to be deceptively difficult. Most of us think it takes the earth twenty-four hours to rotate on its axis. Not so. The sun does take twenty-four hours to return to a point intersecting the meridian, an imaginary north-south line that bisects the sky into eastern and western halves; this is the "solar day." Yet for the sun to make a complete circuit, the earth—since it is advancing in its orbit—must actually rotate about 361 degrees to catch up to where it was yesterday with respect to the sun, which takes around an extra four minutes on average (but with a much wider range than that). The absolute rotation of the earth (the "sidereal day") currently takes 23 hours, 56 minutes, and 4.09 seconds. The earth's spin is slowing gradually, thanks to the friction of the atmosphere and the oceans, necessitating, for instance, an additional second now and then. Five hundred million years ago there may have been more than four hundred days per year, according to evidence from growth rings in fossilized mollusks and coral (the moon's rotation also appears to have once been faster, with a month of about twenty-eight days). There is likewise no universal standard of when the day begins, and options include sunrise, noon, sunset, or more artificial standards, such as our midnight. Nothing is so "everyday" as a day, but it is an entity readily deconstructed as a work of cultural approximation and averaging.

Determining the length of the year is even more complicated.[3] The Babylonians reckoned the year around 360 days, and thus chose 360 as the number of degrees in a circle (thanks also to its easy divisibility by two, three, four, five, and their multiples). Our symbol for "degree," a raised "o," comes from the Babylonian symbol for "sun." Around two thousand years ago in Egypt, Babylon, China, and Greece, it was known that the year takes 365 days and a fraction. The calendar implemented in the reign of Julius Caesar—named "Julian" in his honor—introduced a leap year every four years, putting 365.25 days in the year (in fact, the earth takes 365.24219 mean solar days to orbit the sun). The Julian calendar, which ignored the lunar cycle in contrast to most other systems, was good to within eleven minutes per year. But small differences add up, and the Julian calendar lost a day about every 128 years. By 1582, when Pope Gregory XIII introduced the Gregorian calendar, which omits three leap years every four hundred years, the calendar was about twelve days off. Protestant countries resisted the change for the predictable religious and political reason of not wanting to be seen as taking orders from the Vatican. After 170 years of confusion in dealings with France and the continent, England and its colonies finally made the switch in 1752. Englishmen went to bed on Wednesday, September 2, and woke up on Thursday, September 14.[4] Russia (like Greece and Turkey) did not switch until the twentieth century, with the result that the "October Revolution" of 1917 took place in what we now call November.

The first item printed by Gutenberg was a calendar—that is, an almanac. The Bible came later. Calendars may be as religiously important as scripture. Every religion has a calendar. Jews, Buddhists, Jains, Muslims, Hindus, and Baha'is each have their own. Christianity has at least three, and Roman Catholics, Eastern Orthodox, and Armenian Orthodox can still end up celebrating Christmas on different dates. The chief motive of Gregory's reforms was to keep Easter, the most important of the Christian "moveable feasts," from drifting too late into the springtime. In contrast with Christmas, which always falls on December 25 regardless of the day of the week, Easter always falls on a Sunday, varying widely from year to year (March 22 to April 25 are its theoretical limits). The current definition—the first Sunday after the first full moon after the vernal equinox—was set in the Council at Nicea in 325 CE after long disputes among early Christians. It is a remarkably messy definition, since it requires specifications of (1) the human week, (2) the lunar cycle, and (3) the solar cycle. But the definition succeeded in its overt sociological purpose: to find a date for Easter that would never coincide with the Jewish Passover. The Nicean Council thus drove a further wedge between Christians and Jews, as well as disciplined Christian schismatics such as the Quartodecimans ("fourteenthers"), who continued to celebrate Easter on the fourteenth day of Nisan, the date of Passover in the Jewish calendar. Ironically enough, the Christians had to revert to the lunisolar logic of the Jewish calendar—otherwise foreign to their Roman-Julian tradition—to prevent Easter from matching Passover. In a classic act of repression, Christians fought the foe by internalizing the foe's logic. Calendars are never neutral maps: people signal religious allegiance and identity by the holidays (holy days) they observe.[5]

The Jewish calendar is of particular interest. Jewish scripture starts with an account of the creation of the world in which one of the very first items created was the day itself—which is characteristically defined in the Hebrew style as starting in the evening (Gen 1:5). Moreover, the book of Genesis gives divine sanction to the seven-day week, culminating in the Sabbath or day of rest. Sabbath observance has always been one of the key markers of Jewish identity, as are high holidays such as Yom Kippur (Day of

Atonement), Pesach (Passover), and Rosh ha-Shanah (New Year's), which are also considered Sabbaths, though they may fall on other days of the week besides the seventh. Sabbath observance is perhaps the most intense form of calendrical religiosity. Seventh-day Adventists likewise make an interpretation of the calendar into an article of faith.

The Jews borrowed a lunisolar calendar from the Babylonians, and after diverse refinements, have a calendar that slips about six minutes per year, or one day every 216 years. A lunisolar calendar uses both the phases of the moon and the sun. The Muslim calendar, in contrast, is strictly lunar, with a year of either 354 or 355 days made of twelve lunar months. It makes one complete rotation through all the seasons once every thirty-two Muslim years. Its first year is 622 CE on the Gregorian calendar, and it uses the abbreviation AH ("anno hegirae," in the year of the hegira). Since the Muslim year goes faster, one cannot find its equivalent in the Gregorian calendar by subtracting 622. Doing so would yield a date that is yet to come on the Muslim calendar. Eventually the Muslim calendar will catch up with and pass the Gregorian calendar.

Another historical feature of the Jewish calendar is of general relevance: its governance by central authority. After the destruction of the Second Temple in 70 CE, the diaspora calendar was coordinated by remote control by signal flares and messengers from the Sanhedrin in Jerusalem, which maintained a monopoly control on sighting the new moon and thus declaring the start of the new month. In an era before electric telecommunication, the slow movement of such time-sensitive data was a major inconvenience, and Hillel II ended Jerusalem's monopoly in 356 CE, allowing each Jewish community to determine the new moon. A clear principle in the history of calendar-making is that those in power make the calendar. A key sign of sovereignty is the power to declare a holiday. Astrological prognostications have often served as ideological supports for the rulers. Among the Aztecs, for instance, a priestly class maintained a complex dual calendar of 260- and 365-day years nested within fifty-two-year cycles of the 365-day year (or seventy-three years of 260 days). Indeed, calendars have always been under the control of priestly classes who serve the powers that be.

Every calendar accordingly invites resistance. The Qumran sectaries of the Dead Scrolls, for instance, hated the lunisolar calendar imposed by their Greek conquerors and observed instead what they called the "true calendar." Observing the Sabbath has always been a form of resistance to state and market power.[6] Celebrating the Sabbath on the eighth instead of the seventh day enabled early Christians not only to commemorate the Resurrection, but also to distinguish themselves from Jews. The ancient

Jews, for their part, seem to have made Saturday the last day of the week to avenge their Egyptian captors, who venerated Saturday as the first day. Contemporary Jews and others in turn sometimes resist the Christianity of the calendar by preferring the designation BCE ("before the common era") instead of BC ("before Christ") and CE ("the common era") instead of AD ("anno domini"—in the year of the Lord). Quakers traditionally call the days of the week by ordinal numbers (e.g., Sunday is "first day") to avoid honoring the pagan gods (the seven moving heavenly bodies), whose names the inherited Roman calendar attaches to days of the week—Sun, Moon, Mars, Mercury, Jupiter, Venus, and Saturn. This legacy is clear in the English Saturday, Sunday, and Monday, but obscured for the other days of the week because they take their names from the Germanic versions of the same gods; it is clearer in most Romance languages.

Like all systems of nomenclature, calendars can yield instances of delicious arbitrariness. Consider again the weekdays. In modern Greek, for instance, Sunday is "the Lord's Day," Monday is "second day," and Tuesday is "third day," and so on to Friday, which is "preparation day" (presumably for the Sabbath). In Russian, in contrast, Sunday is "Resurrection Day," Monday is, splendidly, "the day after not working," Tuesday is "second day," Wednesday is "middle" (like the German *Mittwoch*), Thursday is "fourth day," and Friday is "fifth day." Obviously, the Greeks and Russians start counting in a different place, though they both call Saturday "Sabbath." Indeed, when the week ends and starts is as arbitrary as when the day does. The modern weekend is a composite of the seventh and the first day, though to many of us, Monday feels like the first day of the week. Months have a similarly arbitrary quality; how many of us readily remember which months have thirty days and which have thirty-one?

Most calendars possess a deep cultural conservatism—appropriately enough for media that store time. The modern world operates on top of an ancient calendrical infrastructure. Quirks of the Roman world live on in the twenty-first century. July and August, formerly Quintilis ("fifth") and Sextilis ("sixth"), owe their names to the vanity of two men dead for nearly two thousand years, Julius Caesar and Caesar Augustus. We call our ninth, tenth, eleventh, and twelfth months September, October, November, and December, which of course mean seventh, eighth, ninth, and tenth. The calendar gods have a sense of humor. The idea that the course of history has a middle point with a negative direction (before Christ) and a positive one (after his birth), is obviously of Christian origin. The hitch is that when Christian monks figured out this dating, they did not possess the notation or concept of a zero, which leaves us with 1 BC skipping to 1 AD—the reason purists claimed the new millennium began in 2001, not 2000, which would have been only 1999 years after Christ's putative birth date.

Modern reformers sometimes sought to strip away the calendar's accumulated religious content. The French Revolution tried to institute a ten-day week (like that of the ancient Greeks). The Republicans also converted the twenty-four hours into ten, each hour subdivided by one hundred minutes, and each hour subdivided into one hundred seconds; they brought to the calendar the same decimal zeal that led to the metric system of weights and measures, though with less success. The Republicans wanted to weaken the grip of religious holidays and the Sabbath, replacing holidays celebrating saints, for instance, with notables from the history of reason. They also wanted people to work more and take fewer holidays. Napoleon abolished the revolutionary calendar in 1806, doubtlessly to widespread relief. In a similar spirit, the early Soviet Union experimented with a five-day week. The experiment lasted about a decade before it was abandoned. The grip of the seven-day circle is tenacious; some things even the French and Russian revolutions could not change.[7] Every religion may have its calendar, but every calendar probably has its religion, as well, if even the religion of secular reason. As constructs that synchronize earth and heaven, culture and nature, and the periodic events of history and astronomy, calendars remain among the oldest and most important of all religious media of communication.

Clock

As timekeepers, clocks resemble calendars in some ways. In a sense, clocks are fast calendars and calendars are slow clocks. Calendars model time on a macro scale, starting with the day, and aggregate upward to weeks, months, seasons, years, decades, centuries, and indefinitely larger units (the Hindu and Buddhist "kalpa," perhaps the largest cycle in human calendars, takes 4,320,000,000 solar years). Clocks generally model time on a micro scale, starting with the day, and subdividing downward to hours, minutes, and seconds, according to the sexagesimal system, and then—switching to the decimal system—to milliseconds and indefinitely smaller units (a "yoctosecond" is one septillionth of a second, or 10^{-24}). These nether regions are being increasingly colonized by science. There is lots of room at the bottom.[8]

It is easy to exaggerate the differences of these two media of timekeeping, each of which has plenty of internal diversity. There is, for instance, the doomsday clock, which indicates our presumed proximity to thermonuclear apocalypse, and "the clock of the long now," which is designed to run for ten thousand years.⁹ Even so, there is an important difference. Calendars deal in what the Greeks called *khronos*, time as duration or span; clocks deal in *kairos*, time as moment or point. Calendars are chronic; clocks are acute. As a rule, clocks indicate the immediate moment, but lack memory or foresight. Curious automata, strange little personae with their "faces" and "hands," clocks say the same thing over and over again, and yet the information they provide is always fresh. They tell you where the "now" falls in the day. In this locating function clocks do for time what compasses, sextants, and GPS devices do for space. They are compasses whose needle points to the now rather than to the north. While calendar observatories such as Stonehenge or astrolabes can locate you on the calendar, most calendar systems do not provide such data intrinsically; instead, you have to find the "you are here" spot by other means.

Whereas clocks provide ever-fresh data—which is paradoxically always the same message: "it is now"—calendars store and extrapolate data, thanks to their cyclical character. Calendars are literally event-ful, but clocks are relatively barren, their intelligence being used up every moment (when someone asked Yogi Berra "Do you have the time?" his retort was supposedly: "You mean right now?"). Calendars preserve past time and project future time. As compass is to map, so clock is to calendar. Clocks are ultimately pointers of celestial position and today are governed by astronomical calculation.

Among all historical timekeeping devices, the clock is relatively recent. Compared to other small-scale timekeepers, it is distinct by its regular motion and uniform units. The hourglass is ancient: long used at sea, it lives on in board games, but has no standard measure. Clepsydrae (water clocks) were in use in Egypt and Babylon by 1600 BCE and played a role in Greek and Roman courts of law. But these devices too were subject to local variation. The sundial is also ancient, but it traces a longer time span (all daylight) than either the hourglass or the clepsydra, and it has direct legacies for the clock. One is clockwise rotation: in the northern hemisphere, the shadow on a sundial moves from west to north to east, and this motion was retained for the hands on mechanical clocks (the morning hours on a clock face, 6 to 12, indicate that the sun is in the east, and the afternoon hours of 12 to 6 that it is in the west). Another legacy is the dial itself. From the Latin word *dies* (day), a dial is a readout divided into twelve hours: a division of the day that started in ancient Egypt around 2100 BCE. (An even remoter legacy of the sundial may be our twelvefold touchtone telephone dial today.) But its operation can be stopped by a cloud.

The clock, in contrast, works according to an internal mechanism. It ticks away indifferent to light or dark, human want or need. When we say "o'clock," we mean that we are following clock—not astronomical—time. The ubiquity of this expression evinces how the clock has moved us one step away from natural cycles. The historical process by which timekeeping shifted its focus from the natural world to a more abstract system of quantitative constants culminated in the twentieth century. For thousands of years, astronomers or astrologers set the time. In the mid-twentieth century, the duty of timekeeping shifted to physicists, completing the long, slow abstraction of time from the natural cycles. A universal measure of mass and length (the gram and the meter) was more or less settled by 1800; one for time was made official only in 1967, when the second was defined as 9,192,631,770 oscillations of the cesium atom.[10] The standardization of weights and measures began in the French Revolution; it took more than a century and a half to achieve the same thing for time. Today the clock has become an all but completely secular entity.

This was by no means the case in its origins. The word *clock* derives from the Latin *cloca* and is related to the French *cloche* and the German *Glocke*, all of which mean *bell*, and the clock as we know it first emerged in late medieval European clock towers. Bells started to be used throughout Europe in the twelfth century and, as large mechanical clocks developed around the fourteenth century, they took their place in church towers, creating a communications center at the heart of many towns. Bells were not mere timekeepers; they were among the central media of religious and civic communication in late medieval and early modern Europe. Bells were located in either church steeples or municipally owned towers, often with custody battles between church and state (see more on bells below). Again we see the truism in the history of timekeeping: that whoever sets the time controls the society.

As Wolfgang Ernst shows in his own chapter in this book, the clock is a religious technology, a machine that mimics the harmony of the cosmos and orders the hours of monastic observance. Clocks are data processors. Unlike a metronome, which has a regular beat but says nothing cumulative, clocks interpret the time. The minute hand, which started to be used in the sixteenth century, only became practical after Huygens perfected the pendulum in 1656, and the second hand followed by the end of the seventeenth century. It is difficult for us to imagine a world without a minute or second hand (this is the world we moderns seek on vacation). Sport, science, schedules all depend on such fine gradations of time.

The clock, argued Lewis Mumford, was the key technological invention of industrial society—even more so than the steam engine.[11] The clock is a power machine whose achievement is not principally in tracking minutes and hours, but in coordinating the cumulative actions of people. As clocks grew smaller and more personal, they became ubiquitous on wrists, telephones, computers, cars, and ovens, among many other devices. Though the wristwatch seems to be fading (three quarters of my undergraduate class at the University of Iowa in fall 2008 did not own a watch; they used their cell phones instead), clocks remain at the heart of media convergence today. Every new device, from iPods to digital cameras, has a clock in it. Indeed, every computer is a kind of clock, calculating its central processing unit in microscopic fractions of seconds.

The clock's origins, as noted, were largely religious: the need of European monks to observe the canonical hours of prayer. But in eleventh-century China—where horology was much more advanced than Europe, and where the first mechanical (water-powered) clocks were developed—the main context for timekeeping was political. The emperor's power was bound up with his declaration of holidays and calendars, since he was supposed to operate in tune with nature according to the "mandate of heaven." For debated historical reasons, advancements in Chinese clock technology stagnated, and Europe became the world leader in clock technology from the late thirteenth century onward.[12]

Since eighteenth-century Europe the modern clock's chief motive has been neither religious nor political, but economic—that is, secular. In Ben Franklin's words, "time is money." Critics of industrial capitalism ranging from Karl Marx to Charlie Chaplin have seen the clock's strict time discipline as a cruel distortion of human existence.[13] The clock for some represents a world deserted by God. Deists in the eighteenth century found in the clock's indifferent but constant mechanism a model for the universe: God had wound it up in the beginning and now was letting it run down without further supervision. All timekeeping devices implicate questions of time and eternity. Sundials were long decorated with lapidary mottos such as "ultima multis" (the last day for many) or "lente hora, celeriter anni" (slowly the hour, quickly the years). Clocks, too, have produced their share of existential poetry. Robert Frost's haunting lines point to something melancholy about the clock:

> And further still at an unearthly height
> One luminary clock against the sky
> Proclaimed the time was neither wrong nor right.
> I have been one acquainted with the night.[14]

For Frances Cornford (Darwin's granddaughter), the watch spoke a death wish. Read it out loud:

> I thought it said in every tick:
> I am so sick, so sick, so sick.
> O death, come quick, come quick, come quick,
> Come quick, come quick, come quick, come quick![15]

No one who wants to be part of the modern world can defy the clock's incessant beat. It is a prime symbol of modernity, of our Faustian mortgage of ourselves to things we did not choose, but will not give up. It stands less for religion than for secularization, for the standardization and integration of the world. The clock helped smooth out space on both land and sea by creating the grid necessary for global transportation and communication. The synchronization of remote clocks, for instance, answered the problem of calculating the longitude at sea. By creating a clock so accurate that one could know the precise time in England even on a ship in the middle of the Atlantic, the British clockmaker John Harrison made it possible to reckon precise location on an east-west axis.[16] Poseidon lost some of his terror. "Minutes" and "seconds," of course, are not only intervals of time, but angular measurements of distances on the surface of the earth that can be measured with a sextant. They preserve an implicit orientation toward the heavens.

On land, too, the clock helped grind away local claims to be connected to the heavens. Prior to the railroad and telegraph, every town set its noon hour by the sun, by the point of the shortest shadow. It did not matter if Dover, Brighton, Portsmouth, Plymouth, and Penzance, for instance, stretching from east to west along the southern coast of England, each had a successively later noon hour. By the mid-nineteenth century, the crazy quilt of local times in industrializing countries was causing serious problems in railroad traffic, and diverse nation-states sought to synchronize to a single clock. Greenwich Mean Time (GMT) was first broadcast visually in 1833 and by telegraph by 1852 in Great Britain. By the late 1850s, the country was covered with a network of time balls, cannons, bells, and needles designed to spread the news of when exactly 1:00 P.M. was (GMT did not become the official national time until 1880). By 1848 Dickens had already observed the drift away from natural zeitgebers: "There was even railway time observed in clocks, as if the sun itself had given in."[17] Time coordination in the air followed that over the wire. In 1924 the BBC started its six pips signal on the hour, followed in 1936 by a speaking clock service. All radio and television programming remained intensely gridded into national and regional time schedules until the early twenty-first century, providing something like the hours of observance for the modern industrial world.

The cosmic meaning of the clock could not stay hidden forever. In 1905, in a country known for its clocks (Switzerland), a young patent clerk was thinking about standard time. Albert Einstein discovered the principle of special relativity while daily inspecting designs for telegraphically synchronized remote clocks. He wondered, in essence, if standard time was possible on a cosmic scale. Noting the finite speed of light, he concluded that there can be no universal clock, no absolute "now" valid for all points in space, a revolutionary insight whose consequences range from quantum mechanics to cosmology, art to theology.[18] What did relativity mean, for instance, for the old claim of the omnipresence of God? The same means (trains and telegraphs) that brought us standard time on earth revealed its impossibility in the universe. Einstein proved Augustine's point: that time seems obvious until you ask what it is. If the fundamental question of media is the management of time,[19] then perhaps the fundamental question of religion is the management of time and eternity.

Tower

From the Tower of Babel to the World Trade Center buildings toppled on September 11, 2001, towers have long been symbols of communication. They have also been targets of resentment (by God in the first case and al-Qaeda in the second) of efforts to extend dominion over space. Like calendars and clocks, towers mediate between heaven and earth: they point upward to the sky, but thereby gain more advantage over the earth's surface. Towers concentrate and focus power, both divine and secular. Like temples, they mark the binding point of heaven and earth, the *axis mundi*. They are artificial mountains, often built on top of preexisting heights. Every tower implies a network of communication, whether horizontal or vertical.

The key fact about towers is leverage. Give me a place to stand and I will move the earth, boasted Archimedes. Towers provide such a point optically and acoustically. Every unit of increase on the vertical axis enormously multiplies the reach of the horizontal axis, thanks to both the principles of trigonometry and the curvature of the earth. The "Babel complex" that fires our ambition to scale the heavens has a sideways, earthly payoff.[20] A tower is an optical fulcrum, providing mechanical advantage for the eye and favorable acoustics for the ear. Towers are power technologies par excellence, and thus have always been key relays in networks. The leverage they offer is threefold: seeing, being seen, and being heard. Let us take each in turn.

First, towers extend the range of vision. They suppress space and extend the horizon. Viewers on towers have a natural telescopic advantage. Towers are privileged spots from which to observe happenings above and below. Indeed, like ancient temples, they are observatories in the strict sense: places for auguring celestial and terrestrial signs. They set the time and date (it is atop a turret in the castle that Hamlet declares: "the time is out of joint"). Towers are places for the religiously *observant*. As the tower is the classic place to conduct a watch or vigil, it retains a potent hold on the religious imagination. *The Watchtower* is the publication of the Jehovah's Witnesses, a name evoking biblical imagery of military surveillance, evangelical warning, and millennial expectation. According to Vitruvius, the Roman architectural theorist, temples to the gods who protect the city—such as Jupiter, Juno, and Minerva—should be built at the highest point possible so as to oversee the city walls. In the Greek and Roman worlds such temples linked worship, civic festivals, and military reconnaissance. The Athenian acropolis, for instance, was at once an awe-arousing device, an instrument of tax collection, and a fortification. The Bible expresses similar views: "The name of the Lord is a strong tower," says Proverbs 18:10. Yet two biblical towers are also symbols of futility: the Tower of Babel and the tower whose cost you must count in advance, lest you start to build and can't finish (Luke 14:28).

Towers are the fundamental media of surveillance, which explains their long history of military use as posts for sentinels and guards (Bentham's Panopticon had a tower at its center) and launch pads for projectile weaponry (stones, molten lead, arrows, guns, and artillery). The discovery of the vanishing point in fifteenth-century painting in Italy and Flanders might owe something to the points of view rendered by towers and ramparts. The great painter Albrecht Dürer wrote a treatise on fortresses, the *Befestigungslehre* (1527), in which the linkage of ballistics, early modern optics, Renaissance art, and military surveillance from secure positions is crystal-clear. Renaissance perspective and artillery both arose in the fifteenth century; both depended on the analysis of straight sight lines from a central point.[21] To see is to draw is to design is to target is to fire; this sense of armed vision continues in ordinary talk of *shooting* pictures today (a look can be a projectile weapon). Orhan Pamuk attributes a similar revolution in Muslim miniature painting to a tower's-eye view. Ibn Shakir, the legendary calligrapher in Baghdad, witnessed the city's destruction by the Mongols while he was hidden in the top of a minaret and drew it while he could, leading to a revolutionary new depiction of the horizon line from "an elevated Godlike position."[22]

Second, not only do towers allow seeing at a distance, they are also easily seen from a distance. They are often among the most visible objects on any horizon. Towers are always designed to be looked at and are often exercises in conspicuous expenditure (the phallic dimension is too obvious to dwell on). The tallest building in any city usually says something about the city's character. Towers often are synecdoches for a city. In Kiev, Ukraine, the Rodina Mat—a socialist-realist monstrosity that looks like a metallic Green Giantess—was supposedly designed to be just slightly shorter than the tower of the Lavra monastery, which sits behind it on a hill and marks the symbolically laden birthplace of Russian Orthodoxy. Modernity's most important tower, the Eiffel Tower, is certainly symbolic of its city. Guy de Maupassant, who detested the tower, liked to breakfast at a restaurant at its base—since, said he, it was the only place in Paris you didn't have to look at it. The Eiffel Tower has long been a platform for publicity and advertising, being decorated at times with a large clock (of course) and as a giant thermometer. Once it was hung with lights that spelled "CITROEN"; the Nazis in 1940, with a less developed eye for line, hung a horizontal banner on it, announcing, "Deutschland siegt auf alle Fronten." More recently the Eiffel Tower served as a beacon of the countdown to the year 2000, a huge digital readout announcing the remaining days of the millennium, down to the second. Towers not only signal civic identity, but convey vital intelligence (such as via Paul Revere's lanterns), weather, news, and above all, the time. As magnets for public attention, towers dictate, at least to some degree, public space and time.

These two sorts of leverage—vision and visibility—work together. Roland Barthes calls the Eiffel Tower "an object that sees, and a gaze that is seen." It transgresses "the ordinary divorce of seeing and being seen. It achieves a sovereign traffic between the two functions: it is a complete object which unites, if one may put it thus, the two genders of the gaze."[23] Uniting "masculine" vision with "feminine" visibility is of course not unique to the Eiffel Tower; it is characteristic of all towers.

This ease of sending and reception makes towers essential media for line-of-sight communication, such as signal fires in antiquity and modern optical telegraphy. Aeschylus' *Agamemnon* famously begins with a primal scene of communication at a distance: Queen Clytemnestra divining the fall of Troy via a system of signal fires linking Troy to Argos. The play opens with a bored watchman on a tower, tired of waiting for a signal to appear, who jubilantly at long last spots a flickering light on the horizon (he must first decide whether it is a celestial or terrestrial event).[24] The optical telegraph developed in late-eighteenth-century France falls in this lineage of line-of-sight tower-to-tower communication, as do cities that still have a "beacon hill" or "telegraph hill." Towers always establish lines of communication, real or symbolic, that otherwise would not exist.

Third, towers are acoustic devices that enhance the propagation of sound. Carillons, minarets, pulpits, and broadcast antennas all show that a small vertical investment yields major circumferential dividends. Towers and turrets have always been used for proclamations and decrees. Lighthouses—with their searchlights, radio communication, and foghorns—unite all three functions of the tower perfectly.

In European history bells are the key historic acoustic media connected with towers. Bells are key proclaimers of the Christian calendar of Easter, Christmas, and other holidays. They are major timekeepers and day-shapers. In nineteenth-century rural France, for instance, bells summoned people to Mass, weddings, funerals, emergencies, assembly, and battle, and often rang with a distinctive dialect unique to each village.[25] Similar practices took place earlier and elsewhere in Europe. One of the main functions of bells is mobilizing bodies into assembly—either soldiers to battle or Christian soldiers to church. Indeed, Longfellow's phrase "the belfries of all Christendom" has sound comparative religious footing. The Muslim rulers of the Ottoman Empire, for instance, prohibited the ringing of church bells in conquered areas, properly recognizing the great communicative and mobilizing force these media can hold for Christians. Amos Oz reports that his Aunt Sonia, growing up in Poland in the early twentieth century, found the sound of church bells scary, the signal of a pogrom.[26] In the Philippines the Spanish conquistadores ceremonially placed native populations "bajo las campanas" (under the bells). Once people could hear the church bells, they became subjects of both the crown and church. Sound defined the space of Spanish dominion. To hear the bells was to acknowledge the twinned sovereignty of Spain and the Roman Catholic Church. Audition was assent—or at least conscription (here is the ancient link of hearing and hearkening, listening and obedience).

Bells demarcate a space of local identity, allegiance, and belonging. In Italian "campanilismo" (literally "bell-tower-ism") means parochialism, as does the French term "de clocher." To be a true Cockney, as the old saying goes, one must be born within the sound of Bow Bells—the church called St. Mary-le-Bow in London's East End. The BBC's signature sound for decades was the chimes of Big Ben. Lord Reith, the founder of the BBC, said that he wanted "the clock which beats the time over the houses of Parliament, in the centre of the empire, [to be] heard echoing in the loneliest cottage in the land."[27] Parliament-cottage, center-periphery, empire-village, urban-rural—the sound of Big Ben was to the British Empire what the local clock tower was to a village, its pulse of common life. Bells, like fireworks, are public displays that collectively mark local space and time as festivals and holidays. They hail us as political or religious subjects. As Corbin argues, as bells were displaced by other systems of sound production and community media, the one meaning they retained was a sacral one: their sound is of deep time, death, and the echo of history.

Jewish and Muslim practice makes differing use of acoustic media from heights to order the time and announce key events. The Hebrew *shofar* or ram's horn has an ancient array of uses that include alarm, summons to battle, and call to repentance. Josephus says that it was sounded from the ramparts in the battle against the Romans. The Talmud says it should be sounded when a boat is sinking or when a famine or drought is looming. It was an important part of the sound-and-light show atop Mount Sinai as recounted in Exodus, chapters 19 and 20. The new year—Rosh-ha-Shanah—cannot be brought in without it.[28] In Muslim cities, in contrast, *muezzin* (criers) are now electrically amplified to sing the call to prayer five times per day. The shofar is a rare and sacred sound from which women and children were once shielded, but everyone is supposed to hear the muezzins' call. Their invariably tenor voices, broadcast from the thin minaret towers attached to mosques, summon the local populace to pray (with limited success, in my experience of cosmopolitan cities such as Cairo, Istanbul, and Jerusalem). The typical volume of amplification without strict clock or musical coordination means that one can hear competing or contrapuntal muezzin over the city as if in a Muslim beehive. It is hard to know which voice to hearken to, but there is no question about which religion saturates the air at that moment. The muezzin's function is much closer to the bell (everyday time ordering) than is the shofar's (marking states of exception).

The culmination of electrically aided sound from artificial heights is, of course, the radio tower. Television broadcasting and cellular telephony likewise depend upon networks of towers, and perhaps satellites are the ultimate tower, with their "footprint" of continental reach. Even the Eiffel Tower has an acoustic side as the "cradle of French broadcasting."[29] It was central to the conquest of the airwaves. In 1899 Marconi succeeded in sending a radio telegraph "wire" across the English Channel from the Eiffel Tower. Airplanes guarding Paris during World War I were directed from it, and in 1915 it was the vehicle of transatlantic contact. In World War II it was an important military target, enough for Adolf Hitler to pose sentimentally before it, a conqueror awed by the object of his conquest. Barthes rightly notes that the Eiffel Tower is a symbol of both communication and our dreams of ascent. But it is also a channel of communication, its top still bristling with transmitting and intercepting devices.

Finally, towers are catastrophic places of danger, emergency, and death. They are the spots from which the news will come and places at which gravity works most pitilessly. Clocks and calendars can provide intimations of mortality—sundials alert us to our fleeting hours, and watches tick like death—but towers far outshine them in sheer awesomeness. In *Hamlet*—like *Agamemnon*, a play about adulterous parents and avenging children that opens with uncanny sightings atop a watchtower—Horatio warns Hamlet with an acrophobic description of the edge of the tower's platform:

> The very place puts toys of desperation,
> Without more motive, into every brain
> That looks so many fathoms to the sea
> And hears it roar beneath....[30]

The Eiffel Tower, like its cousin the Golden Gate Bridge, is one of the world's premier destinations for suicides. With their "unearthly height," towers put the fear (or allure) of death into us all. They enable a rendezvous of the living and the dead. Like bells, they draw their sublimity from communicating between the mundane and the urgent. Towers stand between heaven and earth, height and expanse, the sacred and the secular, and they are primal extensions of our eyes and ears. In the twenty-first century they have lost none of their ability to put "toys of desperation" into our brains, anchor communication networks, and bind heaven and earth.

Logistical Media

Calendars, clocks, and towers are different in several ways, and towers are more different than the other two. But all three establish basic coordinates of time and space. They are all data processors. They establish the central points around which culture rotates. They belong to a neglected category of media that are so fundamental that they rarely come into view. Logistical media arrange people and property into time and space. They stand alongside more obvious media that overcome time (recording) and space (transmission) and produce messages and texts. Logistical media do not necessarily have "content." They are prior to and form the grid in which messages are sent. Calendars, clocks, and towers are not the only logistical media; others include maps, names, addresses, archives, museums, census, stamps and seals, compasses, astrolabes, the shofar, and money—perhaps the paradigm case. McLuhan's claim that the medium is the message is especially apt here.[31] Logistical media establish the zero points of orientation, the convergence of the x and y axes. They often seem neutral and given—something that gives them extraordinary power.

Though logistical media such as calendars, clocks, and towers are ancient, their relevance is urgent, thanks to new media such as Google—whose power owes precisely to its ability to colonize our desktops, indexes, calendars, maps, correspondence, attention, and habits. New media return us to old media. The fundamental problems that media face are both old and new: time, space, and power. Media record, transmit, and organize; they have memory, networks, and processors; they embody the institutions of temple, market, and palace; and they fill the three main functions of recording, transmission, and logistics.[32] As devices that organize space and time and orient us to the cosmos, media such as calendars, clocks, and towers are partners and competitors with religion, as designers of both ultimate things and the texture of everyday life.[33]

Ticking Clock, Vibrating String

How Time Sense Oscillates
Between Religion and Machine

Wolfgang Ernst

Not to Be Confused: Media (Theory) and Religion

When examined from the viewpoint of media archaeology, the relation between media and religion can be seen as concerning regimes of nondiscursive technologies. Are technologies, once in operation, indifferent to whether or not there was a religious bias in their installation, especially if this bias has left an imprint in their technical form? Is there any association between procedural forms such as liturgy and algorithm? What differentiates the general cultural engineering of symbolic, even transcendental systems, such as religion, from genuine media technologies—namely, those based on the laws of physics or mathematics? Is there a noncultural, autopoietic element at work in technical media that escapes any transcendental notion? In this chapter I will demonstrate how religious metaphors both create and obscure media practice by examining the origin of the oscillating mechanical clock in the monasteries of late medieval Christian Europe.[1] The results will put into question the epistemological discontinuity supposedly separating Pythagorean cosmology from the electrotechnical and technomathematical media age and religious timing from time-based media processes based on differential oscillations, as observed by Huygens, Mersenne, Leibniz, and others.

The oscillating mechanical clock rests on principles of musical harmonics and mathematics, insight into which was first triggered by the ancient Greek notion of cosmic order. The invention of the phonetic alphabet provided one model; the development of letters to represent vowels and consonants individuated poetic oral articulation into distinct syllables, and in so doing created a sense of measurable prosodic "beats." However, it was only in the context of the medieval Christian European monastery that the cultural engineering of timing processes began to be implemented technologically. Monastic practices were imbued with a Christian sense of temporal linearity and stimulated by a religious idea of infinity, which enabled the question of time to be defined by the regulation of technical media. Monastic prayer routines and working practices were closely tied to a sense of periodic beats—not just cycles of the day or year (which vary in their duration), but also the prosody of liturgical chants or the rhythm of the gestures of work. Rolf Nohr states that "With the division of the day into distinct parts, each one fixed within an ordered framework of work and prayer, the order of monastic life became conceivably one of the points on which the framework of the rhythmic was established."[2] However, the development of such mechanisms had the paradoxical effect of emancipating Occidental culture from its dependency on cosmic religious time. The attunement to periodic beats precipitated a decidedly nonreligious development based on the growing knowledge and familiarity with oscillating mechanisms present in vibrating strings. This same awareness led to the notion of "frequency" developed by modern acoustics and other forms of wave analysis, culminating most recently in the development of modern electronic media and in the timing mechanisms of computers. Deconstruction is technologically at work here; the escapement mechanism of the ticking, cogwheeled clock was a direct outgrowth of monastic rhythms, but that very technological development ultimately became a provocation to the liturgical world. Once the framework of monastic rhythms was transferred to a technological order—that of the ticking clock—the bells no longer tolled for traditional cosmic time.

Before describing further the development of the oscillating clock as a "nonreligious takeoff," let us note here some confusion concerning the terms *media (theory)* and *religion*. For Ernst Cassirer, religion is a variety of "symbolic" form and action, alongside myth and art: "the specific media created by mankind in order to dissociate itself from the world and thus be re-united with the world the more firmly."[3] But the relationship between religious phenomena on the one hand and technical media on the other is an uneasy one. Leaving aside topics such as Jesuit Counter-Reformation media strategies or Marshall McLuhan's inherent (and sometimes explicit) media Catholicism, the media-archaeological method employed in this chapter is intended to keep those phenomena apart and distinct. One instance of religious encounter with a technology is the numerical measurement of time. Time is an existential category to which both religions and technologies have been giving decisively different answers (and they still do). Remarkably, though, the origin of the oscillating clock stems from the medieval monastery at the climax of liturgical practice. This coincidence provides a unique opportunity to dispense with simplistic accounts of the antagonism between religion and technological development and to challenge the deeply entrenched assumption that religion and technology exist as two discrete arenas of knowledge and action. Media archaeology seeks to develop frameworks that avoid falling prey to such simplifications by examining the shifting relationships between humans and machines in diverse regional contexts and distinct cultural traditions, including religious ones.

Time-measuring media are more than simply an assemblage of technologies (tools and material artifacts) in that they depend upon the existence of a wide range of sensorial techniques that drive and modulate their specific development. Historically this ties them to religious systems of coordinated action as part of a broader nexus of cultural practices (such as theatrical drama) and epistemological practices (such as philosophy). We therefore require a double-edged approach. Modern technoscientific practice cannot be fully reduced to the instrumental designs and functional properties of specific technologies. But their specific mechanical and mathematical capacities to compress or accelerate time or to erase distance and reproduce sameness display features that could develop only in differentiation from "religious" experiences of time. In the face of the workings of an imperceptible natural order, media separate themselves from religion, just as the oscillating clock grew out of, then away from, the medieval monastery. Indeed, however much at first glance it might seem that European natural philosophers (such as Newton and Leibniz) adopted a purely mathematical approach to the physical world, they also grounded themselves in firm religious beliefs concerning the order of the world. Nevertheless, their technomathematical work autopoietically developed into a world of its own, culminating in what Leibniz had already divined: the binary computer.

Media (like the ghostly presence of the dead, incorporated in the wax cylinders of Edison's phonograph) question the precarious lines dividing humans from nonhumans, the living from the inanimate, or nature from the supernatural. Such distinctions have long been at work to keep culture going, but they have become increasingly blurred through the development of advanced technological systems. As with genetic engineering, the category of time itself is challenged by current sampling techniques (e.g., digital signal processing) or by artificially setting a time base. What used to be a mutually determinative relationship between religion and technology turns out to develop into extremely divergent cultures of practicing time.

From Cultural Techniques to Media Technology

Media archaeology shares a preliminary assumption with other chapters in this book: namely, that the technological past exists as an inherently ambiguous archive of techniques and material conditions for seeing, doing, imagining, and timing. Exploring this archive means defamiliarizing the present through an uncanny remembrance: in this case, the oscillating clock, which started as a nonhuman machine but ended up as a technique of conditioning the rhythm of human bodies and minds, thus replacing religious time. In order to analyze the ticking, wheeled clock as an epistemogenic artifact, therefore, it is necessary to differentiate carefully between religion and media—that is, between cultural techniques and media technologies. One criterion for understanding how cultural techniques become medial is revealed in the moment when time measurement breaks loose from natural temporal perception and becomes a matter of the automated setting of time in a rhythm freed from allegorical interpretations. The difference between letterpress and handwriting can be used as an analogy for the transformation enacted by the wheeled clock. As a mechanical instrument, both the letterpress and the wheeled clock possess a central characteristic of technological media: the identical reproduction of elementary units of measurement. In contrast to rituals and liturgy, mechanized time is no longer symbolically performative, but rather technically operative. It is not time per se that is operative here, but its implementation in a material artifact.[4]

What Gutenberg's casting process for letters achieved for the standardization of characters and their readers, the wheeled clock achieved for the automation of time. Medieval Christian monasteries were characterized by a peculiar interweaving of the representation of cyclical time (the liturgical year, the division of days into rhythms of prayer) with the specifically Christian idea of temporal linearity. The two intersected in the need to regulate forms of living into liturgical algorithms via precisely quantified measurements of time in the form of hours of equal length (equinoctial hours). Oriented to Judgment Day, earthly time had to be used economically.[5] The introduction of temporal beats is thus an epistemologically fundamental inheritance of monastic culture, yet it resulted in technically mediatized time, which was then employed to undo cyclical time so that the temporal beat became a criterion for separating medieval from modern time. Time, in this case, is both subject and object of a media-archaeological moment.

The Abstraction of Time: Monastic Worlds

Whose will was manifested in the mechanical innovation of the "verge-and-foliot" escapement, the key technology that directed the motion of the late medieval wheeled clock? In the monasteries there was at first no compelling interest in standardizing time through mechanically reproducible synchronization. Up until the early modern period, Christian rites were based above all on the principle of temporal hours—that is, on the uneven lengths of daylight, which varied according to the four seasons. Thus, for instance, the Rule of Saint Benedict (540 CE) dictated a regularity of prayer to God, but not its isochronal synchronization. Throughout the medieval period, monastic time was divided according to the canonical hours (the Horae—the old temporal division of the day according to quarter solar days, as well as twelve hours between sunrise and sunset. This spiritually oriented aesthetics of time was set against the agrarian perception of time, where the rhythms of work varied according to the amount of daylight. Even in darkness, when the natural world lay dormant, life in the monastery called for the division of time, and through its practices thus arose the possibility of a time abstracted from nature. Initially water clocks were used for this, though for a long time their equinoctial hours were still converted into temporal hours.

Chronology, Clock, Rhythm: The Monastic Planning of Time

In cultures based primarily on oral communication, traditionally handed-down formulaic chants served to establish real-time prosody, though they did so with a high degree of variance. With the development of external forms for storing the voice, such as phonetic writing, other means of transporting information became possible. Wherever tradition was accompanied by written records in the form of diaries, calendars, and annals, technologically repetitive functions competed with diffusely memorizing humans. Religious canonical action did not permit deviation, and thus required mnemonic techniques such as writing and regulations. The monastic rules and liturgies in early medieval monasteries thus led the way in decoupling natural and artificial ways of determining time; only in this way was a midnight Mass possible, at a time one could be reasonably certain was midnight.[6]

According to the Bible, it was in the first act of creation that God set time in motion as a binary through the division of night and day. Leibniz may have subconsciously heard the analogous binary pulsing of the ticking clock when he formulated his theological-mathematical dyad: "The wonderful origin of all numbers from 1 and 0, which offers a beautiful model of the mystery of creation, for all things originate from God and otherwise out of nothing: *essentiae rerum sunt sicut numeri.*"[7]

The timetable is a legacy of monasteries, writes Michel Foucault in *Discipline and Punish*.[8] Unlike the ascetically eremitic monasticism of antiquity, medieval monastic communities developed rhythms and rules governing both ritual and mundane activities. The stringency of the factory age was rooted in this sense of rhythm: whole armies exercised "the perfection of monasteries."[9] Time measurement as a critical facet of military decision-making can thus be traced back to the monastic rhythm of hours and minutes. In order to become quasi-mechanical, bodies had to be disciplined and manipulated on the temporal axis; this yielded a "cellular" microphysics of power in the form of temporal rhythm. Only synchronized time measurement (as in the coupling of clockwork and photography—e.g., in chronophotography) ultimately facilitated a form of media-technical analysis of movement that would finally produce a resynthesis in the form of cinema.

Starting in the second half of the thirteenth century, the wheeled clock, equipped with a verge escapement (a mechanism that controlled the advancing gear train at regular intervals or "ticks"), put into practice a negentropic dissection of the flow of time analogous to the spatialization of the printing press (see Figure 1). In lieu of the constant analog character of the sundial indicator, the pulse of the mechanical clock was balanced through even intervals of the taut (and thus stored or potential) energy of a weight. As the verge escapement forced time constantly to expend itself, the seeming continuity of time was subdivided into even segments, a folding together of the analog and the digital. This represented an early form of the binary implementation—or indeed the informatization—of mechanical processes as they had been known ever since mill wheels. In

Ticking Clock, Vibrating String   49

it, regulation is based upon an interruption: a kind of penetration of zero at the temporal level.[10] This was no coincidence: once zero was calculated as a gap (a condition of the positional notation system), the clock ticked at regular intervals.

According to Marshall McLuhan, only highly literate communities could imagine accepting the fragmentation of life into minutes and hours.[11] There time came to be conceived as something radically discrete: a virtual differential. However, "it was not until printing extended the visual faculty into very high precision, uniformity, and intensity of special order that the other senses could be restrained or depressed sufficiently to create the new awareness of infinity."[12] Only Gutenberg's media-technical discovery—the process for casting identical letters—made possible the precise reproducibility of visual information. That achievement accompanied the idea of the research experiment, as well as the "concept of indefinite repetition so necessary to the mathematical concept of infinity," which ultimately culminated in Leibniz and Newton's infinitesimal calculus.[13]

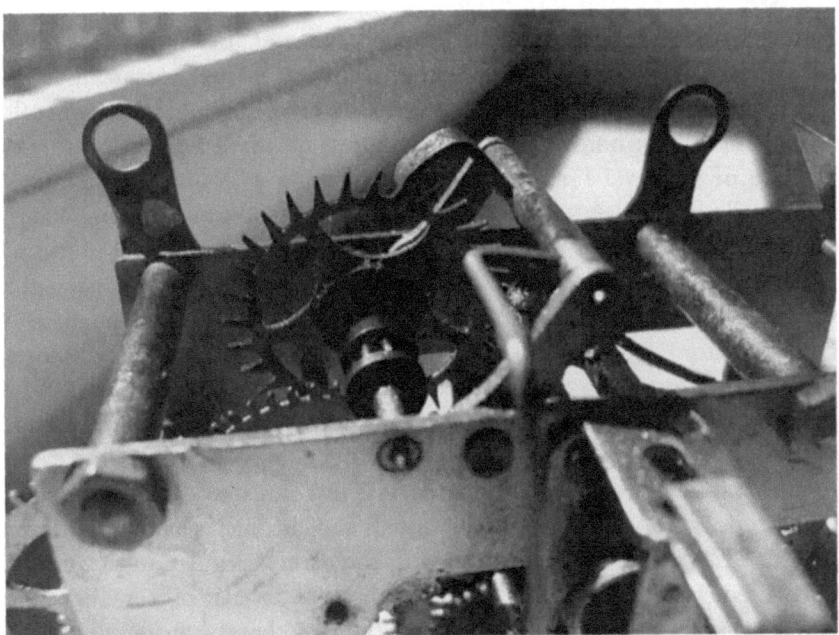

Figure 1. Verge- and Foliot Type Anchor Escapement Mechanism in a Clockwork. (Photo by W. Ernst.)

What was once a static aesthetic of order in the concept of the cosmos became a dynamic wheel with a wheeled clock. The bishop Nicole d'Oresme (1323–82 CE) was preoccupied with the relationship between uniform and nonuniform movement, directly anticipating the infinitesimal calculus that transferred every type of space or movement into a continuous space. With advancing precision, temporal intervals infinitesimally converged on zero. Temporal perception was thereby mechanically specified and later cast by Newton and Leibniz into mathematics. In our day the computer is clocked by the ultra-fast oscillations of an electrically activated quartz crystal—down to units that escape human perception and that allow infinity to reappear in the infinitesimal.

Macro-Clock-Time: The Medieval Annal

Numerical calendrical reckoning had long preceded the mechanization of time through the advent of ticking clocks. Aristotle had already speculated on the relationship between time and number, and his writings on mechanics read like a description of a clockwork: a *kyklophoría*. But the mechanical clock and, more importantly, the ticking, wheeled clock signified that numbers were turning into machines (or that machines were becoming numbers), starting to prepare us for the advent of the Turing Machine, the modern computer of the twentieth century. In the Roman imperial era, *computare* meant "to count on one's fingers," and Roman numerals were modeled on human hands.[14] Counting on one's fingers led to the practice of medieval holiday calendar reckoning as found, for example, in Saint Bede's *De temporum ratione* (725 CE). One literally "elementary" (in the ancient sense of Euclid's *Elementa*) challenge to medieval liturgical understanding was the problem of determining the date of Easter, for which mathematical calculation was obligatory. In this case we might ask: Did the historiographic form of the medieval annal foster an epistemology, a thought pattern for a temporal aesthetics of discrete steps?

The study of arithmetics was primarily an *arithmethica ecclesiastica*, a privilege of the church, above all for calculating the date of Easter. Just as the wheeled clock originated in the context of the Benedictine monasteries, the prehistoriographic annals and chronicles had their origins "in the Benedictine preoccupation with the careful regulation of time."[15] Early medieval annals set the stage for a discrete, tabular processing of the perception of time and reality. Might we then say that the mechanics of the wheeled clock had already been established in the temporal aesthetics of the "list format" that we find in the medieval annal? The annal suggests a form of perceiving reality wherein all events that occur are noted down in serial form as what has been perceived—has been given, that is, as data— and what does not occur appears in the notation as voids. Every year is like a variable in computing, waiting for its "annalistic" entries. In this context the Christian Easter festival gained its near-medial determination through ritualistic annual repetition, and the calculation of the dates of Easter led to the creation of the annal as a series of marginal notes on the tables needed for that calculation: a game of redundancy and information. However, we are not yet dealing with a medium in the sense of "telecommunications" as defined, for instance, by Claude Shannon in his mathematical measure for information: "specifically for the purpose of detaching and making measurable the novelty, and that means the improbability, of a message from the multitude of repetitions necessarily implied in every code."[16] By contrast, the medieval annal was located on the margins of the ritualistic, and thus endlessly repeating, Gospel, and it was in this context that the notation of the uniqueness or the improbability of history as a dynamic system developed. The very anonymity of the annal thus provided the model for a nonnarrative, nonsubjective kind of temporal processing. As Werner Faulstich writes, "Only a medial function remained for the historiographer of the Middle Ages; he was reduced to a simple instrument."[17]

The time of the chroniclers was that of the ticking clock, unlike the narrative time of history. "The historian proceeds diffusely and elegantly, whereas the chronicler proceeds simply, gradually and briefly."[18] Reflecting a mathematical aesthetic, a genuine aesthetics of data that draws no distinction between human ("historical") and natural events, annals are a "dated series of events recorded for the guidance of a monastic house."[19] They constitute not an interpretation of the past, but rather a function of the needs of the present. The wheeled clock transformed this annalistic macro-time into a microphysics of time.

Clocks and Oscillations: The Cosmic Clock

For the ancient Greeks the world was primarily a cosmos; its nature was iterative. Yet, as Heidegger states, "history, too, belongs to world."[20] By breaking open the cyclical thought of mythic time and introducing a teleological vector into the temporal order, Christian theology prepared for the idea of a progressive history. Within the Christian theological concept of time, the figure of the end of time indicated a dynamic concept of time.[21] But the notion of exact, experimental science, coupled with a time-counting machine, was introduced only in the Renaissance. Though the concept of "the machine" originated in classical Greek antiquity as an independent form of physis turned to praxis, "Greek science was never exact, precisely because, according to its essence, it neither could be, nor needed to be, exact."[22] The epistemological concept of exactitude was attached to the clock only in later times. Aristotle for his part rudimentarily equated time and number, but did not divide motion into exact time ratios. Time measurement was associated with poetry and poiesis, not with mathematical numbers. Timing for the Greeks thus remained a function of prosody and the alphabet. Whereas the phonetic alphabet still served musicality and the rhythm of oral poetry, the mechanical division of time served the algorithm itself—that is, the regulated sequences that we also find in the modern computer.[23]

Classical Greek philosophers understood motion as a change of place and were capable of assigning numerical values to it, but they distinguished no motion or direction of movement from any other. It was Christian teleology that introduced the concept of an estimated vanishing point, which—in alliance with zero—produced a new temporal perspective. With the advent of the wheeled clock, a medium began subliminally to massage (in McLuhan's sense) the human sense of time, and its message came to be that the world could be perceived in terms of frequencies. The precise countability of time as movement (beginning with the ticking clock) eventually yielded world images such as those of film and electronic television. Based on frequencies, the cathode ray is a "ceaselessly forming contour of things limned by the scanning-finger."[24] Not until this point did a mathematical sense of time come into play. McLuhan correctly associates this with infinitesimal calculus, but it first appeared in rudimentary form in the fourteenth-century writings of Nicole d'Oresme, was later developed by Leibniz and Newton into the concept of calculation, and finally was related explicitly to the electronic media by Norbert Wiener.[25]

Robertus Anglicus sketched a wheeled clock in the year 1271. Did he have any models? The mechanization of the clock involved the interweaving of an ancient technique with a modern concept of time: not "time discovered," but "feasible time." It is possible that just after 82 BCE a wheelwork sank along with the wreck of the *Antikythera*, but it remains unclear whether that was truly an astronomical instrument. Its construction, whose fixed gear train allows us to count backward in a media-archaeological sense, indicates that it mechanized the metonic cycle, in which nineteen solar years corresponded to 235 lunar years.[26] Johannes de Sacrobosco (1195–1256) ascribed the field of calendrical reckoning to astronomy. But through their empirical measurement of the movement of stars, the ancient astronomers had already increasingly come into conflict with the prevailing cosmic-harmonic world image. In fact, cosmic-harmonic calendrical reckoning always stood in opposition to the empirically exact measurement of time, and for this reason technical experiments were seldom carried out. According to legend, when the Pythagorean Hippasus of Metapontum followed out the trail of incommensurability, he was drowned at sea because this knowledge did not conform to the Pythagorean ideology of harmonic order.[27] Planetary motions are in fact incommensurable with one another and can never cross in identical constellations—a physical truth that was only recognized by the scholastic astronomy of the late medieval period.

Humans experience regular motion harmonically. At the end of Plato's *Republic*, the Sirens sing on the planets to produce the music of the spheres; in the older Pythagorean teaching, the oscillations induced by planetary orbits produced sound.[28] The harmony of numbers established the law applicable both to tonal oscillations and to planetary motion, and this law eventually converged with the development of the pendulum clock as a metronome to measure time. With its mechanical escapement, the wheeled clock produced precisely such movement in the form of a pulse, one that returned at the same time, always segmented in the same way. On the basis of this oscillating pulse, it was possible to generate audible sounds not in mythic, but rather in technical form.

With this movement, existence came to take place as being in time. In Wolfgang Scherer's words, "ringing gradually begins to break away from the geometry of monochord proportions; music begins to leave the space of Greek mathematics, to plunge into the eventful dimension of time."[29] This dimension can be called "media time." In his *Syntagma Musicum* (1614–1620), the organist Michael Praetorius related the symbolic order of the length of notes to the mechanical beat of the wheeled clock.[30] With the metronome of Johann Nepomuk Maelzel (Vienna 1814), musical beat found its own medium, setting the terms on which the micro-time of physical acoustics would later become comprehensible through electrotechnical measurement, "the necessary greater exactness [of which] is obtained by the electric current itself."[31] Ultimately the electronic oscillatory circuit released the beat of time from all cosmic-religious remnants in order itself to radiate in the ether.

In 1377 the theologian, mathematician, and physicist Nicole d'Oresme compared the movements of the celestial bodies with a wheeled clock in his *Libre du ciel et du monde*.[32] There he specified the decisive element of the wheeled clock as the mechanical correlate to the ancient harmonic theory of the cosmos. Once set in motion by God, this system runs automatically. Even Leibniz conceived of his monads as clocks wound up by God: they "continued to keep time with one another like separate clocks, so that they appeared to communicate with one another; but this appearance is merely a deceptive consequence of their synchrony."[33] Monads were thus conceivable only via the wheeled clock as a standardized and standardizing instrument of measurement that also produced comparability in time. Norbert Wiener writes: "As a matter of fact, the automata made in the seventeenth and eighteenth centuries were run by clockwork," and today, more than ever, computing demands highly sensitive preexisting temporal harmonies.[34]

The Epistemogenic Artifact: The Wheeled Clock Escapement

The verge escapement of the wheeled clock aptly illuminates how a media element can be an epistemogenic matter. At the same time, the description of the escapement's media-historical moment provides a suitable occasion to reflect upon some of the methodological implications of media archaeology. Here technically precise explanations carry epistemological weight, and the art of media-archaeological—or better, archaeographic *ekphrasis*—comes into play. We see this in the description of how the escapement works:

> Without such a brake, the rotation of the axle would steadily increase in speed. The escapement works as follows: A crown wheel with an uneven number of teeth, mounted onto the axle or linked to it via a gear train, . . . alternately blocks and releases the verge by means of two pallets attached to the verge at a right angle to each other. . . . The duration of the oscillation of the inertial mass of the verge and the foliot can be adjusted by moving regulating weights on the foliot. . . . This to-and-fro, oscillating movement inspired terms for the device such like "restlessness," "foliot" (from a word describing a quivering leaf, first used by J. Froissart around 1370), even most metaphorically "women's temperament."[35]

The culture of the early modern period thus grappled not only with a new technology, but also with a new language for describing things. The classical art of description had originated in rhetoric, based on linguistic figures. In contrast, the new type of technological objects that emerged in early modern Europe demanded a new type of representation: the language of mathematics and of the technical diagram.

The decisive feature of mechanical clockwork was that it contained stored-up energy. The spring tension produces pressure on the escapement mechanism, distributing minimal energy quanta into equal oscillations, which were then transformed mechanically into beats, placed on the border of pure information. Despite such a radical departure from existing clock technologies, the introduction of the verge-and-foliot escapement was barely mentioned in contemporary sources. Only in retrospect was it described as "significant but mysterious," precisely because its mechanism could not be perceived at the interface of the clock face.[36] Technical media achieve their effect by dissimulating their mechanisms: "In contrast, the appearance of striking clocks was registered instantly, and was felt to be technologically sensational and socially momentous."[37] Whereas the clock face can immediately be seen and heard, generating the effect of an advancing time, a glance at the escapement suggests an alternating oscillation rather than linearity. The escapement thus constituted the first binary mechanism of positive/negative polarity, which ultimately became operative in electrical clocks and electronic clocking devices.

Medial artifacts are worthy of investigation in terms of their epistemic implications for media culture. Every operative technology can in fact be applied to media theory. On account of their material substrates, media, like the science that studies them, are not purely discursive events. But in contradistinction with the objects of classical archaeology, medial-epistemic matters are logical as well as material artifacts. Media manifest themselves only through their operation, placing logic next to hardware and making the term *techno/logy* meaningful.

The former wheel clocks ticked rather imprecisely because the uniform oscillations of the horizontal pendulum (the foliot-escapement with verge) were independent of the precisely wrought wheelwork of the clock. Improvements in the accuracy of time measurement were achieved only with Galileo's discovery of the laws of pendulum motion in 1641 and with their application to the design of a free, vertically oscillating pendulum by Christian Huygens in 1656. Huygens's pendulum escapement established a new basis for measuring time: the periodic oscillation itself, which as a unit of measurement remained valid through to the invention of the atomic clock in the twentieth century. An oscillatory clock seems to be at work even within the sensory data processing in the human brain.[38]

The ticking wheeled clock is not an allegory of time, but a time machine. Its presence is acoustically indicated by the striking mechanism. Precisely because its technical mechanism in most cases remains hidden from the gaze of the observer behind the clock face (the *dissimulatio artis*, or concealing of technology, is the basis of all media effects), it requires media-archaeological attention. The principal work of such a clock was called, in a telling *terminus technicus*, "timework." From there the hour-striking mechanism—and often, deriving from it, musical compositions programmed via a cylinder with pins—was controlled discretely (or digitally). Otherwise, on the visible surface, the motion of time appeared continuous (analog). In the form of kinetic notation, the clockwork could be portrayed in diagrammatical terms: a kind of programming *avant la lettre*.[39]

On the Ritual and Liturgy of the Wheeled Clock: Media Archaeology versus Media Anthropology

Throughout the Middle Ages, time was not an autonomous object of representation, but a category immanent to theology. The ticking clockwork, however, resulted in an abstraction from cosmic time that could be experienced empirically. The mechanism of the verge-foliot escapement allowed the motion of a weight-driven axle to be controlled in such a way that its uniform rotation became suitable for use as a time standard (such as the equinoctial hour).[40] The wheeled clock thus became a time-giving instrument and established a time abstracted from nature. "For the first time in world history, mechanical reproduction emancipates a work of art from its parasitical dependence on ritual," Benjamin remarks about photography.[41] However, that emancipation had already occurred within the temporal regime, thanks to the invention of the mechanical clock.

To what extent is the precise marking of time a product of religious ritual? Liturgy represents the form and the spatial and temporal average of invariance in religion. Ritual is a cultural form regulated through tradition and law, in contrast with the law of the machine. But not every form of coding should be termed "medial." As symbolic acts, rituals are distinct from technological processes, not least because of their tolerance for blurring and their lack of clarity.[42] Ceremonial, ritual, rhythm, and repetition are all cultural techniques for "steadying time."[43] In fact, culture practices a negentropic expenditure of energy, maintaining order against the second law of thermodynamics, according to which a relentless arrow of time is inscribed into physical processes—namely, the tendency toward disorder.

Only with the wheeled clock did media time emerge in a well-defined sense, analogous to how Gutenberg's technology for producing identical letters generated the printing press as a media technique, in contrast with the cultural technique of writing. Ritual and ceremony already represented a form of instruction, and thus a program: a set of continuous mnemonic practices as an algorithmic—that is, fixed—operation, connected to regular performance. But those instructions were still like handwriting: variable in their concrete theatrical manifestations. By contrast, in the working world of modernity, "ritual is replaced by the precise, technical operation, as amoral as it is unchivalrous."[44] The technological *routine* (from the French for "path of habit") denotes a "fragmenting of work into simpler motor functions that can slowly be combined."[45] Culture is technical in the sense of standardization and ritualization. In analog—that is, human cultic—rule processes, every act is immediately interpreted as meaningful in discrete, digital systems: "Any step is . . . as important as the whole result."[46] For the historian of culture, "a timepiece is much more than a mechanism. To attempt to understand it in isolation from its human setting is to forget that it was made in the first place in response to specific human needs."[47] But once such a mechanical clock is put to work, its functions depend on a genuinely media-governed logic, indifferent to whether it is being applied in a medieval monastery or in a present-day museum. The message of this media mechanism is not only the acoustic signal that human ears decode as an indicator of temporal measurement. It is also a media-physical reminder of frequencies and oscillations, rhythm and repetition, which constitute the basic media-archaeological ingredients in the study of nature. The innovative media-epistemological feature of the mechanical clock, the coming into being of the mechanical escapement in the thirteenth century, is as much bound to moments of cultural history as to techno-logical laws operating in an ahistorical temporal register, and its "tradition" is as much a function of the survival of knowledge about wheel-driven clocks (astrolabes) from antiquity into medieval times as it is part of a techno-logical self-reference that is only partly identical with the discursive variations of human history.[48]

The verge-and-foliot escapement—the decisive mechanism that distinguished the "truly mechanical clock" from traditional astronomical mechanisms—was later replaced by the pendulum. Periods of swing (oscillations), which had long been part of cultural knowledge, but which had been restricted to the observation of planetary systems for agricultural use, suddenly became a fundamental parameter in the measurement of micro-temporal events. The insights of media-operative measuring opened up a world of time-critical operations hitherto unknown to human perception (in the original sense of aesthetics, *aisthesis*). Media archaeology does not aspire to explain the ways in which the oscillatory mechanism used for both measuring time and striking a bell in the thirteenth century were "absorbed into the high ritual of the church," nor does it seek to explain why that development may have been "fitting."[49] The canonical hours of the monastic life—especially according to the Cisterian rules (such as Rule XCIV, which referred both to *horologium temperare* and *facere sonare*)—almost inevitably engendered the demand for some sort of automatic control. With clockwork, control was given over to the time of automata. But the driving energy behind the development of the mechanical clock—the desire to cause a clock to sound on its own—operates on a level that is not restricted to religion. Parallel to the unfolding of cultural logic, something else is at work. Media archaeology pays attention to what was established on a subconscious level prior to culture and religion: the training of a sensibility to micro-temporal events. While ever since Pythagoras the essence of sound had been a favorite topic of analysis in early Greek philosophy and musicology, the media-technological reproduction of sound by oscillatory mechanisms followed a logic of its own. At this crossroad between culture and physics, media archaeology steps in.

The Anachronism of the Ticking, Wheeled Clock

The chronological origin of the time-giving mechanical escapement-driven clockwork itself literally escapes historical narrative: "No entry in a chronicle, no narrative account, no description of the construction makes the invention an event we can date or locate."[50] One early weight-driven clock can be found in the Cathedral of Strasbourg; it was built by Henri de Vick (Wieck) between 1362 and 1370. Around 1320 Dante Alighieri described in the *Divine Comedy* a wheeled clock with a mechanical escapement. Despite those examples, the invention of the verge-and-foliot escapement-driven clock belongs to what Sigfried Giedion describes as anonymous history.[51] Although an astronomical clock furnished with a kind of escapement mechanism had already been introduced into China in the year 1092, Gerhard Dohrn-van Rossum considers the foliot escapement as "in all likelihood an independent European development."[52] His argument is a strictly media-archaeological one. The Chinese clock contained an escapement made by pivoting: "balance levers that stabilized a stop-and-go motion. The principle of the European escapement, which employs the centrifugal force of an oscillating inert mass, does not resemble it in any way whatsoever."[53] Only on a technically close reading does this difference come into view. As Joseph Needham writes, "We cannot rule out the possibility of completely and independently parallel lines of thought occurring in widely separated parts of the world."[54]

Thus another temporal order, one that reacts asymmetrically to the temporal economy of narrative history, must replace the *archē* of the escapement as a moment precisely registered in historiography. Here media archaeology refers as much to the discrete time of machines as to the symbolic time of human culture called "history." The digital beat of clockworks and the discrete series of letters in archival records are different kinds of nonnarrative temporal information.

The wheeled astronomical clock at St. Mary's Church in the city of Rostock is still ticking today. It has been preserved in its original form and has been "fully functional" since 1472, and parts of its mechanics even incorporate a precursor clock from 1379.[55] The constant ticking of this clock questions the temporality of such chronomedial systems: a kind of media time that escapes the discourse of history. Media archaeology involves an effort to capture this media-inherent microcosm of time.

"Nor is it fitly said, 'There are three times, past, present, and future'; but perchance it might be fitly said, 'There are three times; a present of things past, a present of things present, and a present of things future,'" wrote St. Augustine in Book 11 of his *Confessions*.[56] Augustine thereby implicitly describes the condition of an intact clock. Among the peculiarities of technical media is the fact that they behave negentropically toward the flow of time. Technical media reveal their essence only by "taking place," which always occurs in the present. All *archē*, all origin, is dissolved in taking place. In this sense the Middle Ages dissolve into the tick of the wheeled clock as it takes place today.

The escapement-driven wheeled clock is therefore the opposite of a mnemonic medium: its stored energy (the wound-up metal spring) is a physical-energetic memory, intermittently converted into information ("time designation") and comparable to the electromagnetic relay used in binary digital memory. In fact technological time and historical time differ fundamentally. Commenting on paragraph 80 of Martin Heidegger's *Being and Time* (1927), the chapter concerning clocks, Friedrich Kittler notes that Heidegger did not haphazardly switch from a fundamental-ontological description to a positivistic, cultural-historical description. According to Kittler, Heidegger's dilemma was this: "A history, which is essentially time, intersects with another history, through which the machines of time-measurement themselves pass. Clocks are ontic devices, thus subordinated to fundamental ontology, which nevertheless bring about historically different ontologies."[57]

Impeded Time

The abstract, quantitative time of watches and clocks took over the regime of qualitative religious time. As Henri Lefebvre writes, "This homogeneous and desacralized time has emerged victorious since it supplied the measure of the time of work," culminating in chronophotography, the technical measurement of the smallest temporal units in working processes in order to optimize production.[58] The replacement of the model of continuous time by a model of discrete pulsing represents not only a culturally historic, but also an epistemological shift. In the Occident, the time of clocks was literally "introduced bit by bit," this phrase being more than just wordplay.[59]

What appears on the clock face as a smooth temporal progression is in fact digital from a media-archaeological perspective (which is, metonymically, the view of the clockwork itself). In Heidegger's words: "Time is not. There is, It gives time. The giving that gives time is determined by denying and withholding nearness."[60] The infinite or negligible impedance between the two poles of a switch is technically called "hindrance." Its mechanical precursor is the escapement. Through the functioning of the escapement, time counts in binary form. What alphabetic writing accomplished for the phonetic stream of speech, the wheeled clock achieved for time: a radical individuation, a core of occidental combinatory rationality. Ultimately the sampling practice of signal engineering is at hand, in which individuation means the replacement of an infinity of consecutive values with a finite number of values.[61] Such a quantification of values changes its temporal essence: "Between 0 and 1 there is no time.... It is the hindrance that gives the 'discretized' [*diskretisierte*] time."[62] The tick of the clock that originated in the monastic order thus returns in the form of the digital computer. In the guiding principle of the so-called von Neumann architecture for computers, commonly in use today, this sense of time is still operative. "One thing at a time, down to the last bit!"[63]

The Electric Touch Machine Miracle Scam
Body, Technology, and the (Dis)authentication of the Pentecostal Supernatural

Marleen de Witte

Introduction

In July 2007 a Ghanaian preacher was arrested at Entebbe airport in Uganda on the accusation of trying to import from the United States an "Electric Touch" machine to lure people into believing that he could pass on the Holy Spirit. The device is purported to give its wearers an electric charge, which they can transfer to people or objects through the medium of touch. The website of the manufacturer of the Electric Touch machine and other magic tricks—the American company Yigal Mesika—promotes its products as "incredibly innovative, clever and a must for those who want to create miracles anywhere at anytime" and "the realest magic ever seen."[1] The Electric Touch promotional flyer promises: "This amazing new product will create *excitement, mystery, curiosity*, and *supernatural powers* all in one unforgettable experience!" The website tells us how: "Have a volunteer touch any part of your body, and watch them receive a pleasant electric static shock that will amaze them! They will believe you have supernatural powers!" Not wanting to "expose the secret to non magicians," Yigal Mesika did not allow me to reproduce an actual picture of the Electric Touch unit in this book, but was "more than happy to show the advertisement" (see Figure 2).²

The preacher, Kojo Nana Obiri-Yeboah of the charismatic We Are One Ministry, denied the accusations of trying to fake supernatural powers and fool his followers; he claimed the machine was a toy for his daughter. But the

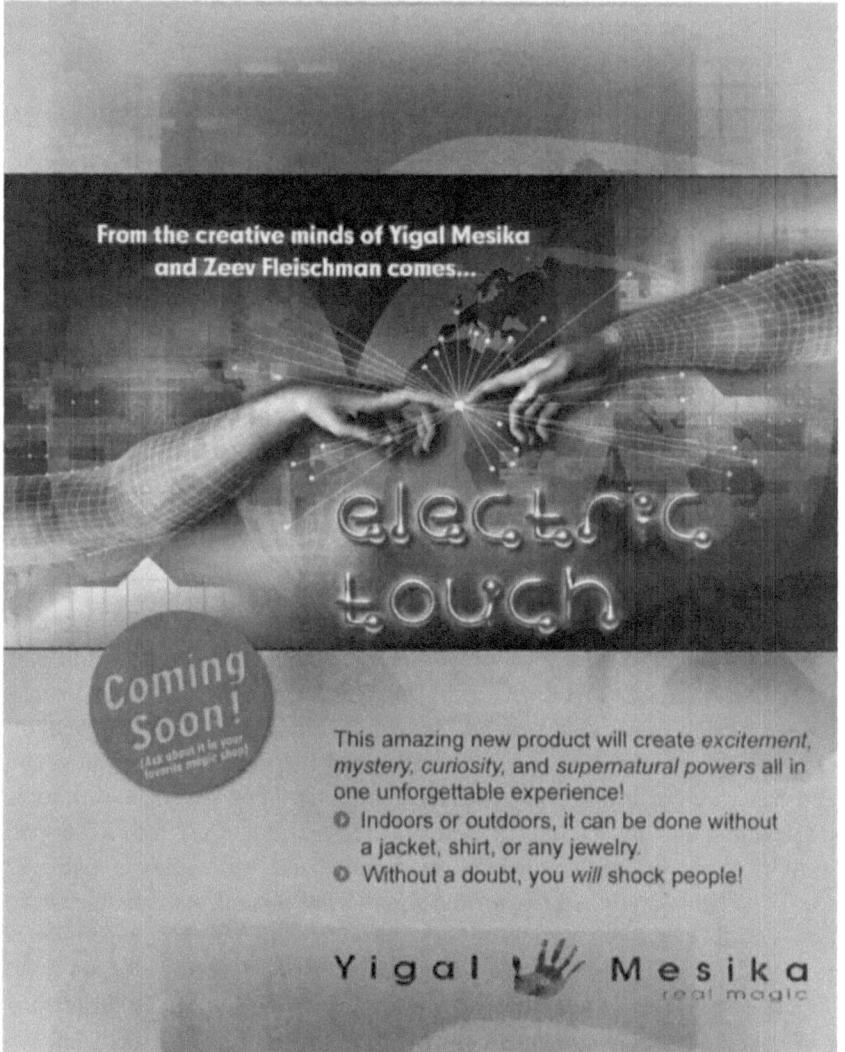

Figure 2. Advertisement for the Electric Touch Magic Trick. (Reproduction courtesy of Yigal Mesika.)

device was seized by the police, and Uganda's ethics and integrity minister, James Nsaba Buturo, started an investigation into Obiri-Yeboah's ministry practices. Global news media quickly scooped the issue, and the story of the "Electric Touch machine miracle scam" started circulating before the machine itself could ever be put to use by the preacher in question.[3]

The brief news story about pastor Obiri-Yeboah and his Electric Touch machine immediately breaks down the distinctions between realms that have long been thought separate in Western hegemonic thinking: that of scientific/technological rationality and that of religious belief or "superstition." It points to the magic of technology as well as to the technicity of experiences glossed as supernatural or religious. In his introduction to the volume *Religion and Media*, Hent de Vries has called attention to the structural resemblance between the miracle and the special effect.[4] Recognizing two elements of the miraculous (and of the transcendental more generally)—its (re)presentation as an extraordinary event and its artificiality and technicity—as two sides of the same coin, de Vries concludes that "the magical and the technological thus come to occupy the same space, obey the same regime and the same logic."[5] This structural and ontological overlap between the miracle and the special effect is not just a philosophical argument. As illustrated by the case of the Electric Touch machine miracle scam and other examples, the necessary element of technicity present in any phenomenon or experience framed as miraculous or supernatural causes great insecurity among believers and a concern with distinguishing true miracles from fraudulent illusions. So while, as de Vries states, "*analytically*, there is no observable difference between true and false miracles," in a religious field marked by fierce competition among religious specialists seeking to convince widely overlapping audiences of their claims to authority and authenticity, this very distinction is the stake in struggles over who can claim access to "real," that is, divine, not human, power.[6]

The story also points to the convincing power of touch in this politics of authentication. Touch and tactile sensations are a key modality of spiritual experience and religious subjectivity in African charismatic-Pentecostalism, and "feeling it in the body" is often taken as an indicator of the true presence of the Holy Spirit. This emphasis on the embodiment of the transcendental should not be understood as alternative or opposed to the "body pedagogics" of modern technological culture, as some authors would still have us believe.[7] On the contrary, charismatic-Pentecostal pastors all over the world are well known for their expansive use of modern technologies, not as instruments of technical rationality, but as means to bring individuals into physically felt contact with the transcendental. From audiocassettes to video compact discs and from broadcasting to podcasting, the Holy Spirit appears to flow through every technological innovation to touch expectant believers. At the same time, the slick media formats, editing techniques, and special effects that media-savvy pastors use to attract people raise suspicions about the authenticity of their claims. The massive growth in churches set up by charismatic preachers in recent years has been accompanied by fears that some could be fraudsters. Especially their fabulous riches and the large sums of money they ask from their followers evoke widespread social criticism, and the mass media carry frequent reports on "fake pastors" using dubious techniques to deceive people into believing that they have supernatural powers. The scandal about the Electric Touch machine was that even people's sense of touch, generally the most trusted of the senses, can be deceived by technological manipulation.

The story of pastor Obiri-Yeboah's Electric Touch machine, then, raises a problem of mediation and authentication,[8] as it is implicated in struggles for and over religious authority, the use of technologies, and bodily and sensory practices. Linked to broader concerns over the authenticity of technologically mediated religious experience, it invites us to explore the nexus of the corporeal, the technological, and the spiritual in African charismatic-Pentecostalism and to ask how electronic technologies intersect with techniques of the body in bringing believers into the presence of divine power. Examining some key techniques and technologies used in Pentecostal practices of mediation as well as concerns over the use of such techniques and technologies and the broader public representation of this movement in Ghana, this chapter shows how technological-bodily mediations are eternally unstable and subject to contestation by both insiders and outsiders.

Religion, Technology, Body

As noted in the introduction to this book, recent years have seen a growing scholarly interest in exploring the intersections between technology and religion, especially in the field of media studies. The most productive focus of attention in this field is not so much on how religion and media technology, as formerly separate spheres, now come to meet as religious groups adopt new—or newly available or accessible—media technologies. Rather than seeing media as new to religion, it is fruitful to see media as intrinsic to religion, understood as a practice of mediation. As an increasing number of scholars emphasize, religion always needs techniques and technologies of mediation that establish links between what is conceived as the physical and the metaphysical worlds and that enable people to experience the presence of divine power.⁹ Modern technologies of audiovisual reproduction and transmission are not external to religion, but facilitate religion's core business of connecting people and spirits. As such they are not essentially different from older, more established technologies of storage and communication, such as painting, writing, or print, or religious techniques, such as prayer, dance, or divination.

The idea of religion as media technology resonates with charismatic discourses in Ghana (and elsewhere) about communication with the spirit world in terms of technology. Various ritual practices are said to "establish points of contact," working as "spiritual electronics" and making the Holy Spirit "flow like electricity." This is not just metaphoric discourse. As media shape people's imaginations of the metaphysical, their experience of connecting to this invisible realm may be channeled through media technologies. Testimonies report of Holy Spirit baptism through a TV broadcast, of healing through a live on-air radio prayer, or of divine anointing through a sermon tape. As Friedrich Kittler wrote, "the realm of the dead is as extensive as the storage and transmission capabilities of a given culture."¹⁰ The available technologies of representation not only make possible (and limit) the religious imagination; they also enable and constrain the expression and experience of divine power. In their capacity of making the divine imaginable and rendering it present, then, modern media technologies such as television and radio are not so different from older techniques of religious mediation. It thus makes no sense to assume that media technologies are some kind of external actor doing something to an already constituted religious formation. Any religious formation is the outcome of particular techniques and technologies of mediation.

The growing attention to technological mediation goes together with a focus on the materiality and sensory appeal of the media technologies employed in religious practice. Resonating with a much broader interest in the body by scholars of religion across various disciplines and inspired by Marcel Mauss's work on techniques of the body, recent anthropological work has explored the ways in which religious mediations employ distinct sensorial (visual, aural, tactile) registers, showing how they are embodied by their recipients and how they contribute to the constitution of religious subjectivities.¹¹

The question of the sensory impact of media technologies has, of course, been debated for some time within media studies, most famously perhaps by Marshall McLuhan. In his *Understanding Media: The Extensions of Man*, McLuhan described television as a touch machine *par excellence*.¹²

"TV," he wrote, "is not so much a visual as a tactual-auditory medium that involves all of our senses in depth interplay."[13] For McLuhan, whereas the invention of photography and radio led to the extension of visual and aural sensory experience, television "is, above all, an extension of the sense of touch."[14] While McLuhan saw this synaesthetic tactility as particular to TV as opposed to other media, I think that all visual, audio, and audio-visual media have a tactile dimension in that they have the capacity to evoke tactile sensations in listeners/viewers and that, in this respect, the differences between television, cinema, photography, and radio are matters of degree rather than of kind.[15] Moreover, whereas McLuhan saw tactility as intrinsic to the technology of television itself, a more anthropological view would posit that what technologies do to people largely depends on what people do to technologies—that is, on how technologies and the encounters with them are culturally embedded and coded.

While avoiding the simplistic technological determinism of which McLuhan has—perhaps wrongly—often been accused, we must recognize that technologies do have specific features that shape human interaction and experience. But we must also ask how the materiality and sensoriality of particular media technologies tie in with cultural, social, and historical subject formations, and in particular with the ways religious traditions discipline the body and tune the senses through conscious learning and rehearsal of bodily and sensory techniques. Attention to the human body and the senses as sites of religious training also implies a shift from a focus on questions of meaning, symbolism, and belief—long privileged in the study of religion—to a focus on how sensory regimes organize relationships between religious subjects and the divine.[16] In a religious culture that pays particular attention to the bodily experience of spirit power and tunes believers' senses to the presence of the spirit, the capacity of media technologies to touch becomes particularly pronounced. The question, then, is how modern media technologies and religious techniques of the body interpenetrate and inform each other in the materialization of religious presence. As I will show in the case of charismatic-Pentecostalism, the sense of touch is particularly well-tuned, and this has important consequences for how we conceive of Pentecostalism's relationship to the sensory regimes of audiovisual technologies.

Charismatic-Pentecostalism and/as Technology in Ghana

In Ghana as in many other sub-Saharan African countries, the popularity of charismatic Christianity has been fast-growing over the past two decades.

With their message of individual success and the miraculous power of the Holy Spirit, charismatic preachers attract mass followings, especially among young, aspiring people in the urban areas.[17] Many scholars have related this exponential growth to the ways this new Christianity addresses the conditions of modernity in postcolonial society while being firmly rooted in indigenous religious worldviews.[18] In Ghana the Pentecostal boom took place in the context of—and to a large extent depended on—the country's return to democracy in 1992 and the subsequent liberalization and commercialization of the media. The rise of privately owned commercial FM radio and TV stations enabled prosperous charismatic and Pentecostal leaders to buy airtime and to establish a strong public presence. Televised church services led by celebrity pastors, commercials for healing crusades and prayer summits, radio preaching, phone-in testimonies, gospel music charts, and video clips make up a large portion of urban airtime. These media are first of all considered effective channels of evangelization, of spreading the gospel of Christ to the masses. But they are also used to enhance images of success, prosperity, and modernity, to boost the charisma of the leader and manage his public personality, and to visualize God's miracles and the church's mass following for an outside audience. With their extensive and compelling media output, charismatic-Pentecostal churches have captured broad audiences beyond their membership as traditionally defined, exerting a powerful influence not only on other Christian denominations, but also on non-Christian religions and on public and popular culture in general.[19]

From the very onset of the charismatic revival in Ghana, this movement was closely tied to mass-media technologies. Since the late 1970s newsletters, books, cassettes, and television programs by faith preachers such as Kenneth Hagin, Oral Roberts, Morris Cerullo, and Benson Idahosa have been coming to Ghana and have fed a new Christian enthusiasm.[20] Local prayer groups evolved into churches that started growing exponentially, and that continue to flourish today. Many of those new churches started recording their services on audio- and videotapes right from the beginning. Such tapes circulated through local markets, lending libraries, and hand-to-hand exchanges among friends. This cassette culture provided an effective circuit for spreading the messages and the renown of new charismatic preachers or—in Pentecostal terms—for spreading the Holy Ghost fire. When in 1992 the broadcast media were liberalized, the airwaves gradually became accessible. Many of these churches made use of the possibility to buy airtime and started broadcasting their recordings on radio and, if they could afford it, television. Inspired by the vision that "churches have to use all new technologies available, because the Devil is also using all technologies,"[21] most charismatic churches now have a "media ministry": a church department entirely devoted to the production, sales, and broadcast of radio and TV programs, audio- and videotapes, and PR material, including radio and TV commercials. "Live" church services and crusades are also mediated by technology. This includes mass events that use public-address systems, closed-circuit television, and videos projected onto huge screens in order to connect the crowds to the preacher on stage or even, through satellite connections, to charismatic crusades on the other side of the globe. People's encounters with and experiences of charismatic-Pentecostalism thus always happen partly via technology. Clearly this is a religious movement that cannot be thought of as prior to or outside of technological media. Technology is constitutive of the charismatic movement itself.

But there is another dimension to this close intertwinement of Ghanaian charismatic-Pentecostalism and technology. Pentecostal thought and teaching often frame the operation of and communication with the spirit world in terms of technology. In his book *Invisibility to Visibility*, pastor Richard Gyamfi Boakye explains the working of faith as "the principal device needed to transport invisible things" comparable with technologies of "remote sensing," such as satellites. Like a satellite, "faith has the ability to gather the energy of the spiritual realm and send signals into the physical in the form of solutions."[22] The same pastor uses the recurrent image of the spiritual working like electricity:

> When you put on light you are confident it will brighten even though you do not see the electric current. The bulb lightens because when you touch the switch you close the circuit and the electric current is therefore able to flow through. When faith is released it will complete the circuit of the spiritual and the physical and as a result spiritual resources will be transported into the physical.[23]

In another Pentecostal publication, Pastor Emmanuel Abrahams of the Power of God Mission explains how money offerings work as "spiritual electronics:" "Electronics is a system in which we use electric current through created devices that perform the things we want. Spiritual electronics is the usage of our financial resources to produce results in our life."[24] Similarly, the practice of speaking in tongues is described as "a direct communication line to God in the spirit." Praise and worship help believers "tune to the power of the Spirit," and prophecy, "seeing powers," is likened to radar or X-ray technology.

Not limited to Ghana, or indeed elsewhere in Africa, such discourse is found across global Pentecostalism.[25] In the Ghanaian setting, however, it resonates with a much wider discursive religious field, in which the presence and working of a range of invisible powers—witchcraft, spirits, the devil, the Holy Spirit—are explained by turning to electronic technologies. Witchcraft and magic ("juju") are commonly termed "African electronics." Traditional healers compare the realm of spirits to radio or television airwaves and divination to computer technology.[26] One "spiritual scientist" described his work as follows: "It is spiritual science, because it is a matter of putting the right things together in the right way for the power to enter and the thing to work. It is like a mobile phone, if it is not arranged well, it will not work. Or a TV and the remote, there is a power working between them, which you don't see."[27]

Pentecostals not only imagine the working of the spiritual realm as electronic technology, they also talk about their experiences of the power of the Holy Spirit, or the "anointing," in terms of electricity. In the context of an ethnographic study of the International Central Gospel Church (ICGC) in Accra,[28] one of Ghana's largest and most media-active charismatic churches, I talked with one of the church pastors, Pastor Dan, about the anointing. Explaining the concept to me, he said: "the anointing of God is like electricity." Had I not felt how, during the anointing service, the church auditorium was "electric with the presence and power of the Holy Spirit?" Christians who say that they have been baptized in the Holy Spirit often say "it was like a jolt of electricity." Pastor Dan told me that when, after such a baptism, he would put his hand next to the person, he could "feel the power, like heat or electricity, radiating off their bodies."[29] This image of electricity is part of globalized charismatic discourse. In *Good Morning, Holy Spirit*, a book that I bought in the Lighthouse Chapel's Vision Bookstore in Accra, the American evangelist Benny Hinn describes an experience he had at the age of eleven: "Suddenly my little body was caught up in an incredible sensation that can only be described as 'electric.' It felt as if someone had plugged me into a wired socket."[30]

The image of the Holy Spirit as electric power is not just a metaphor that is good to think about and understand spiritual matters. Part of a broader religious imaginary of connectivity, circuitry, and immediacy, it informs ritual practices and helps tune the believer's senses to the working of this invisible power. In other words, such images do not remain on the level of representations, but become literally embodied, thus producing bodily sensations. Sometimes such sensations are expressed in general terms of tactility, as "being touched by the spirit" or "feeling the power of the Holy Ghost"; sometimes they are referred to more specifically as a sensation of heat, coldness, heaviness, or goose bumps.[31] Pastor Dan continued: "The anointing is tangible. It can be felt. Just as electricity is tangible, so is the anointing. And not only is it tangible; it is also transferable. You can communicate it, you can give it away. You can store it up and you can give it away."

This transference of the invisible power of the anointing is wonderfully visualized in the giant stage backdrop in the International Central Gospel Church, which served as a visual marker of the church's 2009's theme "Supernatural." A creative charismatization of Michelangelo's *Creation of Adam* on the ceiling of the Sistine Chapel, Figure 3 dramatically shows the touch of the divine hand as it transfers the spark of life to the first man in the shape of a lightning bolt. Note the striking resemblance to the promotional flyer of Yigal Mesika's Electric Touch machine (see Figure 2). The structural likeness described by Hent de Vries of the miracle and the special effect can hardly be better illustrated.

Being invisible, yet tangible and transferable, Holy Spirit power—like electricity—does not touch you out of the blue, however. You need to "plug into a socket" before you can feel the shock. As Pastor Dan explained, "electricity may be flowing all around us in the walls of a building. This electric power can bring wonderful appliances to life, but only if we plug into a receptacle and bring the electric power into contact with the lamp or

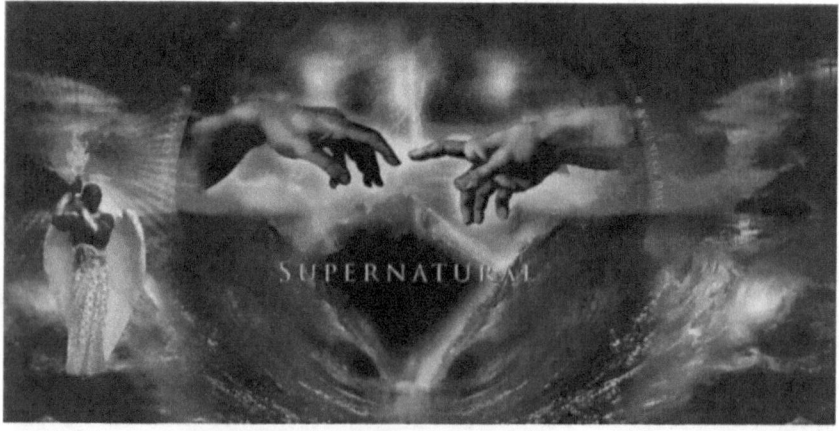

Figure 3. Stage Backdrop to the International Central Gospel Church, by Nana Kwadwo Duah (Accra, 2009). (Reproduction courtesy of the ICGC.)

computer we want to use. When the anointing touches you, you become different. Anointing upon your life will set you alive and break the sickness of spiritual inactivity." Charismatic-Pentecostals thus call upon the language of electricity and electronic technology to describe the supernatural realm as immediate and tangible. Such a conceptualization of Holy Spirit power as electric current—as something to which we need to be plugged in before we can receive it and come to life—informs techniques of the body found in Ghanaian charismatic churches.

Techniques of the Body and the Touch of the Spirit

In charismatic Christianity the personal experience of the Holy Spirit forms the center of religious attention and desire. In contrast with the Catholic tradition, Charismatic churches promise believers a direct relationship with Jesus Christ and access to the power of the Holy Spirit unmediated by ordained priests. God calls everyone, and every Christian can and is expected to embody his Holy Spirit without any intermediary. Despite this theological emphasis on immediacy, however, Ghanaian charismatic Christianity increasingly emphasizes the role of a supernaturally gifted "man of God" to overcome problems and achieve success.[32] Certain people (mostly, but not only, men) are perceived as being chosen by God and endowed with a special "anointing" that enables them to transfer the power of the Holy Spirit to their followers. The body of this man of God is authorized as an important instrument for the operation of the Holy Spirit on earth. It is part of the spiritual "wiring." In the context of charismatic-Pentecostal ritual, this is taken so literally that the touch, and especially the pastor's touch, features centrally as an effective mode of connecting to the realm of supernatural power. Touch the wire and get the shock. In a variety of ritual performances, physical touch closes the spiritual-physical circuit through which the Holy Spirit can flow like electricity and touch an expectant believer.

During the weekly Solution Centre, a healing and miracle service at the ICGC, pastor Dan engages the congregation in intimate physical contact. Laying his hands on people's heads or on sick body parts and shouting in their ears and into the microphone, he casts out any demons that may be causing their sickness or failure in business or marriage, commanding the power of the Holy Ghost to come upon them, and prophesizing victory in the form of a visa, a villa, a pregnancy, a husband, or a job. Sometimes anointing oil is applied on the body, either by the pastor or the believer herself, so as to create "points of contact" with the Holy Spirit. The drama of the performance is intensified by music or sound effects by the church band and loudly amplified glossolalia (speaking in tongues) by the prophet. Spiritual mediation thus happens most effectively through touch and "haptic sound," whereby it is not the symbolic quality of sound (the meaning of words spoken or sung), but its physical quality (uttering meaningless sounds, the sheer volume of shouting, the rhythm of music) that makes the Spirit flow. Technology is already constitutive of this total sensory experience of plugging in: sound amplification, surround-sound technology, musical instruments, cameras, closed-circuit television, and PowerPoint projections all contribute to people's sense of divine presence. The presence of the Holy Spirit in the individual believer manifests itself in the body or in bodily sound: involuntary spinning, shaking, jumping, falling down, crying, screaming, and speaking in tongues are all interpreted as signs of the touch of the Spirit.

What is important to stress here are the technicity and artificiality of this extraordinary experience of the miraculous touch of God and, in particular, the bodily techniques that mediate this sense of spirit power. Consider the example of glossolalia. When people are praying aloud together and speaking in tongues, at first hearing it seems purely spontaneous and unruly, and this is exactly how it is understood to be in charismatic doctrine: a spontaneous manifestation of the sudden presence of the Holy Spirit within an individual. At such a moment the Spirit is claimed to be speaking through the believer according to the will of God. But in practice it is the pastor who subtly indicates when to start and when to stop praying. Moreover, glossolalia is something you can learn by practicing, and some people are clearly more advanced in it than others. Some people told me that as children they were taught how to speak in tongues by saying "I love Jesus" more and more quickly until the words became unintelligible. Similarly, when people fall down upon the touch of the pastor's hand on their head, this is interpreted to be a spontaneous response to the touch of the Holy Spirit. But such events occur within a format of bodily posture and choreography that inexperienced newcomers acquire with the help of church ushers or by mimicking others. Such bodily and sensory formats for the reception of Holy Spirit are acquired and gradually embodied through participation in religious performance. Through bodily techniques the senses are tuned in to the touch of the Spirit, which is at the same time authenticated as something that occurs spontaneously. The experience is thus attributed to divine, not human, agency.

Despite this emphasis on spontaneity and divine agency, the fact of practicing and acquiring techniques is not necessarily seen as contradictory or fake. Rather, conscious and directed action on the part of the spirit-desiring believer is deemed necessary in order to be able to receive the Spirit. One needs to actively plug in and not sit and wait unplugged for the power to come. And yet the technicity of the miraculous touch does create a tension. It is not obvious when a performance genuinely exhibits "divine touch" and when it fails to become so, remaining an instance of "mere acting." Critics often dismiss charismatic bodily practices as "mere performance" or "just pretending." For their part, many pastors are concerned that the increasing mass-mediatization and popularization of charismatic Christianity merely attract people to an outward style of charismatic worship and Christian appearance without instigating the deep, life-transforming experience of being born again. Such criticisms should be understood as a particular religious concern with authenticity that privileges depth over superficiality, content over form, spirit over the body, spontaneity over ritual, immediacy over mediation, and divine agency over human agency. However, we can escape such dichotomies by arguing that experiences authenticated as deep, inner, spontaneous, and immediate and as generated by the Holy Spirit are necessarily mediated by bodily forms and performances. As mediating forms, techniques of the body such as glossolalia or laying on of hands are just as prone to disauthentication—that is, to be identified as simulated or fake—as are media technologies such as video or television broadcasting. Conversely, such technologies are also just as likely to be authorized as conducting wires for the power of Holy Spirit as is the physical touch of the anointed man of God.

Miraculous Touch Machines

While prospective converts are often urged to "visit this church on a Sunday to really feel the Holy Spirit at work," it is also possible to have this experience over a great distance through electronic media technologies. The text on the dust jacket of the religious videotape *Miracle Days Are Here* proclaims: "Join Bishop Dag Heward-Mills in the powerful miracle service captured on this video and experience the miraculous touch of God which is able to heal, deliver and restore! As you receive the Word of God about the Anointing and the miraculous, may faith be stirred up within you to receive your own miracle!"[33] The dust jacket thus promises an experience of "miraculous touch" through the audiovisual medium of a videotape by one of Ghana's biggest celebrity preachers. Indeed, testimonies abound in Ghana of people having received the *touch* of the Holy Spirit through a media broadcast or tape recording.

Some preachers solve the problem of media technologies' transcendence of embodied proximity by calling their listeners, viewers, or readers to create a "point of contact" by laying their hand on the radio set, the TV screen, or the book page. Asamoah-Gyadu writes, for example, that Bishop Agyin Asare of Word Miracle Church International often opens his palms and asks viewers to place their own open palms into his on the TV screen as he prays for them, in the belief that "there is transference of 'healing anointing' to the sick through the screen."[34] In other cases viewers may be asked to place a bottle of oil on their television sets in the belief that the oil will be infused with anointing power as the pastor on the screen prays.[35] Media preachers thus make use of the materiality of the media device much in the same way that the materiality of the body is used to create "contact points" during anointing services. The television set or the radio receiver, Asamoah-Gyadu argues, thus "acquires a talismanic status as a medium for effective anointing."[36] But even without physically touching such devices, people can receive the touch of the Holy Spirit through their eyes and ears.

In order to understand how such an experience of audiovisually mediated divine touch comes about, two things should be noted. First, in Ghanaian charismatic-Pentecostal thought, sounds and images possibly contain spirit powers (good or evil) that may affect the listener or the viewer.[37] Second, particular practices of listening or watching can enable (or block) the spirit contained in the sound/image to enter the person's body. Concerning the faculty of hearing, charismatics commonly distinguish between listening to the word of God as an educational exercise and as a spiritual event: between "learning" and "catching," in the words of Dag Heward-Mills. He writes about "the art of soaking in tapes" in his book *Catch the Anointing*, which has a revealing cover photo of a hand literally catching an audiotape (see Figure 4).[38]

> "Soaking" in tapes simply means to listen to the words over and over again until it becomes a part of you and until the anointing passes on to you! When a tape is fully "soaked," both the Word content and the Spirit content are imbibed in your spirit. The anointing is not something you learn, it is something you catch. Do not assume that the "soaking" in of the tape is just an educational exercise. It is a spiritual event. [. . .] The Spirit enters a person as he receives the Word of God. That is why many people experience a radical transformation by just listening to a powerful message from the Word of God.[39]

Heward-Mills thus advises his readers to listen to tapes in such a way that one no longer just hears the meaning of the words, but embodies their

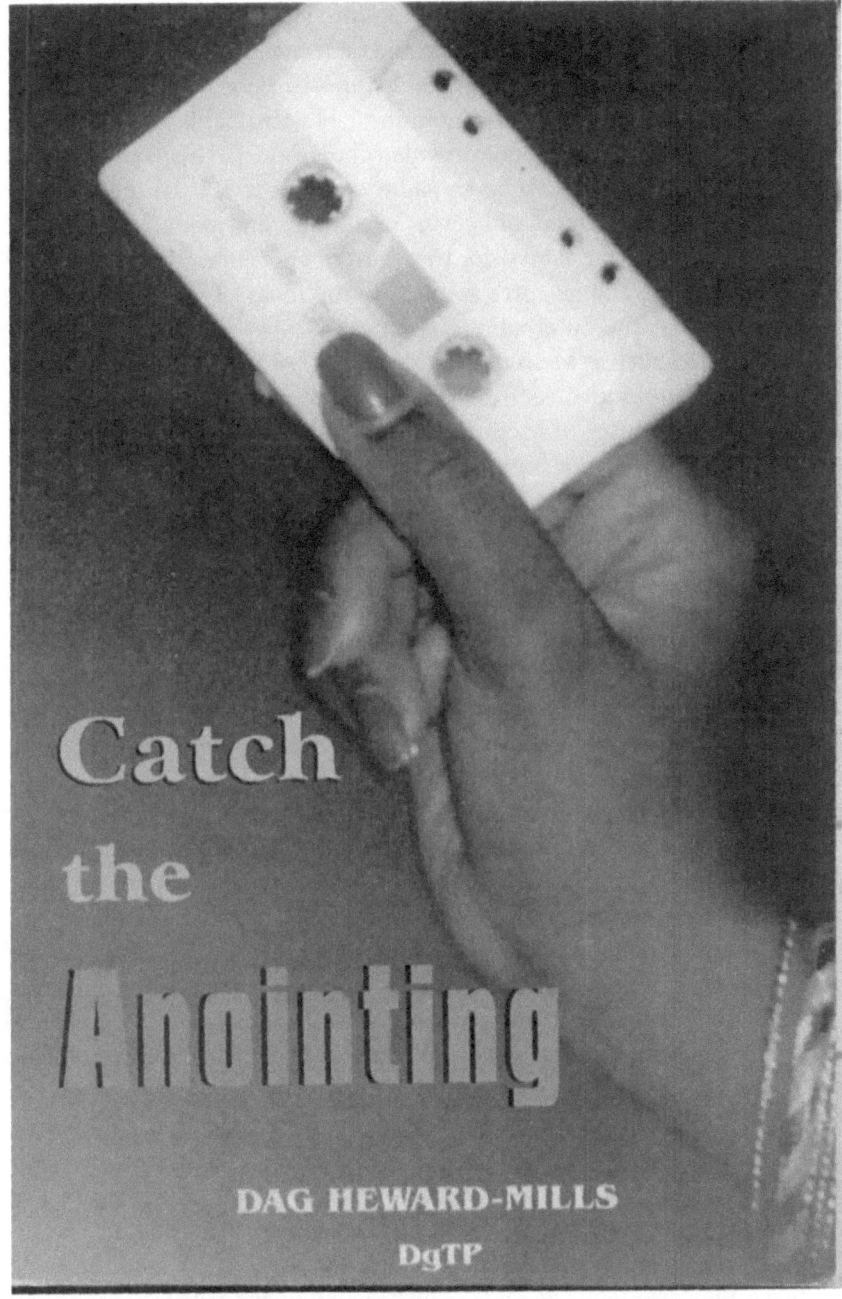

Figure 4. Book cover, *Catch the Anointing* by Dag Heward-Mills (Accra: Dag's Tapes and Publications, 2000).

spiritual quality, and the anointing "comes into you." One may listen to the message only with one's ears and brain and understand it, but it is only when one also absorbs it into one's material being—like porous matter absorbs liquid—that one can "catch the anointing." Heward-Mills also tells us to "avoid the mistake of leaving out the video dimension. [It] helps you to catch things that you cannot catch on an audio tape: posture, attire, gestures."[40] The technologically stored and reproduced voice and body image of the pastor thus become the vehicle for the Spirit to enter into the person.

Posture, attire, and gestures are exactly the focus of the editors in the media studio of the International Central Gospel Church. Producing television series such as Mensa Otabil's *Living Word* and Korankye Ankrah's *Power in His Presence* involves extensive editing of the spoken content as well as the images in order to maximize the intended effect of the broadcasts on their spectators.[41] For both the aforementioned programs, the editors have developed a format that enhances the pastor's specific ministry gift: in Otabil's case, teaching, and in Ankrah's case, the manifestation of Holy Ghost power. *Living Word* thus visually represents the nonverbal interaction between Otabil and his congregation during the sermon, with images highlighting Otabil's charismatic authority and audience shots depicting individuals responding to his words, agreeing with him, admiring him. *Power in His Presence* not only includes Ankrah's sermons, but dramatic images of worship, deliverance, and people shaking, falling down, and rolling on the floor in reception of the Holy Ghost. In both cases the camera operators and studio editors make creative and skillful use of camera angles and editing techniques in order to highlight the spiritual power embodied by the pastor and to suggest its transference to their audiences. For instance, they select particularly impressive shots of the pastor, showing his powerful gestures and facial expressions interspersed with expressive and emotional, but always appropriate audience cutaways in which unflattering shots of the pastor as well as any improper audience behavior—such as chewing gum, looking distracted, or walking about— have been removed.

Talking with the editors about their work, it became clear to me how the visual representation of a flow between pastor and audience onscreen also serves as a technique to transfer the spirit power contained in the message to viewers at home. The editors explained that people at home have a tendency to identify with the people they see on TV, and the body language they see depicted shapes their viewing experience.[42] If they see people agreeing with a statement, they also want to agree. If they see people captured by a message, the message will capture them. In line with media theory that emphasizes that this process of audience identification takes place not strictly on a symbolic level, but on an embodied one,[43] the editors deliberately show the bodily regimes necessary to receive the word of God and with it the Holy Spirit. Bodies that do not appear to be listening appropriately—and thus are not receiving the Spirit, but only hearing mere words—are edited out of the scene. The *Living Word* format thus strongly suggests a bodily way of listening to Otabil's message that is needed for "catching" the spiritual power embedded in it. The editors hope that by mimetically identifying with the televised bodies of the church audience, the TV viewers will similarly subject themselves to Otabil and partake in the anointing he embodies and radiates.[44] Sometimes the editors "cheat" in order to produce a desired effect, such as by cutting an audience shot from the footage of one service and pasting it into another. They also alternate effectively between wide-angle shots and strategically placed close-ups in order to evoke a sense of close association with the anointed man of God.

Charismatic-Pentecostalism is first of all concerned with the coming into presence of spirit power. Media images and sounds must "touch" their viewers, and the experience of being touched while watching or listening is attributed to the power of the Holy Spirit. Just as the bodies and voices of "anointed Men of God" mediate the presence of the Holy Spirit in church services, their technologically mass-reproduced body images and sounds are intended to transfer Holy Spirit touch over distance. Blurring the boundary between onscreen and offscreen and between representation and presence, editing techniques make the television screen a conductor for the Holy Spirit to touch the viewer. In the hands of Ghanaian Pentecostal pastors—or rather their media staff—video cameras, television, radio, cassettes, compact discs, and other media technologies turn into "electric touch machines" of a kind, closing the circuit that enables the power of the Holy Spirit to flow and to manifest itself in believers' bodies as physical sensation. It is in this sense that the technological and the spiritual merge and "God is in the machine." Pentecostals have made it their core business to get God's spirit into the body via the machine. They embrace media technologies as effective channels through which to connect physically to the realm of spiritual power. At the same time, the awareness of the enchanting power of technology and the acknowledgment of the mediating role of bodily techniques and media technologies cause anxiety about inauthenticity and the specter of "fake pastors." The Electric Touch machine's promise to "create supernatural powers" by technological means is so unsettling for Pentecostals because it points to the possibility that miracles are merely human artifacts.

"Fake Pastors" on the Airwaves

The case of the Ghanaian charismatic pastor and the Electric Touch machine described at the beginning of this chapter should be understood in a broader religious field in which the "fake pastor" (*osofo moko*, in local parlance) or "false prophet" is a recurrent figure: one who seems to have gained prevalence and moral importance with the new accessibility of communication technologies since the liberalization in the 1990s. As Jesse Shipley has also observed, electronic mediation has accelerated fears about spiritual trickery and generated a public obsession with assessing genuine spiritual power and unmasking fakery.[45] Time and again one hears about the activities of fake pastors trying to capitalize on the widespread craving for miracles and making huge sums of money from unsuspecting individuals, who call on them for spiritual solutions to their problems. Local FM radio stations are seen as particularly susceptible to such fraud. Easily accessible and hugely popular, radio is an effective medium for people to claim to possess miraculous powers and to support such claims with personal testimonies of miraculous healings. One Christian radio station in Accra, Channel R, has been criticized for broadcasting "false prophets." It denied the allegations, claiming that all pastors are thoroughly screened before they are allowed to go on the air.[46] A popular talk show host in Kumasi, Kwabena Asare, aka "Otsunoko," has made it his mission to expose fake pastors live on air on his radio program, which is aired on Nhyira FM on weekdays from 7:00 P.M. to 10:00 P.M.[47] Similarly, in Nigeria, the authenticity of media pastors became such a matter of public concern that in May 2004 the Nigerian National Broadcasting Commission imposed a ban on the depiction of "unverified miracles" on its television stations.[48] In Ghana such remarkable steps have not been taken, although the fervent use of broadcast media by charismatics is being watched with suspicion by the National Media Commission.[49]

The point is that Ghana's religious marketplace is increasingly constituted by mass-media technologies. The liberalization and commercialization of the Ghanaian media have allowed new actors, including religious ones, to enter the public sphere and to capture new audiences, not only on the basis of rational-critical argument, but also through the visceral power of visuals, voice, rhythm, and volume. Modern technologies, spectacular imagery, and dramatic sounds have become novel markers of religious authority and authenticity. The attraction of followers—or, from the perspective of the critics, victims—to the new and often self-proclaimed men of God depends to a large extent on media and marketing strategies and personality creation.⁵⁰ People's awareness of media technology's power to manipulate, however, gives rise to insecurities and contestations over the authenticity of claims to spiritual authority. Charismatic pastors always risk being accused of faking supernatural powers and just performing tricks to mislead people with false claims in order to get rich quickly and to lead extravagant lifestyles. No pastor is totally immune from such criticisms, and the legitimacy of particular pastors' claims to anointing is much debated in charismatic-Pentecostal circles and beyond. Even established celebrity pastors such as Mensa Otabil constantly need to authenticate the implicit message that they are not mere media creations, but rather embody real and effective anointing from God.

As I have argued, religious authority always needs a certain degree of technicity or artificiality. It is therefore very hard to distinguish between a genuine man of God and a charlatan faking divine inspiration for material gain. Such concerns with discerning fake and real spiritual power are of course characteristic of a type of religion that locates religious authority not in institutionalized hierarchies and formal education, but in divine inspiration and charisma. As such, the false prophet is a global Pentecostal figure. But in Ghana the politics of religious authentication and dis-authentication between competing men of God are also rooted in much older, pre-Christian forms of religious power and competition among religious specialists offering access to spirit powers. Indeed, present-day traditional healers and priests are prone to very similar accusations of fakery. One of the leaders of the Afrikania Mission, a neotraditionalist organization representing "African traditional" religious practitioners in Ghana, told me that one of the problems they faced was that one cannot always be sure who is a genuine priest or healer and who is a quack: "Priests and priestesses can use tricks and pretend to be possessed, because they know the signs of being possessed by a particular divinity. That is a false prophet. The majority of them are quacks."⁵¹

The opening up of the airwaves to the public strategies of religious leaders has given a boost to the old figure of the fake priest/pastor/healer. As a result of their eager exploitation of the power of media technologies to enchant the masses, charismatic pastors have become particularly susceptible to suspicions of fakery, and the fake pastor has come to be associated with charismatic Christianity more than with any other religion. With large photographs and bold headlines, popular tabloids carry all kinds of gossip and allegations about pastors' sexual escapades, criminal activities, and other immoral behavior, thereby spectacularly exposing the hidden evil in these "false prophets." A popular theme is pastors' consultations with traditional shrines and "juju men" and their indulgence in "juju" rituals in order to attract crowds to their churches and get rich quickly. Given the Pentecostal condemnation of "traditional" religion, such revelations of pastors' secret power sources constitute serious charges of hypocrisy. Clearly, while pastors have successfully adopted media technologies, they do not fully control their representation in all media. As media technologies enhance spiritual authority as well as fears of spiritual frauds, pastors' media strategies require a sensitive balancing act on the tightrope between genuineness and fakery and between morality and immorality.

Conclusion

The ethnography presented in this chapter has shown that technologies do not have universalizing effects everywhere, but rather have particular effects and affects in local contexts of adoption. Ghanaian Pentecostals ascribe to modern media technologies the power to connect people not only to each other, but also to spirits. Television sets, radio receivers, and audiocassettes are thus put to use not only as media of representation and communication, but also as "talismanic" objects for tapping into the sources of supernatural power. Incorporated into religious bodily and sensory regimes, they are felt to have the capacity to transfer supernatural power into viewers' and listeners' bodies and thereby to affect their being.

The ascription of magical qualities to media technologies is certainly not unique to the African or, more broadly, the "non-Western" context. The transmission of miraculous healing power through the television screen is in fact a familiar phenomenon in global televangelism. For example, the American charismatic faith healer Ernest Angley is known for his televised faith-healing services that end with a shot of his open palm, projecting the image of an enormous hand into American living rooms, and inviting viewers to bring any afflicted body part into contact with the screen. In the hands of Ernest Angley, David Chidester writes, "television truly became a tactile medium, a medium for establishing a kind of physical contact that manipulated unseen powers of healing."[52] In the Ghanaian context, charismatic-Pentecostal engagements with audiovisual technologies show a remarkable continuity with traditional religious practices, where images and sounds do not so much represent or symbolize the divine as embody and convey spirit power.[53] Objects, images, and sounds—including technologically reproduced ones—can be used to bring spirits into presence. As traditional believers take an effigy or a drumming rhythm to make a deity present in the ritual context of a shrine or a possession ceremony, they may also ascribe to a photograph or video shot of that effigy or a sound recording of that drumming the ability to make the deity present in the context in which the image is viewed or the sound is heard. Charismatic-Pentecostal media practices, then, are much closer to African religious traditions than their ostentatiously cosmopolitan outlook would at first sight suggest.

But also in the West, the association of media technology with supernatural powers is much more widespread than Pentecostal and "modernist" views of technology would presume. In *Haunted Media* Jeffrey Sconce gives a historical account of the persistent association of new communication media (from telegraph, radio, and telephone to television and computers) with spiritual powers and related phenomena in American popular culture.[54] Examining stories of ghosts in televisions, spirit voices heard through radio, and communication with the dead through telegraphy, Sconce and others show how such discourses are connected to the dominant understanding of media in terms of liveness, network, and flow.[55] Throughout history the idea that media have a "living presence"—that they can transcend space and time and put us into direct contact with realms outside our normal sensory perception—has included the live presence of spirit worlds.[56]

The magic of electronic communication technology enchants people worldwide. There is a certain uncanniness about the working of technology that springs from a combination of a sense of awe and wonder inspired by impressive technological advance and performance and a lack of control and predictability—an experience of technology displacing our agency. In certain contexts this "technological sublime" is marginalized by dominant collective representations that favor rationalist scientific approaches to technology and deconstruct its magic.[57] In other contexts, however, the awesome power of technology may tie in with particular religious imaginaries and sensory regimes, thus enhancing its prominence and exploiting its religious potential. When the mystery of new communication technologies meets the mystery of religion, the intersection of religious and media ideologies of liveness, presence, and immediacy may generate experiences of being in touch with a spirit power or powers. The charismatic-Pentecostal ideology of immediacy and the living presence of God appears to fit particularly well with television's suggestion of liveness, thus producing in Pentecostal audiences a feeling of being touched by the Holy Spirit.[58] This again has acquired a particular resonance in the Ghanaian context of traditional beliefs about the presence and direct influence of spirits and the practice of communicating with these spirits and embodying their power.

At the same time, this chapter's focus on Pentecostal uses of media technology in Ghana has revealed a more general and basic tension inherent in charismatic-Pentecostalism: the problem of mediated immediacy and the authentication of religious experience and expression. As a religion that places strong emphasis on personal experiences of spiritual power, it depends on media for contact with the invisible realm of the Holy Spirit. Drawing on bodily techniques and media technologies in order to produce in people experiences of divine touch, Pentecostals at the same time need to mystify the mediating work of these techniques and technologies so as to authenticate a religious experience as immediate and real. That is, technology has to be naturalized, to appear unnoticed in a way, in order for the divine to be identified as the true source of power. The Electric Touch machine could indeed be perfectly suitable to this end, since it remains invisible during the moment of transfer of electricity/Holy Spirit power. When exposed, however—as in the case of the Electric Touch machine—the power of technology risks disauthenticating the sensations evoked as being not spirit-induced, but rather human-produced, and thus "fake."

Despite their structural resemblance, then, modern media technologies cannot be assumed to be unproblematic extensions of older techniques of religious mediation. On the contrary, technologies and the mediating work they do are always possible sources of caution and conflict. Media technologies may be taken to counteract an ideal of authentic, immediate religious experience. But the repetition of bodily techniques may pose the same challenge, as we have seen. It thus makes no sense to associate the body with authentic religious experience and technology with fakery and fiction. The immediacy of the supernatural as an extrasensory presence always depends on techniques and technologies, including bodily ones, to find material form and to be sensed. Immediacy is thus a fiction. And yet some technologies are felt to provide immediate access to the divine, whereas others are experienced as standing in between. Clearly the powers of particular technologies are not intrinsic. Rather they are attributed via a process of religious authentication that invests them with authority—or denies them authority—in the context of relationships between religious subjects and the divine. Recurrent debates and occasional scandals about religious uses and abuses of technologies indicate that this process is never final.

The Spiritual Nervous System

Reflections on a Magnetic Cord Designed for Spirit Communication

Jeremy Stolow

In 1853, in a decade that witnessed the precipitous rise of the modern Spiritualist movement, one of its leading intellectual figures, Andrew Jackson Davis, penned a set of instructions for the organization of séances. Successful communication with the spirit world, he argued, depends on the presence of a proper balance of positive and negative elements and forces. To that end séance-goers were advised to form a "harmonial circle"; those whose negative temperament was signaled by cold hands and "a mild and loving disposition" should be placed in alternate seats with "positively tempered" individuals, distinguished by their physical warmth and their intellect.[1] The balance of forces required for communication with the spirit world could be further enhanced, it seems, with the preparation of advantageous environmental conditions. Participants were directed to meet in darkened rooms, "retired from all noise and interruption . . . so that the persons present, not having their minds attracted and diverted by external things, may the more easily concentrate their thoughts upon the *object* for which they have met together."² Lastly, and most remarkably, Davis proposed that séance-goers

> provide themselves with a fine magnetic cord. . . . Get about five yards of a three-quarter-inch rope; cover this rope with silk or cotton velvet; and wind around it, parallel with each other, two wires, one of steel and the other of silver or copper. Have the space between the wires about one inch and a half, and let them be wound around about a quarter of an inch apart.³

Sitters were instructed to assemble around the table, holding onto the magnetic cord in their laps in order to establish "an equilibrium of vital electricity and vital magnetism throughout the entire circle."⁴ Once the circuit has been completed, Davis explained, "the one which is constitutionally most susceptible to spiritual influx of emotion and influence will feel a throbbing in the hands; and ultimately, by repeated experiments, some one among the company may be rendered clairvoyant."⁵ But even with the arrival of these initial signs of contact with the supernatural, sitters were advised to continue holding the cord for at least one hour, and only then cast it aside and reconstitute the circle through the joining of hands. By that point the magnetic cord will have served its purpose. A truly harmonious human circle having been established, "the members may rest assured that guardian and affectionate spirits will descend, and sometimes come personally into the room."⁶

The historical record offers no confirmation of whether Davis's readers actually took heed of his instruction to build their own magnetic cords and incorporate them into their séance activities. Spiritualists themselves were chiefly concerned with the revelatory messages that were enunciated once contact with the spirit world had been established, and had much less to say about the equipment they used to make those links.⁷ But Davis's text offers a uniquely detailed account of the techniques and instruments at least some Spiritualists must have deemed useful for engaging with the spirit world. His description of the magnetic cord provides a striking example of what we might call a Spiritualist technology for supernatural communication: an instrument whose function was to generate a circuit that linked minds, bodies, physical spaces, and immaterial forces within a shared network of thought, speech, and action. As a medium for transducing different forces and energies within this networked circuitry, the cord seems to have been designed to perform such varied tasks as causing séance participants to experience throbbing sensations, facilitating visual or auditory apparitions, and even providing spirits direct access to the minds and bodies of the living in order to speak and act through them.

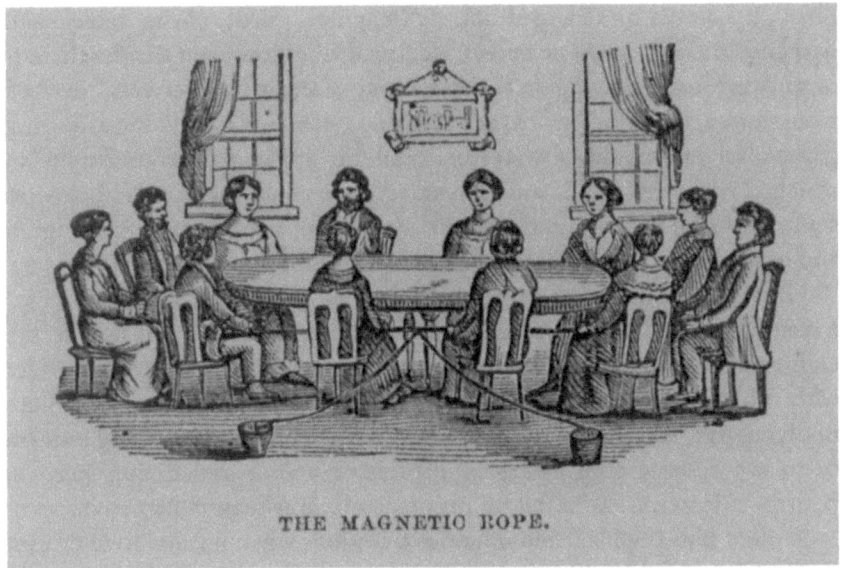

Figure 5. "The Magic Rope." Andrew Jackson Davis, *The Present Age and Inner Life; Ancient and Modern Spirit Mysteries Classified and Explained* (Boston: Colby & Rich, 1886), p. 101. (Reproduction courtesy of Rare Books and Special Collections, McGill University Library.)

In all these ways Davis's cord throws into sharp relief some of the key terms on which Spiritualists contributed, in their own way, to a technologization (ought one say "retechnologization?") of the supernatural order. For twined around the cord one finds not only strands of silk and copper and steel wires, but also deep ontological and cosmological assumptions about the survival of the human soul after death, the physiological constitution of "sympathetic souls" capable of communing with the spirit world, and the amenability of human bodies, material objects, and immaterial entities to a common set of operative principles, modeled on the physics of electromagnetic conductivity and induction. Because it could be plied into a circle and thereby was able to enclose objects within its "circuit," Davis's magnetic cord joined company with other phenomena becoming newly visible in nineteenth-century public discussions, including telegraph cables, railway lines, and the ganglia and fibers of bodily nervous systems. In the context of rapidly expanding bodies of knowledge and practical experiences involving electricity in particular, nineteenth-century Spiritualism presented a vision of the body, the social order, the natural world, and the uncharted beyond, all linked together through a nexus of arranged objects (magnetic cords, chairs, tables, and darkened rooms), sensitive nerves, electrical vibrations, and slender threads of spiritual force. Playing on the etymology of the word "nervous," derived from *neuron*, the Greek word for a tendon, a sinew, or a cord, the following pages offer an account of what I shall call the "spiritual nervous system" in which Davis's instrument was embedded: an account that hopefully invites some further reflection on the shared semantic space within which religion and technology come to be named as distinct entities.

Of course, Spiritualists were hardly the first "theologians of electricity," a term that could be applied to numerous actors going back at least to the eighteenth century, when it was not infrequent to equate electrical wonder with Biblical miracle and, accordingly, to describe electricity as a medium of divine will, manifested in such things as lightning strikes during a storm or in the ecstatic convulsions of Protestant bodies undergoing spiritual rebirth.[8] Moreover, as noted by Bret Carroll, Spiritualists had recourse to even older philosophical and religious traditions when it came to their uses of the figure of the circle—an ancient symbol of order and harmony—in their descriptions of the cosmos (in which both the spirit world and the physical world were aligned into a series of concentric "spheres"), in the way they organized ritual activities (seating themselves around circular tables), and in their discussions about social harmony and republican virtue (in which circles appear as metaphors of familial intimacy, religious fellowship, and national belonging).[9] But for mid-century American Spiritualists, it was now possible to account for the power of circles with reference to the language and exemplary behavior of an electrical circuit. Their liberal use of the lexicon of electrical circuitry thus marks a deep commitment on the part of Spiritualists such as Davis to the procedures and authorizing discourses of modern science, medicine, and engineering. Even more fundamentally, perhaps, it marks their shared conceptualization of communication itself as the outcome of successful reception of a signal located within a linked system of generative forces, transmitting media, terminal points, and feedback loops. As we shall see presently, this *logic of the signal* lies at the root of what was presumed to make a device like Davis's magnetic cord efficacious within the context of séance practice. More generally stated, the circuitous work of signal processing provided a key discursive ground for the articulation of Spiritualist ideas about spirit communication writ large, thanks to a gathering consensus about the nature of electrical transmission that was being formed around the Spiritualist community, in rapidly evolving scenes of scientific experiment, industrial engineering, and medical research, and in the representation of those expert knowledges in the broader terrain of transatlantic public culture.

Davis's magnetic cord thus merits attention on account of its location in an intellectual, cultural, and commercial space somewhere on the borderland between "proper" and "amateur" sciences. This was a space for the circulation of instruments and technical procedures often (but not always) initially developed for scientific inquiry, but now routinely reproduced for pedagogy, entertainment, and domestic consumption. It was also a space for the circulation and hybridization of discourses and practices of scientific observation and knowledge-gathering among a company of interlocutors that today we might too hastily divide into professionals and amateurs, since, in Davis's time, that very distinction was only in the process of being formed. In this respect it is worth dwelling on the fact that not only was the functional operation of Davis's magnetic cord relatively straightforward (hold on and concentrate!), it was also easy to build, requiring what for Davis's middle-class readers would have been readily available materials. By thus lowering the threshold for participation in séance ritual, the cord could be said to offer a means of democratizing the terms of access to transcendent powers. Davis's instructions for the construction and use of magnetic cords echo what was in fact a recurring theme in Spiritualist writings throughout the nineteenth century: that there should not exist any institutionally circumscribed gateways to the spirit world, certainly not ones that conferred a monopoly of knowledge onto priests or other kinds of ritual experts (notwithstanding the celebrity mediums, stage managers, editorialists, and others who had their own symbolic and economic interests to protect). In company with many other Spiritualists, Davis never tired of proclaiming that the spirit world was in principle accessible to all. This is nowhere clearer than in his contention that any properly formed circle has the potential for success, and no one can determine in advance which member of the circle possesses a sufficiently "sympathetic" constitution to be the first to register a sign from the spirit world through the cord's electrical vibrations.[10] What democracy pertained to the organization and performance of séance ritual was also assumed to pertain to Spiritualist intellectual work at large, in the midst of a public culture energetically consumed by news of the latest scientific discoveries and the marvels of modern engineering. Having been chosen by the spirit world to deliver new knowledge about the human body, mind, and soul, the natural order, and the cosmos beyond, writers such as Davis worked alongside, beneath, and sometimes against what in their day were only beginning to become clearly recognizable as professional forms of science, engineering, and medicine.

Despite the misgivings of numerous historians, it is still regrettably common to come across a hackneyed picture of the nineteenth century as a period marked by a widening gap between religion and science, with the rise of an increasingly specialized and fundamentally "secular" scientific community organized into professional bodies that delineated clear criteria for weighing evidence, endorsing theories, and measuring expertise.[11] But Spiritualist intellectuals such as Davis do not fit within the expected mold of "men of science" who supposedly lost their faith along the path toward unfettered scientific inquiry. Nor can their writings so simply be relegated to the margins of popular culture, a domain sometimes disparagingly described in terms of its ignorance and distortion of the "real" scientific discussions taking place elsewhere. Such accounts not only exaggerate the passivity of nonspecialist writers as mere conduits of scientific knowledge, they fail to get at the root of popular science as an arena of public discussion and practical engagement.[12] Paying attention to this arena requires, in the first instance, that we resist all temptation to treat Davis's cord as simply the idiosyncratic invention of a marginal autodidact (if not a religious crackpot), just as we must not allow ourselves to hold accounts of the spiritual nervous system in abeyance at the margins of nineteenth-century technoculture. On the contrary, as an instrument that both mimicked and competed with the kinds of technological apparatuses elsewhere required for the activities of scientific measurement and observation, or for the construction and technical coordination of electrically mediated communications infrastructures, Davis's magnetic cord invites us into the very heartland of transatlantic modernity.

Technoscience and the Spiritualist Imagination: The Spiritual Telegraph

As a religious movement, a cultural fad, and an object of public controversy, American Spiritualism came to fruition in the third quarter of the nineteenth century, a period of intense social restructuring and technological revolution in the domains of communication, transportation, and knowledge production and in the formation of everyday habits among steadily urbanizing and industrializing populations.[13] Many of the ideas set forth by Spiritualists about the survival of the human soul after death and about the ways spirits make their presence known can, of course, be traced back through a much longer history of metaphysical speculation and ritual conduct, stretching back to the founding of the American Republic, if not much further—into the depths of ancient European traditions of Hermeticism, neo-Platonism, and the occult arts, as documented most recently by Catherine Albanese in her magisterial history of the American metaphysical tradition, *A Republic of Mind and Spirit*.[14] One might also concede that the business of talking directly with the dead is endemic to most societies throughout history, and that nineteenth-century American Spiritualism constituted a local variant of what was surely a far more universal cultural desire to communicate with the dearly departed or to receive special knowledge and gifts from beyond the grave. But Spiritualism's prominence and its remarkable geographic spread is just as attributable to the fertile soil of sensational inquiry, popular wonder, and international newsmaking that was feeding the emerging public culture of transatlantic modernity of the mid-nineteenth century. By the same token, when Spiritualists explored the possibilities of human existence beyond the grave, they most often did so by traveling along the grooves of industrial development and scientific inquiry of their day. To those extents, the movement reflected a much larger "kinetic revolution" that was placing new priorities on motion, transformation, and progress in all facets of civil, cultural, and social life in the Jacksonian era.[15] Nowhere was this emphasis on mobility and connectivity more evident than in Spiritualist appropriations of nineteenth-century technoscience, beginning with the electromagnetic telegraph.[16] Indeed, the telegraph functioned within the Spiritualist imaginary as a metonym for the much larger wave of new technologies and institutional arrangements to which they were bearing witness in the factories, transportation routes, lecture halls, public spectacles, and mechanized homes and offices springing into existence around them.[17]

I shall say more presently about the particular figure of the telegraph in Spiritualist discourse. But first, a few words are in order about the widespread reliance among Spiritualist writers on metaphors and causal arguments borrowed from science and industry. It is crucial that we situate such writings in the historical context of an as-yet incomplete process of "purification" of scientific discourse and technical practice, lest we end up mischaracterizing nineteenth-century technoscience with recourse to more contemporary distinctions and definitions.[18] Indeed, the nineteenth century marks the period when the business of science was for the first time moving out of the hands of aristocratic amateurs and into those of an increasingly professional cadre of "scientists": a term coined in 1833 by William Whewell (1794–1866) that by the mid-century had begun to refer to those who worked in the controlled environment of laboratories and whose discoveries were subject to the authorizing scrutiny of peers versed in increasingly specialized branches of scientific expertise.[19] This historical process of intellectual and institutional purification helped to distinguish an emergent scientific establishment from a range of popular, entertaining, and lucrative activities and a range of interpretive frameworks that could henceforth be rejected as "nonscientific."

But at this very same time, transatlantic bourgeois public culture was being reshaped through a parallel growth of interest in scientific knowledge and information circulating through local, national, and international print media, including newspapers, almanacs, pamphlets, and increasingly inexpensive books in which journalists, politicians, theologians, and other public figures commented extensively on new astronomical, geological, and medical discoveries, new feats of engineering, and other wonders of modern science.[20] By Davis's time, science in the New World—and especially the science of electricity—had already been shaped by a long history of public commentary, commodification, and domestication through the transatlantic circulation not only of scientific texts, but also of increasingly affordable instruments and devices and forms of public demonstration that straddled the worlds of formal experiment, pedagogy, entertainment, and commercial enterprise. Most famously there was the example of Benjamin Franklin, but he was only one among a diverse cast of university professors, demonstrators, inventors, instrument makers, booksellers, electrotherapists, itinerant medical showmen, and other entrepreneurs of the transatlantic electrical economy of the eighteenth and nineteenth centuries.[21] Whereas such circulations were in Franklin's day largely the preserve of a genteel elite, by the mid-nineteenth century the franchise had been expanded considerably. This is evident in the United States, at least, in the burgeoning lyceum lecture circuit, which at its peak in 1850 was enlightening and entertaining audiences estimated at 400,000 people per week. New York City alone hosted over 3,000 advertised public lectures from 1840 to 1860, while throughout the rest of the country in even the smallest towns, lectures were being organized by young men's associations, library societies, mechanics' institutes, and other civil institutions.[22] Periodical authors, lyceum lecturers, and commercial agents of electrical devices for amusement, edification, and medical therapy thus comprised a growing class of lay popularizers of science: figures who appeared conversant in the latest advances of the professional scientific community, even as their modes of discourse and activity were being marked as merely amateur, commercial, or crudely "unscientific."

Spiritualists were hardly removed from these expanding circuits of scientific visibility. Andrew Jackson Davis (1826–1910), the "Poughkeepsie Seer," was arguably the foremost of such public figures. A self-taught polymath, trance writer, and committed Fourierist, Davis was dubbed by one of his peers as the "John the Baptist" of the Spiritualist movement.[23] Although Davis himself had an uncomfortable relationship with some strands of Spiritualism (he reserved his sharpest criticism for flamboyant stage mediums, whom he did not hesitate to denounce as frauds and charlatans who were imperilling the legitimate Spiritualist community), his influence on the movement as a whole is hard to exaggerate. Davis's publishing efforts were by any measure gargantuan, spanning four decades and encompassing literally dozens of books and pamphlets; in addition, he had a leading role as publisher and editor of Spiritualist periodicals such as *The Univercoelium and Spiritual Philosopher* (from 1847 to 1849) and *The Herald of Progress* (from 1860 to 1864).[24] No topic of interest to Spiritualist readers escaped his pen: marital advice, proposals for political reform, commentary on recent scientific and medical discoveries, and his seemingly endless descriptions of the afterlife and its inhabitants, or of the flora and fauna of distant planets that Davis had visited while in a trance state. In all these endeavors he presented himself as a sort of modern-day oracle, channeling knowledge and wisdom that emanated from beyond the world of everyday experience in the form of gifts, warnings, and revelations about the true conditions of our mortal existence and our immortal souls. Even more striking, however, is the way Davis's writing is shaped by a "scientific" syntax of discovery, observation, description, and causal explanation.

Davis was not the only Spiritualist who always seemed conversant in the latest discoveries and achievements of energy physics, physiology, astronomy, and electrical engineering. As keen followers of scientific news, numerous Spiritualist writers were well-positioned to take advantage of the expanding circuits of both popular and professional scientific publication that distinguished the mid-nineteenth century as the birthplace of what was to become a truly mass market for popular science writing.[25] One can therefore speak of a class of intellectuals whose task was to draw conclusions about the "true" lessons being revealed by advances in science and technology with respect to the unseen order of humanity, the world, and the cosmos. This class included figures who straddled both the academic world and the Spiritualist public sphere, such as the chemistry professor Robert Hare (1781–1858), who "converted" to Spiritualism late in life, and the geology professor-cum-psychometrist, William Denton (1823–1883). It also comprised popular itinerant science lecturers and preachers, such as the Unitarian minister and trance speaker John Murray Spear (1804–1887), a recipient of detailed instructions set out by spirit agents for the construction of numerous technological wonders, including a perpetual motion machine, an electric ship propelled by psychic batteries, a vehicle that would levitate in the air, and a sewing machine that would work with no hands.[26]

As a member of this larger cohort of mediators of Spiritualist knowledge, Davis offered formulations that were not unique, but that nevertheless stand out as exceptionally lucid and compelling engagements with the scientific discoveries and technological developments of his day. Consider, for instance, Davis's intense engagement with telegraphy, a technology whose history of birth and expansion precisely parallels that of the Spiritualist movement itself (as many Spiritualists themselves did not fail to point out). Telegraphy was, for Davis, a master trope. In response to one reader's inquiry printed in an 1860 edition of *The Herald of Progress*, he expounded on the relations among spirits and the living in the following way:

> The sublime science of spirit telegraphing is yet hidden in the laws of *action* and *reaction* which pervade, and more or less obviously govern, all forms and gradations of matter. Every organ in the brain, and every ganglionic center in the visceral department, has its own peculiar sympathies. These sympathies are distinct and available. The superior organs generate exalted and expansive influences, which radiate over all other organs in the same body, and outwardly also, to immense distances; and these influences positively touch and affect in a similar manner, the corresponding organs and centers in other persons, whether they be absent or present.[27]

For Davis what makes the telegraph "sublime" is the underlying presence of a fundamental set of laws of action and reaction that govern all manner of possible contact, communion, and sympathetic union between parts of the body, between near and distant interlocutors, and even between the living and the dead. "There is not *one law* designed exclusively to govern mind, and *another* to regulate matter," Davis implores. "For the law of mind and the law of matter, is ONE; and souls and stars are moved and regulated by the same great general Principle. Attraction governs all."[28] I shall return to consider at greater length what Davis might have meant by the term "attraction," but for the moment let me underscore Davis's decision to refer to the rapport among human bodies, minds, and spirits as *telegraphic* links. This choice of words reflects Davis's keen awareness of the effects of emergent media technology on existing boundaries of space and time at a historical moment when telegraphic operations had already begun to open up new ways of conceiving scientific objects and to suggest new possibilities of communication and action within a universe increasingly understood to be governed by the laws of electrical flow. In response to one inquiring reader, Davis elaborates this "law of attraction" with reference to a wide range of telegraphically mediated relationships:

> What is true of two individuals will apply equally to any two kingdoms or nations. The psycho-telegraphic law of *one* isolated soul, in the secrets of its own dual constitution, is the law of telegraphing between any two souls through any distance. What is the law, and what the conditions of its operations, in the individual? Briefly these: Feet telegraph their sensations to the brain. There are hundreds of material obstacles and prominences between them, yet they sympathize and converse. Foot says: "I am lame and sore from over-walking." Brain receives the telegraphic message and responds: "You shall be comforted." Foot replies: "Thank you—hope you'll keep your promise." In this familiar manner each organ converses with every other organ, and then they all, individually and collectively, report at head-quarters—at the universally acknowledged seat of government—the *mind*, which is enthroned at the mountain top of all organizational existence.[29]

Just as the foot and the brain are "in conversation" only thanks to the presence of "subtle cords of sympathetic contact," comparable bonds can be forged "between two congenial souls."[30] Conversation thus consists of "a melodious concert of sweet sympathies . . . after which, notwithstanding the immense distances, the twain may commune on the principle of the magnetic telegraph."[31] Telegraphy serves here as much more than a *metaphor* for spirit communication; it is a *model* for orchestrating and coordinating actions between and among sympathetically linked bodies, minds, and souls. In another text, Davis explains how such spiritual telegraphy actually works:

> Suppose a mother, residing in New York, prays for news from her son, living in the city of London. He is very sick. She is anxious to learn of his social situation. It will take ten or twenty days to get a letter. But she must know now. But how? She is no clairvoyant, but she is a medium for impression. . . . What does this mean? That is, the organs, situated on the upper part of the head, are only accessible to spiritual influence. Very well. The mother has guardian spirits in the Spirit-Land—so, also, has her son. They perceive and understand the mother's anxiety, and the son's

condition. Therefore, they draw nigh to the atmosphere surrounding our globe. Like the earth's inhabitants, her and his guardians form a circle of sympathy. . . . The supermundane circle establishes lines of sympathy between the mother and the son, as indicated by the pyramidal currents connecting the two cities. Thus, the actual condition of the son is daguerreotyped upon the mother's brain—telegraphed, so to speak, or *impressed*, as perfectly as any object can be painted on the physical organ of sight.[32] (See Figure 6.)

Subsequent sections of this chapter shall try to unpack the clustered themes of supramundane lines of sympathy, distant contact, and the power of vision invoked in the quote above. For the moment let us note that Davis's description of spiritual telegraphy, or for that matter, of the function and purpose of magnetic cords in séance practice, formed only one small part of an extensive Spiritualist discourse about the functioning of nerves, telegraph cables, and other media systems and their underlying electromagnetic principles of circularity, polarity, and linear conduction. In

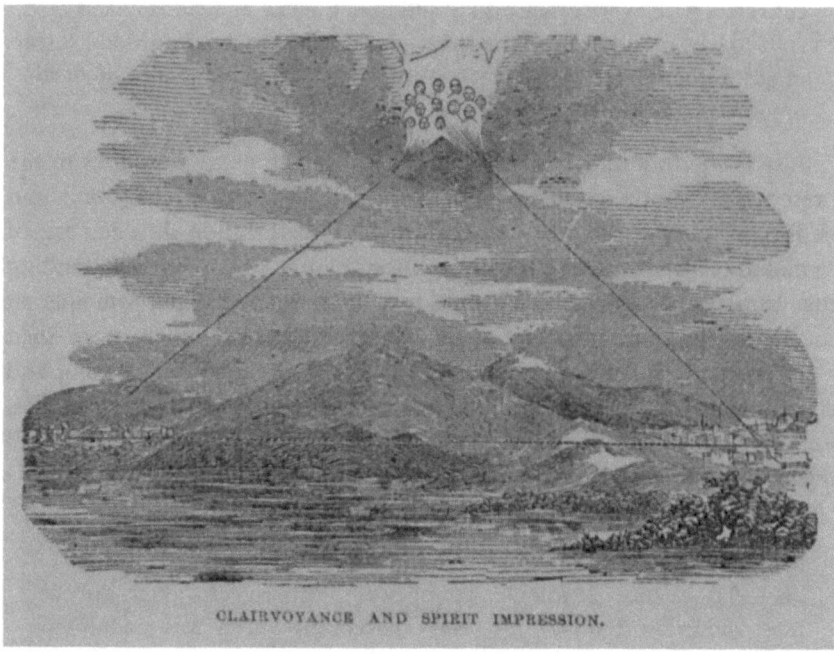

Figure 6. "Clairvoyance and Spirit Impression." Andrew Jackson Davis, *The Present Age and Inner Life; Ancient and Modern Spirit Mysteries Classified and Explained* (Boston: Colby & Rich, 1886), p. 280. (Reproduction courtesy of Rare Books and Special Collections, McGill University Library.)

fact, an appreciation of the elective affinity between spirit communication and electromagnetic telegraphy abounded in the Spiritualist literature, beginning with descriptions of the Morse code–like rappings of the Fox sisters or with the choice of title of the movement's first periodical publication, *The Spiritual Telegraph*.[33] Telegraphically mediated contact between spirits and the living was widely reported throughout this period. James Mansfield, the San Francisco–based "Spiritual Postmaster," was known for falling into a trance state and then tapping out lengthy messages in Morse code with his left index finger, "like the motion of a telegraph key."[34] Practices of mediumistic healing were likewise frequently described as depending on a form of electrical conductivity: the successful coupling of healer and patient and the formation of a circuit of electrobiological forces that could be manipulated in order to stimulate or soothe the body, lift pain, cure disease, or even excite spiritual growth.[35] The trope of nervous fragility might have figured within a long history of orthodox medicine as a pathological condition, but in Spiritualist writings it was the hallmark of a spirit medium's uniquely refined apparatus, acutely sensitive to otherworldly communications—much like the receiving instruments of the telegraphic industry.

From a broader vantage point, the spirit medium's gifts of receptivity and conductivity of spirit forces appear as a single terminal point within a communications system of cosmic proportions. This spirit community was fully interlinked, as the American seer Hudson Tuttle put it, by "sympathetic cords . . . as electric fluid on the telegraphic wire."[36] Heaven and earth themselves are conjoined, in the words of Cora Daniels (one of the most famous American mediums in the nineteenth century), by "constant telegraphy . . . like sensations fired without the loss of the millionth part of a second."[37] And, as reported in a trance communication to the medium Abraham Pierce, it seems that not longer after one's death and arrival in heaven, every spirit is charged with the duty to learn the fundamentals of telegraphy in order to be able to contact those left behind. Even more remarkably, Pierce announced, as the spirits progress through the ranks of the heavenly spheres, their education will continue as they acquire knowledge about such things as the construction of roads and railway systems, until they reach the very highest celestial sphere, where they will embark upon an anatomical study of the nervous system itself.[38] The very idea of a magnetic rope cannot be understood outside the context of this larger discourse on telegraphic rapport, which in the mid-nineteenth century served as a mark of mutual contamination between scientific and nonscientific circles.

Nerves, Cables, and the Logic of the Signal

For Spiritualists, among many other nineteenth-century interlocutors, nerves, telegraph cables, and even homemade magnetic cords belonged together because they all referenced the same fundamental laws of mutual attraction and repulsion that seemed to govern the universe and, more specifically, because they all shared a common set of organizational features that were coming to be seen as essential requisites for the transmission of diverse types of energy and information. In this regard it is not surprising that Spiritualists so readily embraced the telegraph, both as an analogy of spirit communication and as a model for the organization of séance activities. The telegraph, after all, is widely noted for having inaugurated one of the great communications revolutions of the nineteenth century, rupturing longstanding spatiotemporal relations of center and periphery, and of the proximate and the distant, ushering in a new age of global connectivity, hypermobility and supraterritoriality. As the first medium of communication based on electrical transmission, the figure of the telegraph extended from the more sober domains of energy physics, engineering, diplomatic communications, and financial transaction to a very wide terrain of popular culture and public science.[39] As we shall see presently, the telegraph also helped to render intelligible a range of physiological phenomena that seemed to involve connections between the mind and body, most evidently in the case of the nervous system. Like its terrestrial counterpart, nerves seemed to mid-nineteenth-century observers to function indexically: as a signaling system that linked the "immanent" corporeal processes of sensation, impulse, and reaction, to the "transcendent" symbolic processes of cognition, representation, and memory.

Images of networked circuitry derived from the evolving telegraph industry also found their way into the cosmological speculations of Spiritualist writers and public speakers throughout the Atlantic world. Rhetorically positioned as a vehicle of transcendence and of instantaneous disembodiment, telegraphic communication manifested not only the mystery of electricity, but also the more ancient conceptions of mystical union and of the spectral presence of the dead. Indeed, by the time that Davis had penned his descriptions of spirit communication, it had become commonplace to describe the cosmic order as a vast, interconnected web of routes, slender threads, channels, and related lines of communication, and the telegraphic signal provided arguably the most compelling figure upon which one could model the business of contacting and communing with distant things, whether those distances were found within the body, across land and sea, or beyond the threshold of the living world.

Much like a cable transmitting an electric charge, spirit mediumship was frequently described as a means of manifesting forces of distant origin and conveying those impressions to a local receptor. The technological infrastructure required for the reception of spirit messages was the human body itself. For Davis, as for numerous of his Spiritualist contemporaries, the spectacle of spirit mediumship could be attributed to a "kind of spiritual magnetism which some persons of a peculiarly negative temperament and organization are adapted to receive . . . a certain state of mental susceptibility, in which man's nervous system is exceedingly impressible," allowing such individuals to receive spirit communications "by vibrations or waving breathings which pass through the nervous system up to the brain, and awaken there thoughts by impression."[40] Just as "the brain is related to the spinal cord, the heart is related to the arteries, the nerves are related to the organs and muscles, and the whole series of systems are related to the bones," Davis adopted the figure of networked circuitry in order explain the existence of "a connected chain of invisible correspondences . . . ascending the winding flight of stairs leading from bone to brain, [arriving] by finely graded-steps at Spirit, which incessantly elaborates throughout the various systems of powers and relations beneath its control."[41] Spirit communication, in other words, was possible only through the organization of the human body and mind into a kind of telegraphic circuit in which "the Soul, within the brain and spinal cord, and diffused all through the sympathetic ganglia, *feels* instantaneously every transaction in every part of the body."[42] As Davis elaborated:

> Not only is the brain a grand Battery, compounded of innumerable little corresponding batteries, called nerve-cells or nerve-centres: but the brain is also a grand union telegraph office into which pass, and from which proceed, innumerable tubes and conductors called blood vessels and nerve-fibres; and these vessels and fibres connect cell with cell, one little battery with another; also they tie together positive groups of cells or centres with corresponding negative groups of cells, in such a systematic and harmonious manner as to make it impossible to strike one link in the cerebral chain and not at the same moment disturb more or less the entire throbbing chain of feeling and intelligence.[43]

To appreciate how an author such as Davis could so readily move between discussions of telegraphy, the anatomy of nervous systems, and the secrets of spirit communication, it is useful to recall the ways some of these same parallels were being forged in the discourses of scientific and medical professionals over the course of the first half of the nineteenth century. Historians have identified a decisive paradigm shift in the biological sciences at the point where eighteenth-century explanations grounded in vitalist theories of the body, its humors, and its hydraulic systems of pumps and tubes for the circulation of vital fluids were found increasingly wanting.[44] By the early nineteenth century, the nervous system had been, as Laura Salisbury and Andrew Shail put it, "functionally re-invented."[45] Advances in microscopy seemed to indicate that nerves were solid entities, and thus required new explanations of their function and purpose within bodily systems for the communication of sensation, perception, and action. Studies of the functioning of systems of sensory perception, reflex actions, and other autonomic bodily processes pointed to a new model of the human body, at the center of which was placed the nervous system, governed by its own functional rules. Johannes Müller (1801–1858), in his monumental *Elements of Physiology* (1833), argued that there was an entirely arbitrary relationship between stimulus and response and that specific experiences of sensation were simply the outcomes of the organizational properties of the nervous system itself.[46] Such discoveries led to a gathering consensus that nerves should be conceived anatomically and experientially as "media systems," governed by a logic of the signal, the arbitrariness of which depended on the functional separation of sender (or stimulating agent), medium of transmission, and apparatus of reception.[47] Müller's successors, including his most famous student, Hermann von Helmholtz (1821–1894), made this point even more forcefully by explicitly comparing the signaling work of biological nervous systems with the batteries, wires, and receiving instruments of the telegraph industry. For Helmholtz a sensation that passed through the nervous system functioned as a sign of its exciting cause, which, like a telegraph message, was to be deciphered and made meaningful only within the constraints of the representational capacities of its receiving apparatus, the brain. In a famous quote, he summarizes:

> Nerves have been often and not unsuitably compared to telegraph wires. Such a wire conducts one kind of electric current and no other; it may be stronger, it may be weaker, it may move in either direction; it has no other qualitative differences. Nevertheless, according to the different kinds of apparatus with which we provide its terminations, we can send telegraphic despatches, ring bells, explode mines, decompose water, move magnets, magnetise iron, develop light, and so on. So with the nerves. The condition of excitement which can be produced in them, and is

conducted by them, is, so far as it can be recognised in isolated fibres of a nerve, everywhere the same, but when it is brought to various parts of the brain, or the body, it produces motion, secretions of glands, increase and decrease of the quantity of blood, of redness and of warmth of individual organs, and also sensations of light, of hearing, and so forth.[48]

The implication of Helmholtz's comparison is that nerves constituted a kind of signaling system, the arbitrariness of which was based on the fact that the pulses of energy they transmitted were determined by variations in supply and by the organization of a potentially infinite variety of inputs and outputs. As Laura Otis has argued, the "discovery" by Helmholtz and his contemporaries that biological nervous systems were analogically comparable with electrically mediated messaging systems was grounded in a much larger set of discursive convergences among the sciences and technical practices of research in neuroanatomy, energy physics, and electrical engineering in the nineteenth century, occasioning the rise of a common understanding of the functional and operational characteristics of transmission of pulses of energy through alternations in electrical current.[49] What made discrete signaling systems distinct from one another were simply matters of the spatial organization of the network and of the composition of the transmitting medium itself.[50] This similitude between organic nervous systems and telegraph networks was apparent not only to nineteenth-century physiologists such as Helmholtz, but also to electrical engineers and other participants in the evolving telegraph industry. It was in fact exceedingly common to describe telegraphic communications with recourse to the bodily language of vital forces circulating through what were seen as elaborately branched dendritic trees of telegraph cables and railway lines that connected distant senders and receivers within the body politic. Like an organic nervous system, the telegraph seemed to consist of an extensive network of slender, vibrating threads conveying vital information to and from metropolitan centers, linking up regional towns and coastlines, trading partners, and far-flung colonial territories. And, like the functioning of a healthy body, smooth telegraphic operations offered a vision of social harmony that rested on the principles of orderly governance and effective communication within and among empires and nations.[51]

Another point of convergence of both popular and scientific discourses occasioned by the advent of electrically based communication systems can be found in the Spiritualist movement of the nineteenth century. There is a tempting parallel to be drawn between the growing popular fascination with somnambulism, hypnotic trance, and other instances of unconscious activity—a terrain certainly of interest to Spiritualists, who grappled for adequate terms to explain and legitimate séance practice—and the mounting challenge by physiological experts to the commonplace assumption that the conscious mind, seated in the brain, was the undisputed, central coordinating authority for all mental and physical processes. By the time of Davis's writing, an extensive physiological discourse had come into being that treated the nervous system as an autonomous communications system, powered independently of (and in many instances entirely oblivious to) the conscious operations of the mind. In 1812 the Scottish physician Thomas Trotter (1760–1832) had already described the nervous system as a network of sympathetic linkages, whereby "nerves were now seen as communicating with each other, rather than simply running the errands of the brain."[52] By the middle of the century, research on reflex actions and other autonomic processes within the body (such as breathing and digestion) had contributed to a sharpening distinction between voluntary cerebral activities and involuntary motor activities. Rejecting the commonsense notion of the brain as a central coordinating authority, physiologists began to wonder if the organic functions of the body were not more likely controlled by the ganglia of what was sometimes referred to as the "vegetative nervous system," a network of branches emanating from the "great sympathetic nerve" that operated independently of the cerebrospinal nervous network.[53]

At the same time that physiologists and comparative anatomists were isolating the nervous system as an independent entity within organic bodies, the orthodox medical establishment had come to regard the human nerves as a key terrain of investigation for the transmission of diseases from the blood vessels to the brain or the translation of bodily fevers into manic behavior, among other concerns with bodily sensitivity, enervation, fatigue, and irritability.[54] Neurophysiological evidence even provided some doctors with a ready explanation of the "dangers" of religious enthusiasm—including Spiritualist mediumship—understood as a product of mental disorder, rooted in deformities of the major organs, the vasculae, and above all, dysfunctions in the body's most vital communication network, the nervous system. Experiences of bearing witness to spirit manifestations, states of somnambulistic clairvoyance, or the heightened emotions and physical agitation that frequently accompanied such events could now be ascribed to problems of nervous overstimulation or "faulty wiring," occasioning the surrender of the conscious mind to manic behavior.[55]

But orthodox medical authorities were hardly the only commentators on the specter of bodily actions and sensory experiences that seemed to unfold in the absence of conscious mental control. In the context of the print-mediated public sphere of transatlantic bourgeois modernity, their voices were joined by diverse competitors with a stake in the interpretation of the remarkable activities that seemed to be occurring in séance chambers the world over. Spiritualist writers were unsurprisingly the most determined to flout the authority of orthodox medicine. Countering the latter's efforts to align spirit mediumship with madness, they emphasized instead the rarefied sensibilities of spirit mediums and the technical plausibility that revelations from the spirit world could be manifested with the right equipment. The uniquely sensitive architecture of a spirit medium's nervous system was mirrored in the distinct pattern of the séance circle and in the strategic deployment of devices (such as a magnetic cord, perhaps) that could help establish the balance of forces required for the reception of spirit energies. Revelations from the spirit world thus belonged under the sign of a fundamental, cosmic set of laws of attraction, propagation, and reception that governed all possible relationships between bodies of matter and immaterial agencies and forces. In Spiritualist discourse, these laws were typically gathered together around a single term: *sympathy*.

The Architecture of Sympathy

In his brilliant study of nineteenth-century American Spiritualism, Robert S. Cox proposes *sympathy* as a key trope in Spiritualist thought and practice: a term that encompassed diverse connotations of harmonious feeling, connections between body parts, or the exercise of occult powers of attraction between the physical and the spiritual worlds.[56] To many nineteenth-century English-speaking readers, "sympathy" invoked the moral philosophy of Adam Smith (1723–1790), who had defined it as a fundamental principle of harmonious contact and mutual feeling generated among like-minded groups of people.[57] For Smith sympathy depended on the historical process of refinement of human sensibilities—in other words, the evolution of social and cultural restraints of reason, civility, and firm management of the passions. His theory was warmly received among writers of the Scottish and American Enlightenments, where it was often interpreted as an apologetic for bourgeois Protestant Christian modes of restrained piety. Smith's use of the term sympathy also overlapped with the prevailing medical discourses of his day, most evidently with the work of his Edinburgh colleague, the physiologist Robert Whytt (aka Whyte, 1714–1766), who had posited the nervous system as the central bridge between mind, body, and environment and the key condition of possibility for the generation of sensibility and mutual feeling.[58] But as Cox argues, in the context of nineteenth-century America, Smith's theory had become "freighted with a suite of alien connotations," among which figured explanations of sympathetic union rooted in the occult.[59] In the specific case of Spiritualism, experiences of somnambulism, clairvoyance, trance writing, and the manifestation of spirit visions and sounds within the séance chamber provided Spiritualists with occasions to rework Smith's concept in order to produce what Cox describes as

> a theory of community predicated upon the social practice of sympathetic communion, a transcendent nexus of emotion that connected and coordinated all of life and death. Spiritualism provided legibility to life, mapping the cosmos onto a distinctive topography of emotion in which the geographies of the body, heaven, and earth took part in suturing the individual physiologically and socially into the enduring structures that animated the cosmos.[60]

Cox is surely correct that, in their elaboration of this cosmic "topography of emotion," Spiritualists drew just as readily on the authority of enlightened discourses of moral philosophy and medicine as upon occult understandings of the law of mutual attraction. But I would add the discourse of electromagnetism as another key framework for Spiritualist efforts to visualize, locate, and take advantage of the "transcendent nexus" to which Cox refers in the quote above. As I have been arguing in this chapter, the spiritual nervous system operated, not as a system of pumps and fluids, percussive bodies, and diffuse gases, but rather as a kind of electric circuit: channeling signals and linking minds, bodies, and distant things (including those lying beyond the threshold of the grave) through the figural pattern of nerves, telegraph cables, and other electrically mediated networks. For Davis, the condition of possibility for all forms of sympathetic union—among the living or the dead—was electricity. But electricity was simply the name we crudely apply to reference the more fundamental, eternal, and universal laws of attraction that ordered the cosmos into a coherent whole and that provided the universe's supreme divine agency, the "divine mind," with its medium of communication. He writes:

> One modification of electricity we term Magnetism, another Galvanism, another Nervo-vital influence, &c.; yet these terms are merely expressive of the progressive refinement and superior manifestations of the One great principle. The Divine Mind employs electricity as a medium of communication to all parts and particles of the universe. . . . In truth,

electricity is everywhere and in everything. It is the vehicle or medium of divine vitality. It is working miracles in the secret recesses of the earth; it plays in the diamond vaults and chambers under the sea; it flies from point to point in the deepest mineral beds; it penetrates all oceans, and supplies that living battery, the torpedo-eel, with its wonderful power; in a word, it resides in and fills all substances in nature, and it is the immediate cause of all contraction and repulsion, and of all expansion and attraction that occur in the human organization.[61]

As we have already begun to see, in Davis's time it was an appreciation of the rules of behavior of electricity under diverse conditions that provided the greatest shibboleth dividing Spiritualist notions of sympathetic community from those of their eighteenth-century forebears. For instance, both Smith and his compatriot, the philosopher David Hume (1711–1776), had imposed a significant geographic limit on the possibility of sympathetic union; like gravity, sympathy was presumed to decrease with distance. In Hume's formulation, "sympathy, we shall allow, is much fainter than our concern for ourselves, and sympathy with persons, remote from us, much fainter than persons near and contiguous."[62] If, in the eighteenth century, electricity was sometimes imagined to have something to do with these sympathetic connections across space, it was most likely with reference to Benjamin Franklin's widely accepted vision of a self-regulating economy of positive and negative charges. Franklin, after all, had ascribed to electricity an inherent tendency toward the restoration of equilibrium through the balancing of positive and negative forces, proffering a "natural" counterpart to the image of moral governance espoused by enlightened Scottish philosophers such as Smith and Hume.[63]

But the safety of the underlying assumptions about contiguity, proximity, and equilibrium was radically challenged over the course of the nineteenth century, not least thanks to the spread of new telecommunications technologies, beginning with the electromagnetic telegraph, that were dramatically revising received notions of spatial and temporal distance. As we have already seen in the case of Davis, mid-nineteenth-century Spiritualists did not have to look far in order to enlist examples drawn from the expanding telegraph industry, and these writers had no less recourse to evolving scientific scenes of inquiry and experiment with the propagation of electrical forces. One such scene of inquiry, discussed in the previous section of this chapter, was formed around the physiological study of the nervous system, functionally reinvented as an intracorporeal electrical signaling system, and on those terms presenting an incitement even to dispense with the assumption that the brain, as the seat of reason, possessed full mastery over the relations of stimulus and response to which the notion of sympathy pointed.

If Smith might have found it hard to fathom this picture of a functioning human body lacking the reigning authority of the mind and brain, he might have found an even stranger world of invisible connections that was emerging in the context of nineteenth-century experiments and theorizations of electricity and magnetism for which no sufficient guidance could be provided by the Franklinist lexicon of a self-balancing economy, let alone by less learned accounts of electricity as a mysterious fire or fluid. Early in the new century, the Danish natural philosopher Hans Christian Oersted (1777–1851) demonstrated how a magnetized needle could be made to move when placed near a wire conducting electricity, thereby mounting a serious challenge to the widespread assumption that electricity and magnetism were completely distinct phenomena. In the late 1820s the French physicist André-Marie Ampère (1775–1836) sought to determine the exact relationships of current flow and magnetism by experimenting with the circuital forces generated by an integrated magnetic field around a closed loop of electric current. By the 1830s the British scientist Michael Faraday (1791–1867) had established the basis of electromagnetic induction and introduced the concept of "lines of force" as an explanation of the relationship between distant bodies within a magnetic field, although the precise nature of these lines of force remained unclear to him.[64] It was not until the 1860s that new answers to Faraday's riddle were proposed by James Clerk Maxwell (1831–1879), who demonstrated the mathematical equivalence of electricity, magnetism, and light as variants of a single phenomenon—the electromagnetic field—that he theorized to consist of tiny elastic spinning wheels filling the ether and making possible all manner of communication between its parts. What was becoming increasingly evident in the eyes of nineteenth-century physicists was that electricity and magnetism were far more than simply discrete eruptions of energy in a universe otherwise governed by mechanical laws of interaction between massive bodies; electromagnetism was instead a manifestation of a more fundamental flow of forces that was responsible for the very formation of the universe and for the coexistence of all its constituent elements. Within this universe lines of force permeated and operated in ways that often seemed to defy older, mechanistic assumptions about such things as the transfer of energy (such as heat) between bodies or the momentum and inertia of their movements in space.[65]

It is difficult to ascertain the precise degree to which Spiritualists were conversant with these developments in the study of energy physics, but one cannot help but notice the proliferation of definitions of sympathetic union, spirit communication—and indeed, of the deeper workings of the cosmos as a whole—that, instead of relying upon the language of magic, miracle, or impenetrable mystery, marshaled specifically electromagnetic terms of reference. One notion, magnetic polarity, was particularly important for Spiritualist understandings of the organization of both the physical universe and the "higher" cosmic order in which the spirits resided. If sympathy was merely an expression of a more universal law of attraction, the idea of magnetic polarity offered a crucial means of mapping the cosmic forces that allowed for sympathetic communion among its constituent parts, including the rapport between souls of the living and of the dead. Indeed, throughout Davis's works, the Franklinist tropes of electrical polarity and magnetic attraction and repulsion formed part of a broader, recurring structural duality that shaped his many discussions of life, death, and the cosmos. Electromagnetic polarity thus referenced (and could be exchanged for) other binarisms, including those of male and female, reason and passion, or heat and cold. Even the magnetic cord, we can recall, was supposed to be constructed from two elements—one wire made of copper and one made of silver—whose duality was to be replicated in the gendered arrangement of sitters around the séance circle.[66] Polarity likewise provided a fundamental structure governing communications within the body, which was often explicitly described as a binary process of transmission and reception of positive and negative forces. In one meditation on the functioning of the nervous system, Davis writes:

> Every nerve, however thread-like and delicate, is composed of two distinct cords—positive and negative lines or conductors—each having a separate and distinct function to perform in the organic economy. The positive nerve is filled with a conducting substance essentially different from the material within the negative nerve, both lying side by side in one membraneous sheath, and discharging different duties with the most perfect harmony and reciprocation.... This great nerve-system within man's body is the connecting link between lower life and the instinct of the spiritual constitution.... all parts of the body are sympathetically related and tied by the bonds of affection together, forming one brotherhood of interest and mutuality of functions, and making it quite impossible for one member to suffer without disturbing the health and prosperity of all the other parts.[67]

The bonds of affection that constituted sympathy were thus structurally and spatially dependent upon the presence of magnetic poles and upon the lines of force that these poles established within the body. Magnetic polarity also offered the architectural framework through which sympathetic relationships could be extended outward beyond the body: along the "slender, invisible threads" of force that connected human minds and bodies with distant things and places. In one text Davis makes clear how far he and his contemporaries had departed from the eighteenth-century conception of sympathy when he suggests that the laws of attraction and repulsion that governed the functioning of the bodily nervous system can be applied just as readily to the interaction of physical bodies in nature, and even to the gravitational forces that situate the planet Earth in relation to the sun and the other planets and stars in the galaxy. He writes:

> The earth on which we live is a revolving electrical machine . . . an immense magnetic battery. . . . The motion of electricity . . . is spiral. With a swiftness beyond imagination the earth's electricity streams in great ribbons and winds itself upon its own natural spool at the north. The north magnetic pole . . . is an immense magnetic helix, an atmospherically coiled receptacle, for the multitudinous electrical currents arising from all parts of the globe.[68]

The language used here to describe the planet Earth no doubt seems somewhat vague when set alongside contemporaneous writings of professional geologists, astronomers, and physicists, although it should be pointed out once more that Davis could hardly have been ignorant of many of the developments in these fields, given their frequent mention in the Spiritualist press, including in Davis's own newspaper, *The Herald of Progress*. Let us note, however, the reference in the quote above to "great ribbons" of electrical energy and "coiled receptacles" of magnetic force. Here once again, the figure of the slender thread—charged with energy, networked into a larger circuit, and extended across space—provides the architectural framework for conceiving the operation of the cosmos. In Davis's vision, lines of force not only encompass the planet Earth; they extend far beyond it into the furthest reaches of the universe, in the form of "electrical rivers setting toward earth and the various planets in our system from different regions of the Spirit Land [the celestial abode of eternal souls] . . . the orderly method of traveling between the earths and the interior universe is by means of the rivers described. They are the recognized celestial highways connecting spheres and globes."[69] This network of electrical rivers and celestial highways constitutes what Davis

The Spiritual Nervous System

calls a vast "nervo-astronomy" of circulating forces, governed by eternal, ethereal laws of sympathetic attraction. As he explains,

> Terrestrial magnetisms, terrestrial electricities, and whatever else men call "imponderables," constitute the nervous system of this physical universe. The universal nervous system holds the same relation to matter as the nervous system of the spirit to the physical parts of the body.... No, the spirit-world is not remote. We move every moment in its presence. This earthly planet itself rolls in its orbit under the observation of the inhabitants of the Spirit-Land.... Astronomically speaking, the earth is on one side of that vast galaxy of suns and planets termed "the milky way," and directly across this great physical belt of stars, we find the sublime repose of the Summer-Land, and this but the receptacle of the immortal inhabitants who ascend from the different planets that belong to our solar system. These planets all have celestial rivers which lead from them toward the heavenly shores. And [just as] each organ in the human body holds its physical relation to the brain by means of nerves and blood-rivers, so these different planets in the physical universe hold a currental, magnetic, and electrical relation to the Summer-Land, which corresponds to the brain. How is it that strength rises to the brain of a man from what he eats? It is by means of circulation. And this circulation is regulated by the law of attraction and repulsion. How do spirits travel from these physical globes to their homes in the Summer-Land, and reversely, from the Summer-Land to persons and places on the planets? Answer: By circulation. And here, too, magnetic river-circulation is regulated by attraction and repulsion! Thus the analogy may be extended ad infinitum.[70]

A Politics of Vision

It is of course possible to place Davis's theory of "nervo-astronomy" in the context of a long history of occult cosmologies, where sympathetic forces are seen to permeate the universe, accounting for such things as astrological correspondences between the movements of planetary and human bodies and the mystical forces of affinity that enable even the most distant parts of the cosmos to be drawn together. But let us not lose sight of the fact that these sympathetic forces are represented here through the visual and discursive idioms of nervous systems, telegraph networks, and other media modeled on the figure of the electric circuit. By locating sympathy within this nervo-astronomic order, Davis does not simply update the archaic trope of *unio mystica* so much as reconstitute its very conditions of possibility. The soul within and the heavens above were now tied to the tethers of nineteenth-century transatlantic technoscience; sympathy between souls was now something that could be achieved, analogically if not directly, through the medial architecture of electrical grids and through the observable effects of electromagnetic forces on territories and modes of industry, both large and small. It is not so surprising, then, that Davis proposed a magnetic cord, of all instruments, in order to help Spiritualist knowledge seekers navigate the nervo-astronomic cosmos and thereby forge reliable communicative links with the spirit world.

I do not mean to suggest here that, simply because they appropriated the visual and discursive idiom of the electrical circuit, Spiritualists such as Davis somehow joined company with the scientific community of their day. It is one thing to invoke electromagnetic metaphors in one's writings, but quite another to attempt to elaborate findings about the properties of such forces on the basis of controlled observation, among other protocols of experimental practice that serve to distinguish scientific expertise. If anything, Spiritualist cosmology and séance practice seem to fit more closely into the history of public demonstrations of science rather than its formal history of experiment and theorization. Both Davis and his readers likely had at least second-hand knowledge of, if not direct experience with, examples of what by the mid-nineteenth century had already become a venerable tradition among itinerant electrical showmen to invite audience members to hold hands and experience simultaneous shocks in a human circuit.[71] The popular culture of electrical demonstration and widely discussed experiences of electrostatic shock were surely as (if not more) important for the generation of Spiritualist ideas about body, soul, and spirit than the experiments, debates, and other forms of intellectual exchange taking place within the professional scientific community. In this same train of thought, let us also note that through his endless references to electrical "fluids" and "flames," Davis spoke a language more reminiscent of eighteenth- rather than nineteenth-century professional scientific discourse, making his account of the spiritual nervous system sound anachronistic, if not vulgar. Even the construction of a device like the magnetic cord can hardly be said to rival the mechanical and operational complexity of "real" telegraph systems, whose designs were based on expert knowledge about electrical circuitry and whose functioning depended on the coordination of complex processes of metal manufacture and power generation, to say nothing of the considerable sums of financial capital required to feed this expanding industry. Is it not tempting, therefore, to treat the magnetic cord, alongside the familiar stock of Spiritualist technologies, such as planchettes, chalk slates, and speaking trumpets, as little more than amateur toys or crude replicas of the modern instruments of science and industry?[72] Is it not equally tempting to treat Spiritualist cosmology as a fanciful attempt to mimic "real" scientific talk about the fundamental structure of the universe and the behavior of its various residents?

Affirmative answers to these questions presume the legitimacy of a divide between, on the one hand, natural facts, secured by witnesses whose credibility is authorized by a community of recognized scientific experts and, on the other hand, the popular arenas of magic, spectacle, and metaphysical speculation (in which "facts" turn out to be merely ideological representations, attributable to the social and cultural conditions of their believers). But this distinction between matters of fact and matters of belief is itself a historical product of what Bruno Latour famously called the Modern Constitution: a paradoxical arrangement of science and politics, facts and values, and knowledge and power, which are all proclaimed to be epistemologically and ontologically distinct from one another, at the very same time that they have become interdependent in new and more profound ways through the proliferation of technologically mediated representations and coordinated actions among humans and nonhumans.[73] If, as Latour argues, it never was and perhaps never will be possible to disarticulate questions about society and nature from one another, let alone to separate either from more fundamental questions about ethics, origin, causality, or the future that we sometimes designate as the "ultimate" concerns of religion, it would seem that the characterization of nineteenth-century Spiritualist cosmologies, technical procedures, and instruments of spirit communication as "merely popular" is nothing more than the rhetorical fiat of the professional scientific community.

Things were hardly so clear-cut in Davis's time. Over the course of his career, most scientific, medical, and engineering professions were only beginning to take institutional form. Throughout the nineteenth century, for instance, the terms *electrician* and *electrical engineer* were markedly porous categories, designating a congeries of self-taught as well as professionally trained mechanics, motor designers, telegraph operators, and other interested parties. It was only toward the end of the century that electrical professionals mounted a sustained effort to distinguish their own legitimacy as experts against the technological illiteracy of "outsiders."[74] Much the same has been noted in the history of other branches of science, medicine, and engineering, where emerging professional bodies sought to exercise their newly won authority by railing against quackery, magic, collective delusions, and superstitious minds. But no pretender to scientific orthodoxy has ever wielded a total monopoly over the anarchic terrain of medical therapies, amateur inventions, and descriptions of nature or the world that lies beyond. At the time Davis revealed his designs for a magnetic rope, the business of scientific experiment, demonstration, publication, and debate was in fact populated by diverse, often self-appointed authorities who were eager to take advantage of the flexible and still contestable interpretive horizons within which knowledge of the universe was to be located.[75]

The inchoate status of scientific and engineering professions in the nineteenth century was matched by a widespread lack of consensus concerning the interpretation of scientific data, as well as diverging standards for defining and measuring success in the design and implementation of new technologies. One might consider in this regard the long history of frustration among physiologists that the nervous system remained impenetrably mysterious. In 1764 Robert Whytt concluded that "the extreme smallness of the nervous tubes, and the subtility [sic] of the fluid which they contain, make us altogether ignorant of its peculiar nature and properties."[76] In 1812 Thomas Trotter complained that "dissections have not forwarded our knowledge" about how exactly the nervous system operates.[77] Helmholtz, for his part, lamented that physiologists had "hitherto been unable to establish" whether "the actual process of irritation in individual nerves may always be precisely the same, just as the electrical current in the telegraph wires remains one and the same notwithstanding the various kinds of effects which it produces at its extremities."[78] Rather than interpreting such comments retroactively from the perspective of a "more complete," "purified" body of neurophysiological knowledge that we possess today, we might benefit from closer attention to the ways Whytt, Trotter, Helmholtz, and many other scientists, unwittingly or not, were throwing into relief more unresolvable questions about what counts as a useful instrument or technical procedure in the generation of reliable knowledge. Perhaps, one might even suggest, the nervous system provided a basis for heated interpretive debates precisely because its finest endings lay beyond the vanishing point of the nineteenth-century microscope, where speculations were rife, and where it was ultimately impossible to distinguish physics from metaphysics.[79]

What can be said about the shaky foundations of nineteenth-century neurology might just as readily be said with respect to telegraph systems, which were beset by considerable technical and operational difficulties. Grids were prone to power failures. Climates were inhospitable, and cables were often severed (the most famous case being the transatlantic telegraph cable of 1856, which linked England and the United States for the first time, but which lasted only for twenty-three days). There was not even much agreement among nations about how to establish uniform technical standards for telegraphic communication, a problem that was only partially redressed with the formation of the International Telegraph Union in 1865. Indeed, at the time of Davis's writing, we are far from seeing a world enclosed within a circle of reliable and seamlessly interconnected telegraph systems; "the network" was more utopian fantasy than lived reality.

So it seems that in the nineteenth century what most dramatically linked the gigantism of world space and the microcosm of bodily communications were profoundly unresolved questions about the invisible forces that animated the universe: forces that remained difficult to locate or to harness, let alone to fully explain. Spiritualism and professional science thus encountered one another in an indeterminate zone of complementarity, competition, and exchange. Located in this contact zone, Spiritualists and professional scientists shared a common assumption embedded in the promise of scopic observation: to see properly is to know the true order of things. And yet for both, some of the most fundamental things to be known are in fact invisible to the naked human senses, and it is only in their technical mediation that they become visible. Against the dark background of an immense universe of things hidden from natural sight, Spiritualist techniques for registering spirit presence and scientific instruments for registering the effects of electricity were thus shaped by the same principles of a constitutive invisibility that was redefining the very meaning of vision and of sensory perception, turning visible acts and facts into constructed and calculated data, displacing the "natural coordinates" of the human eye, and stigmatizing every visible experience with the taint of provisionality.

Davis was keenly aware of the degree to which his contemporary professional scientists were beholden to this impossible and unfulfillable demand for "unmediated" visibility, and he used the epistemological limitations of scientific observation to great rhetorical effect. If scientists cannot see what Spiritualists know, this is a direct consequence of the technological inadequacy of the instruments that mediate scientific representation. Davis writes:

> It may seem to your imaginations that this spiritual world is afar off—that it must be a vast and remote existence, because astronomers have not peered into it. But it is my belief that astronomers, with their physical instruments, will, one of these fortunate future days, recognize the Summer-Land, and I believe, furthermore, that astronomers will see

landscapes and physical scenes more clearly than those vague images which are now revealed through telescopes, as existing upon the moon and different rolling stars.[80]

Just as astronomers cannot yet locate or visually register the distant celestial abode of departed souls, physiologists have yet to catch sight of the deep animating force of spirit within the body, which "lies sequestered in your least nerves, in your finest points of life and sensation." Davis continues:

> The tissues [of the human body] are built up out of the invisible life of the nervous system. But what makes the nervous system? These physical physicians can trace the nerves. But there is some hidden principle *within* the nerves, *within* the electricity and dynamic life of the nerves, *within* the mellow magnetism which covers the fine electricity—something *within* everything in you that is human and interior—a principle of recuperation known only by the power you feel.[81]

In another text Davis expands on this interplay of scopic observation and invisible force through a "clairvoyant examination" he conducted on his own pneumogastric nerve (also known as the vagus nerve, one of the central cranial nerves, distributed to the pharynx, oesophagus, larynx, lungs, heart, stomach, liver, and spleen, and most of the abdominal viscera), an object of sustained attention among anatomists at that time. Not needing to rely on the limited representational capacities of microscopes, Davis reports how he

> traced its terminations to the intestinal cavity, upon the muscular fabrics of which we alleged its motive influences were easily and freely exerted.... Viewed with the leaden eyes of materialism, and studied from the wholly physiological standpoint, the body presents nothing either "fearful or wonderful." Once open your spiritual eyes, however—fix their analytical powers upon the anatomical structure of the nervous system—and the *wonders of a universe* are instantly unfolded to your understanding. Wheels within organs, tissues within muscles, fibers within nerves, globes within blood, motion within life, sensation within motion, and myriads of beautiful processes going on in the several departments of the temple at the same moment—all impress the spirit-observer with sublime and unutterable truths, and with gratitude beyond all bounds of expression.[82]

In the same way that the "spiritual eyes" of the clairvoyant are proposed here as reliable instruments for the visual representation of spirit energies, the magnetic cord presents itself as a reliable tool for spirit communication.

One can well imagine that the efficacy of Davis's cord would have been denied *a priori* by a scientific establishment that refused to entertain the theoretical possibility of spirit forces, despite (or perhaps precisely on account of) the fact that, at the very same time, Spiritualists such as Davis were seeking to enhance their own credibility by explaining the magnetic cord's functioning in terms of the observable behavior of electrical signals and circuits. But on what grounds can we say which of the interlocutors in this debate succeeded in providing a more "truthful" account of the invisible forces that govern the cosmos? Who was authorized to determine the generation of reliable knowledge about the amenability of invisible forces to technologically mediated modes of representation and action? To assume that the magnetic cord was merely a figment of the Spiritualist imagination is to side with Davis's detractors, both then and today, in the name of a purified technoscientific practice that imagines itself as having been "liberated" from the shackles of metaphysics—at the very same time, paradoxically, that modern technoscience has become structured by new forms of invisibility that render knowledge incomplete, if not inherently uncompletable. In this case, as in many others, it would seem that the separation of technology and religion rests on political decisions. Taking the magnetic cord seriously demands that we revisit the history of that politics.

Bio-Power

An Empowered World

Buddhist Medicine and the Potency of Prayer in Japan

Jason Ānanda Josephson

If you were to travel to the small town of Kotohira on the Japanese island of Shikoku, you might, after strolling past one of the country's oldest Kabuki theaters and partaking of the region's famous Sanuki udon noodles, find yourself at an ancient shrine, the town's central attraction for tourists and pilgrims. There, on the grounds of this old religious site, you would find a dedicatory plaque sporting a very modern image: that of Japan's first cosmonaut, Akiyama Toyohiro, clad in a spacesuit standing next to his craft. Despite its space-age content, however, the plaque gives thanks to Kompira, the so-called god of sailors, for Akiyama's safe voyage through interplanetary space.[1] This confluence of technological hypermodernity and public religiosity is by no means unique to the Kompira Shrine. Analogous examples dot the Japanese landscape, from nineteenth-century mechanical models of the Buddhist cosmos, to websites devoted to prayers to the god Hachiman, to the Buddhist stupa at Hōrinji temple dedicated to Thomas Edison and Heinrich Hertz as the "Patriarchs of Electricity and Electro-Magnetic Waves."[2]

The most striking thing about the modern "clash" between religion and technology in Japan is the absence of conflict. To speak in general terms, neither religion and technology nor religion and science are in public confrontation in Japan today. This détente is not merely a contemporary or temporary truce, but rather a nuanced position, which we should see not as an ahistorical essence, but instead as an architected compromise crafted in the temples, schools, and law courts of the nineteenth century. This chapter will broadly sketch out the history of this compromise by focusing on one of the main issues of controversy—the power of prayer. Situating the debate about prayer's efficacy in its historical context, the chapter will argue that a close look at the concept of empowerment, *kaji* (加持) offers insights into the fusion between the technological and the ritual in contemporary Japanese religious praxis.

I will begin this chapter by demonstrating that, in premodern Japan, before the contemporary demarcation of an autonomous sphere of religion (as distinct from science, the political, and so on), Buddhism was medicine and empowered prayer was an important therapeutic technology. I shall first trace the evolution of the concept of empowerment through Buddhist philosophy and its ultimate embodiment in popular practices in the nineteenth century. Then I shall analyze the Meiji government's attempts to produce a hygienic modernity situated in a hegemonic amalgam of Western medicinal and neo-Confucian ethical discourses. According to the logic of this new hybrid discourse, as embodied in a series of laws, trials, and textbooks, healing prayer was understood not as a treatment, but as a barbaric "disease" that needed to be eradicated in order to heal the body of the nation. In the final section I shall discuss the radical implications of debates about empowered prayer for the Buddhist conception of the cosmos as a whole. I shall conclude by demonstrating that the division between the technological and the religious, held up as a rhetorical ideal in secular modernity, collapses as a rigorous conceptual strategy. Reconciliation can be found, at least in the Japanese context, in an asymmetrical relationship in which technoscientific modernity is seen as empowered by, rather than undermined by, religious praxis.

Buddhism as Medicine: Prayer and Empowerment in Premodern Japan

> The Buddha is the great king of physicians who discerns the symptoms of illnesses and understands the nature of medicines. He dispenses medicines so well suited to the disease that sentient beings take them with joy.
>
> —*Wúliángyì jīng (The Sutra of Innumerable Meanings)*

Throughout Japanese history the Buddhist institution benefited from widespread belief in the practical, this-worldly power of its rituals. Despite later scholarly dismissal of these practices as superstitious accretions or naïve folk religion, the ability of Buddhist rituals to work a range of wonders was a primary component of orthodox Buddhism. A basis for the efficacy of prayer can be found in numerous canonical Buddhist sutras and in the writings of Buddhist leaders.[3] Rituals intended to produce concrete effects played a central role in premodern Japanese Buddhism, and they still do today, despite nineteenth-century efforts to eliminate these practices. The potential benefit of such prayers was limited only by the imagination. Tale collections such as *Konjaku Monogatarishū* attributed a range of outcomes to Buddhist prayer, including better rebirths, accelerated healing, protection from fire, increased rainfall, and even morally ambivalent results such as victory in battle or the drowning of corrupt officials.[4]

Prior to the mid-nineteenth century, the promise of miraculous healing was particularly crucial to the mission of the Buddhist institution. As the Swiss Buddhologist Paul Demiéville observed over seventy years ago, throughout the Buddhist world medical metaphors play a vital role in a tradition that describes the Buddha as the king of physicians (Sanskrit, *vaidyarājara*), and the Buddhist teachings as promulgated in order to heal the world. This healing practice was conceived of as not merely symbolic or "spiritual." In Japan guidebooks such as the *Edo Shinbutsu Gankake Chōbōki* described which temples were particularly useful for the treatment of which malady.[5] Popular printed broadsheets from the same period discussed the miraculous cures performed by Buddhist clergy, advertised Buddhist pharmacology, and repeated tales of the marvelous intervention of healing *bodhisattvas* (post-human buddhas-to-be) in the human world. The attitudes they embodied were not relegated to an uneducated populace. They appeared in elite texts written by intellectuals, government officials, and, of course, Buddhist priests. Many of these works, in addition to making claims about the efficacy of Buddhist ritual, also described specific Buddhist therapies that might benefit a range of illnesses.

A concrete example of the way Buddhist medicine functioned can be found in canonical scriptures such as the *Sutra of the Thousand-Handed, Thousand-Eyed Avalokitesvara Bodhisattva on the Treatment of Illnesses and the Preparation of Drugs*, which includes materials for the diagnosis and treatment of various medical issues, as in the following passage:

> When a woman carries a dead child within her body, take one large dose of apamarga herb (*Achyranthes aspera*), boil it together with two measures

of water, drain the liquid and discard the sediment. The patient then takes one measure of the liquid while reciting the incantation twenty-one times. The child will then be expelled with no pain whatsoever.[6]

This prescription for what Western medicine would call complications of antenatal mortality involves first the preparation of an infusion from an abortifacient herb, *Achyranthes aspera*. This component of the prescription looks rather like contemporary herbal medicine, and the plant involved continues to be used for similar purposes in India today.[7] The second portion of the ritual, involving the repeated recitation of a "magical incantation" or mantra, may strike the contemporary reader as unnecessary or perhaps even distracting. Yet this mantra is central to the Buddhist text in question. As the text stipulates:

> When men and women of pure faith, who accept, preserve and also recite the incantation for the relief of suffering, treat illnesses using obscure worldly techniques, they should nonetheless recite [the mantra] 108 times out of compassion and with an upright mind. . . . After a short period of time they shall rise again in the lotus blossom as Buddha.[8]

Both the repetition of the mantra and the performance of healing practices are connected to the attainment of the power of a bodhisattva and to soteriological aims, as well. As the text reinforces at several different points, one can attain Buddhahood through this particular combination of medicine and ritual. In this sense the text suggests a parallel kind of healing process by means of which the ritual-physician secures his own karmic healing through the healing of others.

Such identification of the aims of Buddhism and medicine is normative in many Buddhist scriptural materials. As Demiéville has noted, Buddhist texts promote a range of therapeutic practices, which he classifies under three broad headings: (1) religious therapeutics (practices of worship, contrition, breathing exercises, and meditation); (2) magical therapeutics (incantations, exorcisms); and (3) medical therapeutics proper (pharmacology, dietetics, and surgery).[9] Further, as Demiéville argues, "the lines demarcating these three fields are not at all distinct. . . . All of Buddhism is a single therapeutic."[10] Thus, before the nineteenth-century demarcation of distinct domains for science and religion, Buddhism was understood as a medical tradition.

In Japan the medical technologies provided by the Buddhist institution (and by semi-affiliated lay practitioners) covered all of the above-mentioned types of techniques, from herbal pharmacology, dietetics, and surgery to prayer ritual.[11] There was nothing about prayer ritual that marked it as in any way less instrumental or less "technological" than any of these other practices. In other words, prayer ritual did not occupy a separate or sacred sphere, but rather constituted a therapeutic technology in the Buddhist medicinal toolkit.

The range of activities I'm referring to as "prayer healing," like other medical techniques, did not represent a single uniform practice, but rather encompassed a wide spectrum of procedures for different types of ailments. A certain outcome could be best brought about by gaining the aid of a particular supernatural entity, through the efforts of a particular priest, engaged in specific ritual at a specific temple, and often with the aid of an efficacious relic. In other words, the likelihood of having a prayer answered depended upon its point of origin: upon the specific confluence of attitude, place, ritual, and specialist. Many such rituals existed before any attempt was made to conceptualize their efficacy according to broader theoretical principles. In other words, in this case, practice preceded theory. Ultimately some Buddhists attempted to fit these diverse rituals into a universal explanatory frame, which functioned in some ways like an emic account of ritual's efficacy. This frame centered on the concept of "kaji," or empowerment.

During the Tang Dynasty (618–907), the Sanskrit term *adhiṣṭhāna* was frequently rendered with a unique calque composed of two characters, 加 and 持, read in Japanese "kaji." The first character meant "adding" and the second "holding." The translators who produced this new terminology, which took on a life of its own, seem to have understood *adhiṣṭhāna* to mean the ability of a buddha or bodhisattva to "augment" and "sustain" someone or something.[12] This term "kaji" also took on diverse meanings in a number of the Chinese-language Buddhist texts imported into Japan. However, an additional technical usage, independent from the original Sanskrit *adhiṣṭhāna*, was reinforced in the writings of Kūkai (774–835), the founder of the Japanese Shingon school of Buddhism.[13] In one text, *Sokushin jōbutsu gi* ("The Principle of Attaining Buddhahood in this Body"), Kūkai writes:

> Kaji indicates the great compassion of the Tathagata [Buddha] and the devotion of sentient beings. The compassion of the Buddha pours forth on the heart of sentient beings, like the rays of the sun on water. This is called *ka* [adding], and the heart of sentient beings, which keeps hold of the compassion of the Buddha, as water retains the rays of the sun, is called *ji* [holding]. If the practitioner thoroughly understands this guiding

principle, through the inter-correspondence of his three mysteries [with those of the Tathagata] he will quickly manifest and realize in his present body the originally existent three bodies [of the Tathagata].[14]

Accordingly, kaji (as empowerment) was understood to occur at the pinnacle of a mutual relationship between the Cosmic Buddha (*Dainichi Nyorai*) and the devotee, when the compassion of the Buddha merges with the devotion of the practitioner, producing a sympathetic resonance.[15] This act of attaining "buddhahood in this very body," so central to Kūkai's articulation of the goal of the Buddhist path, establishes kaji as a crucial bridge between the devotee and the Buddha, thereby taking on a lynchpin role in Kūkai's larger philosophy.[16] In this model empowerment represents salvation, yet it also explains how an ordinary human being can wield the miraculous powers of the Cosmic Buddha. In the moment of empowerment the devotee is fully interpenetrated by the powers of the Cosmic Buddha, and he can thus direct those powers toward his particular concerns. Kaji, then, is not only the bridge to enlightenment, but also the vehicle for wonders, and as such, explains how particular Buddhist rituals can have their effects in this world.

Ultimately this secondary meaning of kaji, as a method for working miracles, exercised the largest impact upon popular conceptions of the term. In influential literary works like the eleventh-century *The Tale of Genji*, the term "kaji" occurs frequently as a reference to a type of this-worldly ritual especially efficacious in the treatment of illnesses.[17] In this context empowerment was understood as a way to channel the merit of a particular ascetic (or Buddhist monk) for the benefit of a lay patron. Empowerment did not represent the entirety of a particular ritual, but one component of a ceremony that increased the rite's worth relative to the value of the monk's austerities. Kaji thus fit into a system of exchange in which the symbolic capital of the ascetic was converted into traditional economic value. A primary function of empowerment was thus to ensure the health of the patron. It was often invoked when an illness proved particularly intractable or during periods of specific medical concern. In this context, kaji served to enrich or empower other kinds of medical practices with the energies of particular ascetics.

Initially kaji was a Buddhist sectarian specialty, but eventually it spread to a wider range of practitioners. This development is not surprising, given the range of benefits associated with the practice of empowerment. A number of ritual specialists outside of the Buddhist institution added kaji to their repertoire. By the Tokugawa period (1603–1868), kaji was performed not only by Buddhist monks from the Shingon, Tendai, and Nichiren schools, but also by professional Shinto priests and a range of quasi-lay practitioners, including mountain ascetics and other shamanic figures. Increasingly these figures used the term "kaji" in a nonspecific way when advertising their services to indicate the added usefulness of their particular religious practices.[18] In this manner the term "kaji" gradually became detached from the nobility and associated with popular practices and the lower classes.

Despite the popularization of empowered prayer, however, the Shingon school of Buddhism continued to portray itself as the authentic practitioners of this ritual technology. Details about the techniques and imputed meanings of Shingon empowerment appear in a behavior manual for Shingon priests published directly by Taiyūji temple, entitled simply, *Collected Rules of Conduct* (*Sahōshū*). This undated work made public rituals that hitherto were the closely guarded property of esoteric lineages, who transmitted them behind closed doors. The *Collected Rules of Conduct* describes the proper performance of a range of different activities, from alms begging to fire rituals and coming-of-age ceremonies, and it includes a host of different kaji practices.[19] Kaji is particularly important to the empowerment of a range of material objects. Take the following example, "Empowerment of a Pregnant Woman's Belt":

> [The priest should] dip the belt into empowered fragrant water. The belt should then be inscribed with the easy birth incantation.[20] Subsequently, [one should] empower (kaji) [the belt] through the recitation of the mantra of the "One Syllable of the Great Solar Medicine Peacock the Immovable" (*Dainichi Yakushi Kujaku Fudō*).[21]

The text goes on to describe the performance of other incantations and the wrapping of the patient in the empowered belt, all of which are supposed to help secure an easy birth. Also included in this section is another Siddhaṃ mantra designed to be chanted during the performance of the ritual.

Despite the diversity of empowered prayers in *Collected Rules of Conduct*, the intended effects fall into two remarkably consistent categories, one medical and the other apotropaic (warding off evil). In this context kaji either facilitates healing (or childbirth) or protects against malevolent influences, a pattern confirmed by other collections of kaji.[22] However, these texts expand the category of apotropaic rituals to include rites for the general prevention of calamity and the elimination of household pests (the latter performed as a type of exorcism).

In order to achieve these aims, *Collected Rules of Conduct* includes rituals for empowering a range of materials, such as grains of sand, water, and clothing. This transformation of objects is the key to understanding much of the value added by kaji practice. The performance of kaji allows the priest to enrich ordinary matter: to convert a commonplace belt, for example, into a birthing aid; or to turn a series of mundane written characters into a protective talisman. This logic extends to other artifacts, as well.[23] Yet these rituals do not render profane into sacred. Kaji practices do not produce a simple, binary transformation of state. Instead, the root ritual involves the granting of several different kinds of impetus. Objects are not simply energized by a uniform force or by a uniform intent. Rather, they take different energies from a particular god, demon, buddha, bodhisattva, or a combination of entities. In so doing, they are not permanently transformed into sacred things. The types of energy they are granted can be very different to fulfill a range of different functions (from healing to warfare). Empowered objects are flagged temporarily in the ritual space as paradoxically having an additional function. They become multiply indexical, as in the case of the "belt" that comes to represent itself, a medical technology, and a manifestation of the Cosmic Buddha.

The most crucial aspect of this change, however, is the manner in which empowered artifacts, pregnant with new meaning, become components in a ritual technology intended to produce a specific effect. The "belt" is but one cogwheel in a machine intended to change something about the world or, to use a preindustrial metaphor, but one ingredient in an alchemical reaction. Thus, to ignore the intended effect of the ritual, to dismiss its intentional, this-worldly result as epiphenomenal, is to overlook its actual function in Japanese medical technology. Ultimately the healing claims of empowerment ritual would come under greatest scrutiny as changing conceptions of illness developed, especially in the nineteenth century, that gradually eliminated the need for demonic epidemiology, as a new professional class asserted that its methods were more efficacious in the treatment of disease.

Treatment as Disease: Disempowering Prayer

> [Superstitious people] believe in fortune telling, magic, [and] empowered prayer.... When they are sick their superstitions are all the more excessive, and in their hearts they fall ill. Hoping to drive the disease from themselves, they invite misfortune. How idiotic!
>
> —*Ōmachi Keigetsu, Jogakuseikun*

In 1876 in the small Japanese town of Shiba Hamamatsuchō, a Buddhist by the name of Tanaka Hisajirō was arrested and charged with the illegal performance of healing rituals.[24] Before Tanaka's ultimate acquittal on a technicality, the police questioned people from several different villages and fined those who had solicited prayers from him. Hardly an isolated incident, this episode reflected a radical inversion of the status of Buddhist healing from an established medical practice to a criminal "sickness." As is clear in Tanaka's case, the Japanese government not only dismissed the efficacy of healing rituals, but, more importantly, understood them to be dangerous cancers in the body politic.

The first systematic criticisms of Buddhist ritual healing came neither from European observers nor from Japanese elites schooled in Western sciences, as is often assumed. While these stereotypical sorts of "secularizers" would later instigate a legal disenfranchisement of Buddhist medicine in the late nineteenth century, we must look much earlier for the origins of the disempowerment of Buddhist prayer: to a group of Japanese neo-Confucian thinkers whose confrontation with Buddhist medicine originated in the context of local concerns. For the bulk of Japanese history, the majority of medical practitioners were Buddhist monks or individuals otherwise connected to the Buddhist establishment. Yet, starting in the late sixteenth century, independent centers for the study of medicine were established. Many of these schools combined an education in medicine with the study of Confucian and neo-Confucian classics, as was common practice in China. While pre-Western medicine is generally described in the historiography as a monolithic movement called *kanpō* medicine, there were several competing approaches to healing centered around different texts and practices. Yet, by the late sixteenth century, the gradual professionalization of medicine had functionally united these disparate approaches to produce a class of doctors trained in Chinese classics. They embraced professional norms that flew in the face of those accepted by both institutionalized Buddhist medicine and lay ritual healers. This burgeoning group of medical professionals regarded prayer rituals as emblematic of a folk charlatanism incommensurable with their elite approach to medicine.

Antipathy toward "folk religion" was a common theme in neo-Confucian writings of the period and frequently drew its inspiration from the Confucian classic *The Record of Rites, Liji*: "Offerings to those to whom you should not make offerings are called licentious worship (*inshi*; Chinese *yinsi*). Licentious worship brings no blessings."[25] This phrase was often read in conjunction with a later passage from the same text: "It is permitted to kill those who delude the masses through demonic gods, [auspicious] dates, and divination practices."[26] While *The Record of Rites* calls it a mistake to make offerings to the wrong deities, it does not criticize belief in the gods more generally, nor even belief in their ability to provide blessings. It merely cautions readers to choose as a subject of worship entities that bring "positive" results, rather than ineffective or dangerous ones.[27] Later Japanese neo-Confucian thinkers, however, would extend this critique to the whole of the Buddhist medical tradition, which they deemed to be fundamentally misguided.

Although a number of neo-Confucian thinkers criticized Buddhism, folk religion, and other schools of medicine, one of the earliest figures to condemn kaji in particular, rather than prayer in general, was the doctor, neo-Confucian scholar, and natural scientist Chihara Tei (1774–1840). In 1833 he published a collection of naturalist and medical writings, *Bōsō Manroku*, in which he articulated the following critique of folk medicine:

> From the spread of demonic epidemics, beguiling wicked enchanters follow in the wake [of the illnesses]. They speak in tongues and practice other forms of divination, and they engage in empowered prayers (kaji kitō) and call up various kinds of wonders. In so doing, they deceive the ignorant and vulgar, coveting [their] treasures, and misleading the public. They are detrimental to the righteous path for governing the country.[28]

By juxtaposing speaking in tongues and divination, Chihara makes it clear that he associates empowered prayer not with the Buddhist establishment, but rather with a class of ritual specialists, known broadly as *miko*, who engaged in ritualized possession. His distrust of healing prayer originates within this larger context of suspicion of charlatans. Yet Chihara does not completely dismiss the powers of these "wicked enchanters." He understands them to be dangerous precisely because they have magical (or near magical) abilities to beguile. In other words, the neo-Confucian criticism of folk healing does not represent a disenchantment of magical rituals, but rather a revalencing of popular medicine from public good to public ill.

When Chihara wrote these words, however, a new form of medicine inspired by "Western learning" was already taking shape. Ultimately this new form of medical knowledge would become hegemonic by claiming to be the sole legitimate source of the public good. It would eventually attempt to eliminate both Buddhist healing and the kanpō medicine promoted by Chihara and his peers. Central to the "Western learning" approach was a new metaphor about the human body. Whereas the body had previously been portrayed as a site of flowing energy (*ki*), European dissection manuals, with their detailed illustrations, suggested that human physiology was essentially mechanical, functioning like a system of pipes and bellows. The veins were full of viscous liquid, and the bones served as scaffolds for pulley-like muscles. In this conceptualization of the human body, there was little room for the cyclic movement of energy, which was so important to the previous system of medicine.

At first Western medicine was banned as a dangerous type of barbarian sorcery, but early vaccination efforts demonstrated its potential efficacy. In 1860 the Tokugawa Shogunate transformed a small clinic for smallpox vaccination into the first official institute of Western medicine in Japan. Renamed the Medical School (*Ishigakusho*) in 1863, it steadily gained prominence as the national training center for Western medicine. Yet kanpō and Buddhist medicine continued to be the official standard, and Western medicine was closely regulated, permitted only in limited contexts.

During the same period the perceived status of Western technology in general was undergoing a radical shift. Starting in the eighteenth century, the instrumentalist advantages of Western technological artifacts (such as the telescope and cannon) began challenging the various ideologies competing for dominance in Tokugawa Japan. The main rivals, Buddhism and neo-Confucianism (and later Shinto), each claimed to be hermeneutically complete: to be a type of *Weltanschauung* that could provide an interpretive structure for the whole of the cosmos. The ability of European technical knowledge to provide concrete benefits (however slight) challenged the metaphysical totality of these ideologies. The fact that European telescopes could see a world unimagined in Buddhist and neo-Confucian sources posed problems, as did the fact that European guns could fire farther than their Japanese equivalents. Western technology brought with it a new type of discourse that enshrined a set of competing modes and categories for representing the world. As Heidegger famously argued in "The Question Concerning Technology," the essence of technology does not lie dominantly in something technological, but instead in a new type of attitude that Heidegger calls *Ge-stell* ("framing").[29] Although this may be a globalizing Euro-American mode, rather than a universal approach to the mechanical, I believe that evidence for a changed framing of the world can be found in this period of Japanese history, accompanying the importation of Western material culture. With the introduction of Western technical, mathematical, and scientific texts, the claims of the European system to capture the fundamentals of the world, order them in mathematical forms, and then render them instrumentalizable challenged previously held conceptual schemas.

The challenge of the European system in turn led to a competition between different ideologies, but not the conflict between religion and science, as it is ordinarily narrated. Instead, as I have argued elsewhere, there were multiple possible positions in regard to Western science occupied by different actors rather than simply a binary opposition.[30] Neo-Confucians criticized Buddhists, Shintoists criticized neo-Confucians, and so forth concerning which ideology could best accommodate the new data flooding into the country along with European material culture. At the same time each indigenous ideology was forced to undergo radical transformations in keeping with these new Western modes of scientific and technological practice.

Rhetorical reconciliation was found in the writings of neo-Confucian scholar Sakuma Shōzan (1811–1864), who later became interested in Western military techniques and sought reconciliation between indigenous and Western models. His position was embodied in the slogan "Eastern ethics, Western technical learning" (*tōyō dōtoku, seiyō gakugei*). In his writings on the subject, Shōzan associated Eastern ethics with the ultimate world of virtue and Western technical learning with the particular world of form.[31] Although *dōtoku* is generally translated as "ethics," in this case it refers to something broader: an engagement with the true nature of the universe. Shōzan called it "a most amazing fact that, with the invention of the steamship, the magnet, and the telegraph, [Westerners] now appear to control the laws of nature."[32] In so doing he gave Western learning domain over not only the movement of the stars, but also the everyday mechanics of the world. While his predecessors advocated Western studies only in answer to specific problems, Shōzan argued that both Eastern ethics and Western science are indispensable and, to be an ideal person, one must study both.[33] Yet despite this apparent ecumenism, Shōzan insisted on the ultimate supremacy of neo-Confucianism.

While initially Shōzan's vision was sufficiently controversial to justify his imprisonment, from the 1850s onward his views became widely known, encapsulated in the popular slogan, "Japanese spirit, Western technique" (*wakon yōsai*). The expression was coined by reformulating Shōzan's views in the form of a famous phrase popularly attributed to the ninth-century scholar Sugawara Michizane (845–903), which proclaimed "Japanese spirit, Chinese technique" (*wakon kansai*).[34] Originally the latter phrase was used to refer to the Japanese interpretation of Chinese cultural forms, from matters of state to aesthetics. It was not so much a division of the world into two spheres as a description of how Chinese cultural forms could be modified in the Japanese context. But the phrase "Japanese spirit, Western technique" meant something quite different. It represented a public resituating of the locus of civilization from China to the West. Further, it meant not only the preservation of traditional ethics and cultural identity, but also compatibility between Western technology and diverse worldviews promoted by Shintoists, Confucians, and Buddhists. It carried the implication that an ontologically neutral interpretation of Western technology could be achieved or, to put it another way, that guns could be manufactured without manufacturing a new worldview. Yet insofar as the phrase produced a new dualism by separating metaphysics and ethics from scientific observations, it gave Western techniques authority over the superficial world of form while preserving the more important ultimate world of virtue (or in the Buddhist case, "absolute truth") for indigenous ideologies.

In 1868 the massive social upheaval known as the Meiji Restoration brought a new government to power in Japan. As I have argued elsewhere, the Meiji regime enshrined a Shinto secular ideology rooted in Shinto-scientific hybridity that fueled its ambitious campaign efforts to transform the Japanese nation at all levels.[35] This movement, however, was by no means internally consistent. Warring factions, bureaucratic territorialism, and competing political visions produced a shifting ideological terrain. Yet members of the Meiji leadership could agree that a Western-style medical system was vital to the modernization process. Their confidence in Western medicine seems to have been rooted more in its reputation than in its results, since in this period Western medicine had comparatively little to offer.[36] Yet in 1870 the Council of State issued a public proclamation reversing all previous bans on Western medicine, thereby promoting it alongside other types of healing.[37]

In 1873 Nagayo Sensai (1838–1902), a Japanese doctor who had studied in Germany, garnered government permission to establish a Bureau of Medical Affairs within the Ministry of Education.[38] Nagayo advocated a new model for the relationship between the state and the health of its people. In the past health had been the responsibility of the individual. The Tokugawa government had no policy for disease epidemics or public sanitation. In contrast, Nagayo was heavily influenced by the German system, which placed health and economic life in the service of the state.[39] In formulating what would become national policy, Nagayo rendered the German word *Gesundheitspflege* (health care) into the new term, *eisei*, that combined the character *ei* (policing or patrolling) with the character *sei* (life). This new word for healthcare literally meant "policing life."[40]

There are clear parallels between Nagayo's concept of "policing life" and Foucault's idea of modern biopolitics. Foucault argues that in European history, state authority derives not only from the state's power to choose who lives and dies, but also from the infiltration of state authority into the very fabric of life in an effort to regulate or discipline basic biological processes in the service of national agendas.[41] Even before Nagayo took control of the Bureau of Medical Affairs, he described the proposed organization as "form[ing] a single but comprehensive administrative department dedicated to removing dangers to life and ensuring the welfare of the state" and "encompass[ing] all facets of life, whether great or small, that could possibly endanger human existence, including prevalent diseases and epidemics."[42]

Nagayo successfully established a bureau modeled on his idea of policing life, and this organization increasingly influenced government policy. In a significant shift from its previous functions, the Japanese state began to interfere in the life processes of its citizens in order to render them of service. Nagayo promoted public sanitation and the regulation of epidemics, and he encouraged various other measures to produce strong and healthy citizens who would serve as effective soldiers and subjects. Despite having received some training in kanpō medicine, he believed it to be useless as a medical practice. In 1874 Nagayo was partially responsible for the Japanese government's establishment of a standardized system of medical examination based completely on Western medicine.[43] Two years later he authored a regulation that officially required all medical practitioners to study Western medicine. This regulation marked the beginning of the active elimination of indigenous medical practices.[44] Yet it was Nagayo's successors who targeted popular forms of indigenous medicine as an obstacle to the health of the nation. In the writings of policymakers such as Gotō Shinpei (1857–1929), indigenous forms of medicine were described as useless. Individuals who sought treatment according to customary practices were therefore seen as retarding the healing of their bodies and hence delaying the purification of the national body.[45] This sentiment clearly echoed the neo-Confucian ethical condemnation of popular religion. These policymakers treated indigenous medicine as not only ineffective, but also unethical: as a "barbaric disease" that needed to be eliminated for the health of the Japanese nation.

Interestingly, it was not the Bureau of Medical Affairs that launched the official campaign against healing prayers in nineteenth-century Japan. Rather, the first anti-healing prayer ordinance (1874) was issued by a government organ known as the Ministry of Doctrine. Functionally under the control of Shinto scholar Fukuba Bisei (1831–1907), the Ministry sought to assert jurisdiction over the newly autonomous Shinto tradition.

On June 7, 1874, the Ministry of Doctrine issued a proclamation known as Article 22, which stipulated: "Healing by means of magical rituals and the like are obstructing the government and are prohibited henceforth."[46] The terms of the other ordinances issued by the Ministry of Doctrine during the same period suggest that the agency's initial impulse was probably not to eliminate obstacles to Western medicine. More likely it sought to suppress noninstitutional popular religion in general, which Fukuba and his peers, like their neo-Confucian predecessors, viewed as particularly threatening.

While the 1874 regulation emerged as part of a Shinto program to restrict unaffiliated ritual practitioners, its later enforcement was shaped by the government's commitment to Nagayo Sensai's new medical policy of "policing health." Assuming that traditional healing practices (from kanpō medicine to prayer rituals) were obstructions to modern medicine and therefore public health, policymakers worked to eliminate traditional healing practices and promote Western medicine. Yet because the process of training Western-style doctors proved slow, only wealthy urbanites had access to Western medicine. Thus one ironic result of the policy to discourage Buddhist, popular, and kanpō medicine was to give fewer people access to any form of medical treatment. Simultaneously increased urbanization and poverty caused epidemic illnesses to spread, and the need for medical care quickly outstripped its availability. Instead of relaxing the prohibitions against older forms of medicine, increased demand spawned additional regulations, which appeared in successive revisions of the criminal code.[47]

Oddly enough it was a novel that most directly contributed to the acceleration of the campaign against popular healing practices. *The Red and White Poison Dumpling* (*Kōhaku dokumanjū*), which first appeared in serial form between October and December of 1891, had a profound impact on the history of religion in the Meiji period. The author of *The Red and White Poison Dumpling*, Ozaki Kōyō (1868–1903), was arguably the most popular writer of his era, which guaranteed his work a fairly wide circulation even before he chose his sensational topic—sexual impropriety and the distribution of fake "holy water" by a fictional religious group he termed "Gyokurenkyō."[48]

After the novel's publication, newspapers identified the inspiration for Gyokurenkyō as the new religious movement Renmonkyō.[49] Now extinct, Renmonkyō was at the time of Ozaki's publication one of the most dynamic religious movements in Japan. Despite being less than eight years old, it reportedly boasted over 900,000 followers, concentrated largely around

Tokyo. Founded by a former shrine medium and diviner, Shimamura Mitsu (1831–1904), Renmonkyō was very loosely affiliated with the Shinto sect Taiseikyō. The focus of Renmonkyō's teachings, however, was the miraculous power of the Buddhist Lotus Sutra, which Shimamura regularly demonstrated through acts of faith healing. Several scholars have suggested that the sudden growth of the movement was connected in particular with the claim that its precise form of holy water cured a range of illnesses, including the dreaded cholera.[50]

On March 28, 1892, the progressive, labor-oriented newspaper *Yorozuchōhō* published an article called "The Immoral Religion of the Renmonkyō Church." An exposé of the scandalous past of Renmonkyō and Shimamura Mitsu, the article detailed revelations of sexual improprieties and the exploitation of popular superstitions for financial gain. The topic proved so popular that Yorozuchōhō turned it into a ninety-four-part series, which was picked up by a number of other newspapers and reproduced in sensationalistic pamphlets.[51] In short order sectarian Shinto and Buddhist groups publicly distanced themselves from Renmonkyō, speaking out against the movement in lectures and articles with such titles as "The Extermination of a Superstitious Religion."[52] While representatives of Renmonkyō sued for slander, the public outcry prompted an investigation by the Tokyo Metropolitan Police Department. Renmonkyō holy water was confiscated and reported to contain ammonia.[53] Judged unsafe for drinking, its use was banned. After a struggle between the Bureau of Shrines and Temples and Renmonkyō, Shimamura was stripped of her official religious status, and most of the group's preaching and religious activities were curtailed—a death blow to the organization.

Following the Renmonkyō incident, public attention to "evil cults" increased, a trend further exacerbated by popular opposition to a number of Meiji policies articulated by mediums under the influences of fox possession and oracular trance.[54] However, the mere banning of "dangerous" rituals did not seem sufficient to many government officials, so, in the early 1890s, a number of government-sponsored elementary school textbooks shifted their attention from practices to beliefs, and they began to actively discourage specific "superstitions" (*meishin*). This pattern became increasingly widespread after April 13, 1903, when, following a textbook corruption scandal, official textbooks came to be directly composed by government committees.[55]

The new government textbooks continued to provide basic scientific education and to inculcate patriotic slogans, yet they placed a much greater emphasis on the development of ethical sensibilities (*shūshin*). Rather than producing simplistic value distinctions, this new form of ethical discourse, borrowing from neo-Confucian texts, focused on the cultivation of specific virtues such as benevolence and filial piety. For the first time textbooks also addressed a key popular concern largely ignored by their immediate predecessors—namely, the danger posed by "superstitions." From 1903 until the end of the Second World War, elementary school children were explicitly taught to avoid superstition. In essence the textbooks treated the cultivation of a particular kind of intellectual skepticism as a central virtue and as a vaccine for the public moral "illnesses" produced by frauds and charlatans. They featured, alongside stock phrases such as "honor your parents" (*fubo o uyamau*), a new admonition to "avoid superstition" (*meishin o yokeyo*).

Rather than providing a stable definition of the slippery term "superstition," these textbooks took an almost Wittgensteinian delight in the taxonomic enterprise of enumerating different superstitions. Although the lists of superstitions vary from one textbook to the next, one classic version appeared in the first government-sponsored ethics textbook in 1903 and was reproduced, essentially unchanged, in textbooks through 1912.[56] It reads as follows:

1. Do not say that foxes or badgers deceive or possess people.
2. There is no such thing as winged goblins (*tengu*).
3. There is no such thing as curses.
4. Do not believe in empowered prayer (*kaji kitō*).
5. Do not trust in the efficacy of magic or holy water.
6. Do not put your trust in divination, whether by written oracles, physiognomy, geomancy, astrology, or ink stamp.
7. It is wrong to be concerned with omens and auspicious or inauspicious days.
8. Do not otherwise believe in anything that is generally similar to these things [mentioned above].[57]

The inclusion of empowered prayer in this bestiary demonstrates how far it had fallen from its former status as a dominant mode of ritual practice a mere fifty years earlier. Yet, given empowered prayer's association with exorcism, its inclusion is not completely arbitrary. Through such textbook accounts the Japanese government effectively suggested that it had successfully banished the monstrous, and thus that further apotropaic rituals were no longer necessary. Further clues as to the inspiration behind the focus on prayer rituals can be found in an anti-superstition lesson from a government-sponsored elementary textbook published in 1907. In the seventh chapter, entitled, "Avoid superstitions, Number 2 (30 Minutes in Duration)," it states:

> People recount oracles from the gods. They discuss their [experience of] divine possession. There are people who promote prayer rituals (*kitō*) using this language. However, *these people are just thinking about making money* for themselves. As a result, they do not actually do the things they claim. Even today, there are those who, when they are extremely ill and for a long time get no better, believe that it is the result of a curse. Then they pray to receive healing. Some receive prayers and [holy] water, which they drink. . . . No one gets better through spells or prayers. Accordingly, drinking that [holy] water is a very dangerous thing.[58]

As this example shows, textbooks encouraged the suspicion of fraudulent charismatic figures. The ritual practitioner's motives are not described in ethical or palliative terms, but are instead portrayed as the callous pursuit of financial gain at the expense of others. In essence the textbook contrasts selfish interest with the public good and suggests that the children of Japan should not allow themselves to fall prey to the deceptions of religious charlatans.

Despite disagreement on a single definition throughout the late Meiji period, the state continued to ban superstitions in various forms. Article 18 of the new penal code of 1907 read as follows: "[It is a misdemeanor] to obstruct medical treatment through the performance of spells, prayers, or magic for sick people, or otherwise distribute charms or holy water."[59] This ordinance was an expanded version of the Ministry of Doctrine's regulation from 1874 (noted above) that had already increased the number of regulated practices, also including magic and charms. The addition of holy water to this list in the wake of the Renmonkyō controversy suggests that holy water had also come to signify new religious movements, themselves targets of the regulation. Yet, note that the language of offense number eighteen sets up a direct opposition between medical treatment (at this point conceptualized as Western medicine) and folk healing practices, an opposition made manifest in trials relating to this ordinance.

One precedent-setting trial for the interpretation of this offense occurred in 1910, when a fifty-eight-year-old man named Hanada Mataichi was arrested for giving an ill woman some herbal remedies and six grains of rice that had been offered to the Bright King Fudō. Hanada was accused of "obstructing medicine" through the use of faith healing and sentenced to ten days in prison. However, instead of accepting this judgment, he demanded a courtroom trial and presented documents demonstrating that he was a legitimate religious professional of a recognized religious sect. This claim in itself was not sufficient to sway the judge, who refused to interpret the law as a concerted, or even perhaps unjust, attempt to eliminate unaffiliated ritual specialists or the practitioners of new religions. However, Hanada's lawyer argued that for the charge of "obstructing medical treatment" to be applicable, it must refer "either to the interference with someone currently under the actual care of a physician, or else acts which would prevent someone from coming under such care." The lawyer then suggested that, "in the event the individual never demonstrated any intent to receive therapy from a physician, the performance of any faith healing cannot be interpreted as interference with such medical therapy."[60] Although the court eventually dismissed the charges against Hanada on the strength of this argument, such isolated challenges to anti-superstition laws did little to stop the arrests of faith healers throughout the country. The result of these laws, then, was the systematic disempowerment of ritual healers.

A Division or Revision of the World: Empowered Prayer in Buddhist Debates

> One should not try to separate the Cosmic Buddha's dharma-body from the human realm of this universe. . . . The real world is the perfect harmonious form of the Cosmic Buddha's dharma-body, and it is [simultaneously] the realm in which his deeds are made manifest.
>
> —Kobayashi Ubō, "Kaji Sekai no Igi"

Against this backdrop of trials and newspaper attacks on ritual healing, Buddhist leaders began to reappraise empowered prayer. Even as state regulation began to radically circumscribe the practice of Buddhist pharmacology, much of the Buddhist institution persisted in performing traditional healing prayers. Yet in order to avoid running afoul of government ordinances, Buddhist leaders became increasingly cautious about exactly how they promoted their prayers. In this context a number of voices called for the complete elimination of Buddhist healing rituals. Simultaneously, vocal defenders of healing prayer emerged, particularly from the ranks of the Shingon institution. At stake in these debates was not only the role of a particular ritual practice, but the manner in which the miraculous and the mechanical might fit together to form either a whole or a divided vision of the cosmos.

The public face of criticism of Buddhist "superstitions" was lay Buddhist philosopher Inoue Enryō (1858–1919). Although he addressed the topic of this-worldly prayer in several different works, Inoue focused most directly on empowered prayer in an essay entitled *Kaji kitō no koto* ("The practice of empowered prayer"), published in his 1904 *Meishinkai*. There Inoue cites critiques of empowered prayer in neo-Confucian circles, in government-sponsored ethics textbooks, and in newspaper reports of recent arrests for violation of the government's ban on healing prayer. Inoue begins by conceding ground to kaji's critics. He acknowledges that proponents of empowered prayer are motivated not by altruistic devotion, but by fear of "various illnesses and calamities."[61] Inoue further admits that empowered prayer is but one type of this-worldly Buddhist ceremony, and thus not the only suspect variety of Buddhist ritual.

Rather than dismissing empowered prayer completely, Inoue divides it into two aspects. On the one hand he suggests that there is a "justifiable" or "lawful" (*seitō*) portion of the behavior rooted in "sincere whole-hearted devotion."[62] In Inoue's account this authentic aspect of empowered prayer helps to cultivate true faith, and thus should be permitted. However, on the other hand, Inoue strongly condemns what he calls the "unjustifiable" or "unlawful" (*fuseitō*) component of empowered prayer. Inoue connects this aspect of empowered prayer to "licentious worship," which he portrays as both irrational and immoral.[63] Although this might at first appear to be a defense of normative Buddhism at the expense of new religious movements, Inoue's analysis indicates that he regards licentious worship as a potential danger for Buddhists, as well. For Inoue the proper performance of empowered prayer is rooted in the motives of its practitioners. Those whose actions spring from altruistic, or at least devotional, intentions are not at fault, but those whose motives are selfish or focused on this-worldly benefits are acting improperly. However, implicit in this division of empowered prayer into justifiable and unjustifiable aspects is a separation of the world according to an almost Cartesian fracture line.

In his efforts to distinguish the positive and negative aspects of empowered prayer, Inoue asserts that kaji is a meditative and psychological practice unconnected to the miraculous. Thus, he reasons, "what are called prayers in the mundane world have a completely different meaning [from Shingon doctrine]."[64] However, Inoue argues that, over time, monks of the Shingon sect became known for the performance of prayer rituals, in part because their temples intermingled (*kongō*) gods and buddhas.[65] Accordingly, "the confusion that is empowered prayer came about as the result of the confusion of gods and buddhas."[66] Thus, for Inoue, empowered prayer is not "original Buddhism," but rather an unwholesome offspring of the miscegenation of Buddhism and Shinto. Building on this logic, Inoue frames the rejection of empowered prayer not as an imposition from a modernizing state, but as a purifying return to tradition.

The fundamental problem with empowered prayer, according to Inoue, lies in the idea that one could pay for the performance of wonders. At one level "selling miracles" is ethically flawed because it contributes to the avarice of some religious professionals, tempting them to exploit people for money. At an even deeper level practices intended to produce miracles are rooted in an ontological confusion. As Inoue argues elsewhere, there is a fundamental division between the material and spiritual world, and neither buddhas nor gods have control over material existence.[67] Inoue's sharp division of the world into spiritual and material realms allows him to preserve an autonomous spiritual realm for Buddhist philosophy, which does not necessarily conflict with scientific knowledge. But this strategy also makes the material world the sole province of science. This meant that the causes of illness and earthquakes, then, ought not to be sought in curses or demons, but in the laws that govern human health or plate tectonics. Empowered prayer is always superstitious, because it is based upon the belief that something other than universal physical laws governs the events of this world. While Inoue does not dismiss prayer completely, he regards its benefits as psychological or spiritual, not physical. This view has a universalizing function, because it treats all devoted prayer as equal, regardless of its sectarian origins. However, at the same time, it discounts the need to engage in the elaborate ritual of empowered prayer, since it possesses no ability to transform the material universe. By implication, then, empowered prayer does not work as a ritual technology, but at best functions as a psychological palliative: a purpose better served by a range of meditative practices. While Inoue does not seek to ban empowered prayer entirely, he almost completely eliminates any rationale for its performance.

Many Buddhists, however, rejected calls to abolish empowered prayer. Rather than challenging government policy, the majority of the debates about the value of prayer took place in Buddhist circles and focused on the ideal status of empowerment and this-worldly ritual. Some defenders of prayer's efficacy contributed to an aptly named journal, *Kaji Sekai* (*The Empowered World*). First published in 1900 in Tokyo by members of the Shingon sect, *Kaji Sekai* attracted a range of young Buddhist priests who otherwise lacked a voice in their school. The name of the journal itself was meant to resonate on several different levels at once. It referred to a specific Shingon term for the world in which the *nirmāṇakāya* (manifest body) of the Cosmic Buddha revealed itself, and also to the broader context of empowered prayer and anti-superstition policy.

In its first issue *Kaji Sekai* carved out a new position in the debate concerning superstition. An article entitled "Concerning Superstition and True Belief," attributed to the pseudonym Kōon (Hidden-Bamboo-Grove), begins with the contention that "definitively distinguishing between superstition and true belief is next to impossible."[68] However, the article goes on to assert that Buddhist modernists have attempted to do just that. Kōon summarizes this new Buddhist view as based on a fundamental distinction between belief in common sense and belief in the true knowledge that comes from science and philosophy.[69] The author challenges the authority of science by insisting that knowledge is relative and continually changing and thus does not provide access to absolute truth. Kōon implies that Buddhist modernists, in their dismissal of superstitions, have misunderstood Buddhist two-truth theory by mistaking scientific truths for ultimate truth (*shindai*; Sanskrit, *paramārtha-satya*).[70] Kōon suggests that, because scientific truth is being constantly revised, what appears to be true today may be seen as superstition tomorrow. Thus, by challenging the authority of what he understands to be the basis of the distinction between true and false knowledge, Kōon concludes that there is no way to firmly demonstrate that a given belief is really superstitious. He observes that "what we call superstition and what we call true belief are based solely on the criteria of own subjective judgments."[71] Kōon argues against contemporary government policy, writing that "we want the general faith to be as free as possible without damaging society. In the absence of [this freedom] it would probably not be possible to protect [belief in] the divine mysteries of the universe from elimination."[72] Kōon seems to be suggesting that the popularity of prayer rituals stems from the appeal of the universe's profound mysteries and that, without the censorship designed to eliminate so-called "superstitious" beliefs and practices, the true teachings of the Shingon sect would win out in an open marketplace of ideas.

In 1906 an article appeared in the same journal by a Shingon priest named Kobayashi Uhō (1873–1937) that focused explicitly on the meaning of empowerment, but did not address empowered prayer as such. In the article "The Meaning of the Empowered World" (*Kaji sekai no igi*), Kobayashi writes: "Mundane people have a grotesque reaction to what is called kaji. Having come to use kaji to refer to empowered prayer, magic, and divination, they have as a result come to describe the Shingon and Hokke schools as purveyors of superstition and blind belief."[73] Kobayashi portrays this common reaction as based upon a mistaken understanding of the fundamental meaning of the word "kaji." In Shingon doctrine, he explains, all events in this universe result from the manifestations of the dharma body of the Cosmic Buddha. According to Kobayashi, then, this world is none other than the empowered world (*kaji sekai*). Following and expanding upon Kūkai's solar metaphor, Kobayashi says that, just as living things on the earth are dependent on the light of the sun for heat and life, so too are all sentient beings dependent on the Buddha's energies. In other words, in an argument resonant with Bergsonian vitalism, for Kobayashi all life is empowered by the Cosmic Buddha.

Kobayashi responds directly to the popular critique of the Shingon School as superstitious by delinking human intentions from the possibility of the miraculous.[74] He argues that the true meaning of empowerment lies not in the fulfillment of selfish motivations, but in the continual manifestation of the Cosmic Buddha in the universe and in the human world. The Cosmic Buddha is always present, deciding at one moment to heal and at another to allow suffering to continue. Yet, on a fundamental level, the entire world remains the responsibility of the Cosmic Buddha and, as such, everything that happens both subjectively and objectively is a manifestation of his dharma-body.

Implicitly Kobayashi rejects Inoue's division of the world into spiritual and material aspects, for it would quarantine the Cosmic Buddha to the spiritual plane, when in fact the Cosmic Buddha is the whole of the cosmos. Thus empowerment rituals, in their ability to bridge practitioner and Cosmic Buddha, human and world, are fundamental to Shingon philosophy and cannot be surgically extracted without fatal injury to the entire philosophical system. This makes a seemingly peripheral ritual technology central to a total vision of the universe. Without the possibility of miraculous empowerment, the Buddha could not appear to human senses, nor preach his teachings, nor provide us with the mysterious keys to his wondrous unfolding of this empowered world.

Although the debates about the efficacy of prayer raged on both within and outside the Buddhist institution, they were never resolved. Today one can find empowered prayer practices all over Japan.[75] Although the Meiji government succeeded in radically destabilizing Buddhist medicine as an independent institution, it ultimately failed in its campaign to stamp out ritual healing. Empowered healing continues to be practiced in conjunction with modern medicine, but functions only in a supplemental capacity. In other words, the empowered world has become, at best, a mere supplement to the mechanistic cosmos.

Conclusion

> When kaji [empowered prayer] is performed, a cancer patient's white cell count may rise to a level half of normal within a day. This astonishing phenomenon has been measured and documented scientifically.
>
> —Oda Ryūkō, Kaji

A 1963 Supreme Court decision reinforced the Meiji-era precedents discussed previously. Accordingly, Japanese law and the Buddhist institutions have maintained a particular compromise—that prayer healing could be practiced as long as it supplemented, but did not supplant the dominant Westernized medical system.[76] In other words, kaji could be added to medical treatments, but could not be allowed to replace them. Just as mantras and empowered prayer were seen in premodern Japan as contributing to the efficacy of Buddhist herbal medicine, kaji is today understood by many as a ritual that increases the efficacy of modern medical care. Thus the logic of empowerment has been displaced from the traditional techno-ritual component of Buddhist medicine to an analogous function in contemporary healing practices. This pattern is reproduced outside of the medical sphere, where wonder-inducing rituals are now seen as supplementing contemporary technological efforts. To return to the example with which this chapter began, rituals previously designed to invoke the God of Sailors to calm storms are now seen as having the potential to secure the safety of astronauts by, in effect, contributing special energies to the space vessel.

Despite the perceived complementarity of ritual and technology in modern Japan, Buddhism remains part of a demarcated domain called the "religious," which perpetuates an artificial distinction between discrete spheres of knowledge. This partition has contributed to the gradual elimination of most of the Buddhist medical institution. Based on the perceived supremacy of modern medicine over the physical world, material *technai* became the domain of doctors trained in Westernized medicine. Herbal and surgical treatments inspired by Buddhist scriptures have been almost completely eliminated. However, prayer rituals, existing between the frames articulated for the instrumental-technological and the religio-spiritual, continue to be performed for both this-worldly and otherworldly purposes. Yet, as is clear from this section's epigraph, its effectiveness is now measured according to criteria (such as white blood cell count) originating in a modern medical context.

Shingon priest Oda Ryūkō (1914–1993) made it his life mission to promote empowered prayer within the Japanese medical establishment. His books, published in both Japanese and English, made use of the testimonies of physicians to argue that empowered prayer could be an effective treatment for a range of illnesses, from leukemia and malignant tumors to gastrointestinal ulcers and epilepsy.[77] While empowered prayer is not officially recognized by the Japanese medical institution, one does not have to travel far from the noodle shop in Kotohira to find it in contemporary Japan, where a number of Shingon Japanese priests now promote its efficacy.[78] Perhaps you can even find empowerment closer to home if you happen to live near the Royal Forest of Dean in the town of Mitcheldean in Gloucestershire, England, where for ten pounds you can have kaji performed by a British Shingon priest who invokes Oda on his webpage.[79]

Does Submission to God's Will Preclude Biotechnological Intervention?

Lessons from Muslim Dialysis Patients in Contemporary Egypt

Sherine F. Hamdy

In a long hospital corridor in Tanta, Egypt, a middle-aged physician, the attending nephrologist in the dialysis ward, shook his head in exasperation. He had just been counseling Ali, a young man stricken with kidney failure who commuted from his home village via public transportation to receive life-supporting dialysis treatment three times a week. Dr. Sami attempted to explain to the patient that his only hope to return to a "normal life" would be via a kidney transplant. But the patient had refused, saying simply, "The body belongs to God. It belongs to no one else to give away, and it is not for me to take." Dr. Sami let out a long breath and said to me: "It is very difficult, you know, with these patients—the religious fanatical types. They are fatalistic, saying God knows when they will die before they are even born. So they don't accept the idea [of transplantation]."

I spent two years in Egypt researching the heated debate about organ transplantation among patients, physicians, and religious scholars. Egypt—more so than any other Muslim or Arab country—has been home to a lively national debate among legislators, physicians, religious scholars, and journalists around the ethics of organ transplantation. It is not uncommon for physicians or journalists to use labels like "fanatical," "fatalistic," or "backward" in the print media to describe people's reluctance toward organ transplantation. Almost all religious scholars—and all those in official state positions—have declared that organ donation is permissible for Muslims, and the Coptic pope has argued the same for Coptic Christians (who comprise an estimated 10 percent of the Egyptian population). Yet most ordinary Egyptians still express antipathy toward the idea, including many physicians and patients in need of organs. Since Egypt's first kidney transplant in 1976, pioneering surgeons have pushed in vain for the legislation of a national organ transplant program. In the 1980s the national media (particularly the opposition-party newspapers) began to publicize stories of orphan children disappearing for organ theft, a thriving black market in kidneys in Cairo, and body parts surreptitiously being taken from Cairo's public hospital morgues. In trying to formulate a reaction, politicians were unable to agree on how best to define or minimize "criminal" medical wrongdoing. Thus kidney transplants have been carried out for over three decades in Egypt in the absence of any legal framework or national organ transplant program. Brain-death is not recognized as legal death, hence all organ donors are living. Patients like Ali are expected to go "find" their own kidney: from a donor within the family or, presumably, on the black market. When patients refuse, their physicians, like Dr. Sami, and other commentators in the press often read their rejection of a transplant as "fatalist."

In this chapter I demonstrate how the internalized Orientalist trope of Muslim-as-fatalist has worked to obscure complex debates in the field of organ transplantation in Egypt. I argue against the dominant narrative: that religious fatalism obstructs people from pursuing biotechnological intervention. This dominant narrative is an offshoot of the powerful myth that religion always opposes scientific and technological progress. I argue instead that people's understandings of religion and biomedical efficacy are often inextricably enmeshed and together factor into their cost-benefit calculations about medical intervention. Below I offer some ethnographic examples from my work among terminally ill dialysis patients in Egypt. I demonstrate that their religious logics intersect with their assessment of social and medical risks and benefits as they face life-and-death decisions about their medical care.

Sticking with What Works

In the Tanta University Hospital dialysis center where I conducted fieldwork on kidney failure in Egypt (2002–2004), I sat with a group of young men in their twenties who were following a soccer match on a small, grainy television while receiving their dialysis treatment.[1] Many were poor, either agricultural laborers from the countryside or low-income workers in Tanta's factories and service industries. They all received compensation for their dialysis treatment directly from the Ministry of Health, which covers the full cost of dialysis for the poor.[2] One of these men, Muhammad, told me that he was born with only one kidney and suffered from hypertension. One day he took the wrong pill for his high blood pressure, which resulted in acute renal failure. The physicians had later told him that if he had taken *two* pills (the regular dosage) he would have died immediately. But for some reason he only took one and ended up in a coma.

Muhammad was not particularly religious before his diagnosis. But since that time, seeing his young life suddenly and drastically changed, he said that he would never miss any of the five obligatory daily prayers (*al-salat*), nor would he forget to continuously thank God for still being alive. Muhammad had his whole life in front of him and suddenly saw it cut short. His difficulty in managing his disease was not merely in his physical pain and newly acquired disabilities. He told me that the most difficult change he had to endure was the ways his illness had altered his social relationships, such as his inability to get married. His fiancée's family refused him, saying they did not want to see their girl widowed in a few years, essentially issuing him a poor prognosis. He could no longer continue working or spending time with friends, who feared his condition might be contagious. His physician, Dr. Yusuf, also discouraged him from getting married, explaining to me that the physical and sexual side effects of kidney failure and dialysis would render such a marriage "not viable."[3] Shaking his head gravely, Dr. Yusuf told me that dialysis was not really treatment, and that transplantation was the only way out of this situation. At the same time, Dr. Yusuf also related to me his own personal misgivings about transplantation, and questioned whether it was ethically responsible to put a living donor at such an unacceptable risk.[4] Like Muhammad, he also questioned the transplant's efficacy for the recipient. In contrast, Muhammad described his dialysis sessions as "safe"; he told me the outcome of dialysis was more predictable and made his life bearable. In his words:

> Getting a transplant isn't guaranteed. I know my kidney is ruined, so I come [for dialysis] three days a week. Only God knows if I tried to get a transplant whether I would die doing it. There are people who get sick with the transplant; the body rejects it, or they end up with other diseases. So I need to just be content with what I have. If I tried a transplant,

I could die the next morning. So what would I have gotten out of it, just having had myself opened up and stitched back together? Sometimes the operation can last five to six hours—only God knows what could happen during that time. . . . So I need to stick with what is guaranteed. I come here [to dialysis] and can go home after four hours. And that's it. . . . This is a trial from God, most exalted and high. He created me as His servant/slave (*'abd*) and out of all the people that He created, God is thinking of *me*, in giving me this disease. And in my suffering, I am getting rid of my sins. I will still be tried [for my deeds after death] but the punishment will be lesser. . . . I have kidney failure now and could die in five years. Why me specifically? God has ultimate wisdom (*hikma*) in this. It didn't just come to anyone; it came to me. God is saving me [from my sins and heedlessness] because now I remember God all the time. A person has to have his beliefs.

Muhammad narrates his decision-making process in religious terms, saying "God has ultimate wisdom in this," as well as voicing his uncertainty about the efficacy and outcome of the transplant. He does so by calculating the great costs of a donated kidney—no one in his immediate family qualifies medically as a donor, and there is no national registry in Egypt—and his adversity to the idea of putting a living "stranger" at the risk of a major medical operation (extracting an organ), if he were to buy one on the black market. In any case, he does not have the cash necessary to make such a purchase. In Muhammad's calculation, the costs—medical, ethical, and monetary—outweigh the benefits, given that transplant operations are not always successful. His body, he reasons, may reject the kidney in the end anyway. He may die on the operating table. So he decides to "stick with what works" and to maintain his dialysis schedule.

Given that Muhammad relies on a dialysis machine to filter his blood in place of his failed kidneys, it is clear that he is not rejecting all medical and biotechnological intervention. The risks of dialysis are significant, too—many patients have contracted hepatitis C and HIV from infected needles—and the side effects include incapacitating exhaustion. Yet dialysis has now become routine and naturalized for Muhammad. Each session has now become part of a difficult life to endure: unlike the high-stakes, high-technological drama of a transplant operation, where the patient risks everything, the donor loses a vital organ, and the outcome could very well be fatal.

Fatalism is the notion that humans can exert little or no control over their own destinies. The issue is at once theological and, in the medical world, about treatment efficacy: What is the scope of human agency in the realm of an omnipotent deity? And what is the power of a particular treatment in stopping the course of a particular disease? In its early years the outcomes of organ transplantation were grim throughout the world. It was only with the advent of stronger immune-suppressive drugs that patients' survival rates improved.[5] And as the survival rates improved, ethical debates abated (including those in the United States about playing God and resurrecting the dead).[6] In parts of the world with fewer resources, this experimental phase is often more complicated and more extended. This brings up a larger question, which American physician-writer Atul Gawande poses: new medical procedures inevitably pose risks, often fatal, to patients. Yet physicians persist in the hopes that with practice both the new technique and the new technician (e.g., the surgeon) will improve. So what are the ethical implications toward those early experimental patients? This is where ethical religious discourse and questions about medical scientific efficacy meet. Yet this very intersection is consistently ignored and misrecognized, obscured by the "religious opposition to science" narrative.

In Dr. Yusuf's narrative, Muhammad's choice should be simple: clinical results show that a kidney transplant is more efficacious than dialysis for a person in end-stage renal disease. From Dr. Yusuf's perspective, Muhammad's appeal to God's will is religiously incorrect—for God surely would encourage the best medical treatment and the preservation of his own creation. But for Muhammad the risks of a kidney transplant (including falling into financial debt) are less tolerable than life on dialysis. For Muhammad, God has given him the strength to face structural and material constraints that seem to give him no other option than to persevere and endure his fate.

Devout Muslim patients often told me they work actively on their selves to cultivate steadfastness and patience (*al-sabr*). Questions about *when* and *in what contexts* patients appeal to God's will are at once about medical efficacy and religious devotion. Judging the medical efficacy of a treatment has to do with a host of factors, such as scientific literacy, previous experiences with medical care, trust in the medical profession, access and affordability of treatment, and one's ability to tolerate the disease without treatment. One's ability to cultivate a religious disposition toward suffering has to do with one's social support system, one's understanding of God's will, and one's psychological fortitude at a particular moment in time. Thus when physicians and patients appear to be disagreeing about whether or not one is being "fatalistic," they are often disagreeing about sociomedical calculations of risks, costs, and benefits.

Quest for the Good

The factors that enter into people's decisions—whether to appeal to God's will or to seek treatment—are not only complex and intermingled, they are also constantly changing. Whether a treatment option appears beneficial and accessible, whether the costs seem attainable and tolerable, whether the medical practitioners seem trustworthy and reliable—all these factors are in flux, and could even change for the same individual on the very same day.

Across town from Dr. Yusuf's clinic, in another hospital dialysis unit, stories of death and disease after transplantation circulated among patients. These stories served as reminders that only God can will life and death. Many patients often repeated that a person could not truly "save" another person from his fate, nor could a person "lengthen a life" by donating an organ to someone else. Ali, a young patient in the unit, often said that you might think doctors can help—but if doctors can heal, they are only instruments of God's unique healing abilities. According to Ali, "You might borrow large sums of money to pay a donor to part with his kidney, but you are self-deceived if you think that this will guarantee your recovery. God is the sole Guarantor who heals whomever He wills, and the One who decides who will die when."

Ali once said to me, "What is that particle that Zewail discovered? A femto-sone? We are less than a femto-sone in God's creation!" Like many literate Egyptians, Ali knew well the accomplishments of Egyptian-American Nobel Prize Laureate and chemist, Ahmed Zewail, and his discovery of the subatomic femto-second (which Ali pronounced as "femto-sone" in Egyptian Arabic) has entered into the Egyptian lexicon. Ali said this to me after I showed him the back of my American driver's license, where I was asked to be an organ donor after death. Ali did not approve of organ transplantation even from dead donors. Echoing the justification of many Islamic scholars, most notably the popular Egyptian television figure Shaykh Sha'rawi,[7] Ali argued that God alone owns everything, including human bodies and their parts. Who are we, then, to give something away that we do not own? Ali further stated that those who think they are "saving" someone by donating are presumptuous, for they are less than a subatomic particle when compared to divine powers, and God is the only one who saves.

In the hospital dialysis center, Ali remained the most outspoken opponent of the idea of organ transplantation—for himself, that is. He never discouraged others, but he genuinely struggled against the idea that a transplant would improve his own situation. Ali and his young wife had two small children; the youngest was born, he told me, after he fell ill. Unlike the other patients, who often seemed completely exhausted by the dialysis, Ali could successfully fight off the exhaustion, keeping up his energy and making everyone in his session laugh. Ali and his family lived in the countryside in Minufiyya.[8] Ali had worked in the army, which is why he had the insurance to cover his treatment. Aside from his good humor, Ali stood out from the other patients in the ways that he asserted his politicized form of Muslim identity. The other patients poked fun at his full beard, joking that he would be mistaken for a "terrorist," especially in my "American research." Ali tended to talk animatedly about the current attack on the *umma* (Muslim community) and about the ways Muslims must come closer to God to regain political and moral strength.

Knowing that my topic was focused on transplants, Ali spent many hours with me debating the Islamic stance on donating and receiving body parts. Ali was one of the few patients in the ward who in practical terms could undergo a transplant without too much financial hardship, and since he had fallen into acute end-stage renal failure five years ago, his wife and his many siblings had repeatedly offered to donate their kidneys to him, and his army insurance would cover all costs of the operation in Cairo. Yet Ali was convinced that this was *haram* (forbidden/sinful).

Ali and I continued for months discussing his situation. One day he told me, "Religion is the only issue that is stopping me.[9] Most people in my situation would say it is *halal* [permissible], because they need it. It is very rare to find someone like me who needs it and still says it is *haram*." I asked him, "Why are you not convinced by the *shuyukh* (Islamic scholars) who say it is *halal*?" He answered, "I have nothing to do with them" (*malish da'wa bihum*). Ali asked me to read him what I had written so far. After I did, he nodded and continued, "Write this down: If I got a transplant, I would have to pay *no money*. My wife wants to give me her kidney, and the army will pay for it, and they say that I will get experts from abroad [to perform the operation]. But I am convinced: No."

The army and other employers calculated that the costs of transplantation would be less than years of dialysis treatment. Many employers encouraged their ex-employees, whose treatment they paid for, to seek transplantation. I asked Ali why he was so convinced not to pursue a transplant, and he told me that God did not make it easy for him to accept the idea. I told him, "But you wouldn't have to pay any money, and your wife has offered to give you a kidney. Why isn't this [evidence that] God has made it easy for you?" Ali shook his head and said, "No, but I prayed *salat al-istikhara*" (a prayer for guidance). He pulled out a wrinkled piece of paper that he carries in his wallet. He told me, "Look at the date." The date on the piece of paper was over a year old: April 26, 2002. It was a referral from the army for a fully paid appointment for Ali's wife to be tissue-typed with him. It had taken him four years to make this one step. Ali's wife had been pleading with him to go to the appointment, but Ali had been refusing, feeling that it was not right.

The Arabic word *istikhara* means "seeking the good." Many Muslims, when faced with a choice that they feel they cannot make, perform a special *salat* (ritual prayer) of two *raka'* (prayer cycles) in length, and then ask God directly for proper guidance so that they can make the choice that will be good for them in life and in faith. In Egypt Muslims often pray *salat al-istikhara* before a marriage choice. They believe that your heart must be neutral, that you cannot be leaning toward one decision or another, and that you must truly be committed to doing what is right. God will then answer by making apparent the right choice.

Ali told me that after praying *salat al-istikhara*, he never felt "happy" about a decision to go and get tested for tissue typing. He told me that he did not feel it was the right thing for him to get up, get dressed, and say to his wife, "Let's bring the kids and go get tested now." I asked him, perhaps too cynically, if he felt this way about going to the dialysis unit three times a week. Defiantly, he said yes. Ali explained that he interpreted his reluctance to tissue-typing to be God's answer to his prayer, and he refused the idea of transplantation for the past five years out of fear that it was *haram*. Having articulated a deep mistrust of those state-appointed Islamic scholars who described the practice as "permissible" on state television and in the newspapers, Ali felt that he could only trust his own heart and conscience. That is why he was deeply committed to seeking God's counsel through prayer. When he looked into his heart, he did not find transplant as an option that would bring "the good" (*al-khayr*).

A Change of Heart

Ali spent hours debating with himself, and with me, about why kidney transplantation could not possibly be pleasing to God. He would tell me, "God is trying me with this disease. When we are tried by God, we remember Him and praise Him for everything. God says: 'He who is not pleased with God's will can find another universe [besides the one God created] to live in.'" That is why it surprised me when one day I came to the unit and Ali happily announced to me that he was going to get a transplant. I asked him what had changed his mind. He had gone to Cairo to the military hospital for a check-up, and the doctor who treated him there had himself undergone a transplant operation in the United States. He encouraged Ali, telling him that God had given people their bodies as a trust (*amana*) and that he was therefore responsible to take care of it. Dialysis was slowly ruining his body, the doctor told him, and was not a treatment that would ever make him better. But, the doctor reasoned, God blessed him with the *chance* to have a transplant and the military insurance that could cover it. When I had previously spoken to Ali, he would tell me that his wife had pleaded with him daily to let her give him her kidney, but that he had refused completely, not wanting to hurt her in any way. But his recent doctor's appointment had clearly made an impression on him. Furthermore, Ali said, the son of another patient in his dialysis unit, a military captain, had heard a television program where a respected Islamic scholar said that it was not *haram* to have this procedure done, and that God urges us to seek cures. The scholar on television had said that it was *haram* to leave your body to deteriorate, Ali explained (*ma ta'adish nafsak lil tahluka*), paraphrasing a Qur'anic verse in colloquial Egyptian Arabic.

Ali was happy and laughing that day, saying "May God stand by us." He said that he had spoken to a lot of doctors when he was in the Ma'adi hospital, and that they had said that they performed transplant operations there every day, and that the outcomes were successful. People did fine after transplants, they told Ali. When I spoke with Ali's wife, Wafiyya, she told me:

> I just want him to have the transplant so that he gets better, and so that he can get back to his normal self. But he says that he doesn't believe that transplanting will get him back to normal.[10] I tell him: "Our Lord is with us" (*Rabbina mawgud*). His brothers and sisters say, "[We'll donate], leave your wife. She's so young." But Ali got scared for his siblings, for their wives and their children.

Wafiyya was obviously torn over her position. At least when Ali had refused to even consider a transplant on the grounds that it was *haram*, she had given up feeling responsible. In tears, she said to me, "He is my husband, and if, God forbid, something happens to him, what am I going to do?"

Ali and Wafiyya did eventually decide to return to the Cairo military hospital laboratory for tissue analysis.[11] A few weeks later I was back at the dialysis center when Ali got a phone call in the unit. I could see Ali's face clearly while he was on the phone. It was from Wafiyya, and she had just received the results from the lab. Ali tried to act calm and unaffected: "Wafiyya heard from the [military] hospital. Let's see what will happen now," he announced to a fellow patient, Madame Sabah, before returning to Wafiyya on the phone. There was no tissue match. Ali still sounded unimpressed, saying, "Okay, okay, Madame Sabah sends her *salamat* [greetings] to you," and hung up, announcing to whoever was interested that there was no match.[12] Madame Sabah immediately saw through Ali's attempts to be cavalier about the news. She said: "Don't be upset, Ali, we're better off this way. We won't make other people [the donor] sick with us, we won't get all swollen [from the post-operative treatment], we won't be in the hospital days after days, worrying about some kind of infection. The way we are with dialysis is just better."

Madame Sabah was a widow in her fifties who never had any children. She was so pleasant and well-loved that she had many family members who offered to donate their organs to her, most pressingly her niece. But there was no way Madame Sabah could think of taking this from her. As I discovered in my research, mothers generally refused to take kidneys from their daughters; the unstated presumption was that life should flow from older to younger generations. In this logic, how can an aunt accept a kidney from her niece?[13] Later Ali told me, "Madame Sabah was just saying those things to make us both feel better, so that we would be able to stay patient and steadfast in the face of this hardship (*tasabbar nafsaha wa tasabbarni*). But of course she wants to have a transplant and to get better, just like the rest of us. But what can we do?"

In the months that followed, Ali came to accept this news as a gift from God. God had prevented him from doing something potentially *haram*, he explained. He continued to thank God for the blessings that he was receiving on dialysis. A year later the patients in the dialysis unit were cheered up by the news that Ali's wife, Wafiyya, gave birth to another baby girl, whom Ali described as "sweet as honey."

The hours I spent talking with Ali made me appreciate more fully the complex ways that people embody their ideas about divine will, about how much of their lives they feel they can control, and how much they feel they *should* control. In contrast with the situation in the United States, where kidney-failure patients can be put on a waiting list to receive kidneys from anonymous brain-dead donors, in Egypt patients have to act on their own to "find kidneys" from living donors.[14] The Egyptian case thus brings to the surface a host of ethical questions and dilemmas.[15]

Once, when trying to compare Ali's situation with that of patients in the United States, I asked Ali what he would do if, hypothetically, he could put his name on a list and be told that the hospital would make all the arrangements for him to receive a kidney from an anonymous dead donor. He thought for a while, and then said that he would probably accept it, even if deep down inside he still had reservations. A remarkably insightful man, Ali realized that his refusal, prior to agreeing to the tissue test, was shaped in a particular social situation in which he had to overcome several obstacles in order to proceed with a transplant: to find a donor; to be responsible for the donor's tests; and to bear the responsibility for the donor's sacrifice, pain, and side effects. Already predisposed to mistrust this particular medical practice, Ali lacked the drive to surmount each hurdle, as each of these steps raised for him the ethical uncertainties surrounding organ transplantation. He thus recognized that were he to find himself in an alternate sociomedical setting in which a kidney was somehow made available to him without such constant reminders of risk and cost, he would likely accept it. Given the reality he lived in, though, he turned to God to seek the strength he needed to remain on dialysis for the rest of his life.

In explaining Ali's reluctance to pursue transplantation from his wife in his first five years on dialysis, his physicians described him as "religiously extreme" and "fatalistic." But Ali himself did not think of his religion as something that prevented him from seeking a beneficial treatment. Nor was his reluctance solely determined by scarce material resources inhibiting medical access, since, as we have seen, Ali did have military insurance that would cover all the costs of a transplant and family members who were willing to donate to him. Yet he insisted that he would rather die and "meet God" than be responsible for causing harm to his family members, or for putting his family into debt to buy a (tissue-compatible) kidney, which he saw as clearly *haram*.[16] Ali harbored deep reservations about "using" his wife or siblings as kidney donors—being responsible for their potential illness, suffering, or potential inability to look after their children.[17]

But what are we to make of Ali's sudden change of heart? He had temporarily allowed himself to be convinced by a competing moral discourse about the meaning of the "body belonging to God," in which he should pursue transplantation as a means to respect and care for the body that God had given him. The doctor at the military hospital and hearsay from a fellow patient's son about the proclamations of a television *shaykh* (a type of Islamic scholar Ali had earlier claimed not to trust) were suddenly able to convince Ali that it was part of his religious duty to pursue transplantation to protect the body as a divine trust. This occurred in a new context, in which Ali was shown the fruits of successful transplant surgeries and the routinization of transplantation in a large military hospital in Cairo. While his thrice-weekly routine of hemodialysis in a less-than-ideal hospital setting in Tanta had made him wary of medical services and practices, the state-of-the-art facilities in Cairo had made an altogether different impression on him; he was particularly impressed by the doctor's exhortations that such potentially efficacious treatment (the doctor himself having been a post-transplant survivor returning to daily activities) were within his reach. Perhaps it was returning to the reality of poverty in his rural village in Minufiyya or his return to the drudgery of the regular commute to Tanta and the dialysis regimen that deflated his hopes. When a slim window of hope had opened and transplantation looked like it might be a beneficial solution to his illness, Ali not only saw it as religiously permissible, but agreed with the doctor that it would be a religious *duty* to pursue it if it meant restoring his health. But this hope was fragile, and it was soon crushed with the news of an incompatible tissue match with his wife.

Patients like Ali, who at times seemed the most resolute in their positions, often changed their minds, depending on changing circumstances in their lives. This does not make their religious convictions any less strong or meaningful. Finding it hard to believe the religious scholars who permitted transplantation, and long unable to make this position salient in a situation where he might harm his young wife, Ali had initially turned to supplication and prayer for guidance. Many analysts of religion, appealing to notions of false consciousness, would maintain that such behaviors are examples of religion serving as a "comfort mechanism" in suffering. In Egypt some physicians and interlocutors I encountered would interpret the fact that Ali had believed that transplantation was permissible when his wife was still potentially a donor for him, and later as forbidden/sinful when his wife's tissues were not a match, as a manipulation of religious doctrine to suit his circumstances.

But such an interpretation would miss the point. Religion is not an object external to Ali's self, as something he manipulates to suit his needs. On the contrary, devout patients like Ali embody a religious tradition in which they struggle to cultivate within themselves the disposition of *rida* (contentment with God's will). Ali believed strongly that true submission to God is predicated on the understanding that God's will transcends everything, and that the purpose of worship and remembrance is to bring oneself in utter closeness to God, such that "God is with you wherever you are,"[18] and that "Wheresoever you turn, there is the Face of God."[19] When he felt that he had the opportunity for transplantation, he felt that God had willed for him to seize this opportunity.

And what are we then to understand of Ali's ultimate acceptance of the news of incomplete tissue match as a divine sign to not pursue the transplant? When a transplant appeared to be no longer available after news of his wife's incompatible tissue type, Ali still read God's will favorably. God had prevented him from pursuing something potentially harmful or sinful. In the words of an oft-cited Prophetic tradition, "How remarkable is the case of the believer! There is good for him in everything, but this is not the case for anyone except for the believer. When the believer receives any good, he is thankful to God, and gets a reward. And when some misfortune befalls him, he endures it patiently, for which he is (also) rewarded."[20] As Ali and many patients reiterated, the Prophet Muhammad indeed told his believers to "seek counsel *(fatwa)* from their own hearts." This has led many to the conviction that behind their specific illnesses lay divine wisdom. In their specific struggles toward God and the conscientious development of dispositions of fortitude, they embody the sentiment that their bodies belong to God and that they are preparing for the day when they will be returned to their Creator.

Conclusions

One of the most fundamental ways that religious devotion is held to be "anti-biotechnology" is in its emphasis on submission to divine will. If bad conditions are accepted as a sign of God's will, then why should the faithful develop the technological means to improve them? If illness is a test of faith, then should devotees not seek medical treatment? Social scientists have generally had poor analytical tools for tackling these questions, particularly in their secularist presumptions about human agency and the normative subject who transcends cultural norms and religious bounds.[21]

Faith in divine will has often been interpreted as passivity or inaction that hinders a religious devotee from pursuing a technological benefit. Or, too often, religion is assumed to be a tool of manipulation by the powerful to keep the disadvantaged downtrodden. In Western academia, on the one hand there has been much discussion of Muslims as "passive fatalists," and on the other, there have been attempts to show that this is not the case: that Muslims really do have "agency." One tendency in Western scholarship, then, is to view the cultivation of steadfastness as passive; another is to view it as an active manipulation of religion to provide a comfort mechanism or to placate the disadvantaged.[22] But we should not assume that patients foreclose all treatment options out of their "fatalism," nor should we assume that they merely appeal to God to comfort themselves after the fact in their lack of access to treatment.[23] People embody and experience religions to varying effects. In the case of Ali, his efforts to cultivate steadfastness as he struggled to "find the good path" involved a continuous alignment of himself with what he defined as God's will. He continually asked God to allow him to understand each turn of events as part of God's overall plan of benevolence and compassion (*al-rahma*).

To assume that religious practitioners refuse particular technologies or medical interventions because of their fatalism carries the danger of missing the contingencies that inform when and under what conditions patients work to achieve this disposition. Such a characterization potentially overlooks the rampant problems in medical care that patients seek to avoid. The medical anthropologist and humanitarian physician Paul Farmer has memorably cautioned against the tendency to confuse structural violence, poverty, and inequality with cultural difference.[24] I would add that there is also a tendency to conflate poverty and structural violence with fatalism—a tendency that obscures the ways that forbearance in the face of suffering can be construed as a virtue, as something that can be actively cultivated by coping with suffering, rather than being a direct outcome or cause of the suffering.

Moreover, the perceived efficacy of a treatment plays an important role in shaping one's ethical stance toward it. To understand how patients arrive at complex ethical decisions, we must be attentive and vigilant to their own experiences and understandings of their disease processes and etiology and their own cost-benefit analyses, which may be articulated in religious terms. That said, we should not assume that patients appeal to God's will *only* because a treatment has been deemed inefficacious or inaccessible. In many cases the ethical disposition patients have toward a particular treatment, their assessment of its benefit and harms, and their understanding of disease etiology and specific experiences of the illness are not separate from—nor do they formulaically determine—their dispositions toward divine will.[25]

I have argued in this chapter that religious sentiments, including those that attribute a positive value to steadfastness in suffering, should not be seen as passive, as anti-science, or as constraints to medical treatment. In various ways patients grappled with how to achieve the greatest benefit for themselves and their families, while at the same time trying to conform to what would please God. Reliance on God should not be understood in opposition to seeking treatment. We should not ask whether patients appeal to God *or* seek treatment, since neither of these excludes the other, and we should therefore remain attentive to the interrelations between the two. An appreciation for what it means to embody a religious tradition in which religious reasoning and sentiment are not understood as external to the self, but as *central* to it, can help us broaden our understanding of medical life-and-death decisions and of ethical formations in devout patients' lives.

The Canary in the Gemeinschaft?
Disability, Film, and the Jewish Question
Faye Ginsburg

In the nineteenth century canaries were taken into British mines to detect methane gas, which is odorless but lethal to animals. The sensitivity of this small and delicate bird to an invisible, but deadly substance meant that if it died, a danger was present that humans would not have been able to detect. My title plays with the phrase "the canary in the mineshaft," which evolved from this poignant interspecies situation. In this chapter I explore how scientific and documentary images of disability have served as visible evidence (the "canaries," if you will) of a kind of danger lurking in the Jewish community over the course of the twentieth and into the twenty-first century. The toxic element in this case is the stigmatization of the Jewish/disabled body within a particular Gemeinschaft, a development in which biomedical discourses are deeply implicated.[1] As a counterpoint to this process of exclusion, I examine recent works—primarily documentary films—that are reversing that trend through a process I call "mediated kinship." In these projects relationships among family members with disabilities—which often require rethinking the normative frameworks of the taken-for-granted Gemeinschaft world—are reimagined on their own terms and in ways that recruit relationships outside the biological family into a kinship arena. We might think of these as unnatural family histories, made public through documentaries that become what I call "parables of possibility," thanks to the alternative cultural scripts that they offer viewers, as well as the innovative outreach campaigns that extend this cultural work into the off-screen world, intervening in the biomedical regimes that have too often defined the lives of people and their families who are living with a difference. I argue that these films, most of them quite recent, are technologies through which a current generation of Jewish activists, whom some call "the New Jews," are providing a new Jewish imaginary that is far more flexible and inclusive than that of prior generations.[2]

I focus much of this chapter on the work of filmmakers whose documentaries diagnose the shifting meaning of disability in different Gemeinschaften from the 1930s to the present.[3] In particular I examine recent works that address the human costs of the exclusion and denial of people with disabilities in the past by practitioners of Nazi "science," not only during the Third Reich, but for decades beyond that, even into the 1990s. Other films focus on the denial of disability in the Jewish community in the postwar period. And finally, the most recent work reveals the capacity of Jewish tradition to embrace different modes of embodiment as part of a more inclusive Gemeinschaft in the future, a position supported through idioms of kinship and human rights. I also briefly discuss how new forms of digital media offer unanticipated possibilities for participation in Jewish life by people with disabilities, as has happened in the online world of Second Life.

A Note on the Jewish Question and the Question of Technology

My choice of the German word Gemeinschaft (community)—in addition to its punning effect in the title—stresses a feature that distinguishes Jews from members of other religious communities. While Judaism as a faith draws on particular theologies and practices, the category of "the Jew" also indexes a kin-based cultural world—a Gemeinschaft—as well as a shared (and seemingly inescapable) genetic heritage. As such the question of Jewish identity problematizes more bounded definitions of religion as a community organized around shared beliefs and rituals.

The sociological instability of "the Jewish question" in relation to more standard understandings of religion raises questions regarding the role of technology as well as bio-power.[4] In particular, how can we consider the question of technology in relation to the complexity of the category of "the Jew," which for its part can shift from defining a kind of religious practice to standing for an ethnic/racial/cultural community subject to the forces of what Michel Foucault calls bio-power.[5] To encompass that range associated with Jewish identity, I draw upon Foucault's understanding of technologies as methods that can "permit individuals to effect by their own means or with the help of others a certain number of operations on their own bodies and souls, thoughts, conduct, and way of being so as to transform themselves in order to attain a certain state of happiness, purity, wisdom, perfection, or immortality."[6] In other words, I deploy Foucault's use of technologies as techniques—sometimes imposed via forms of governmentality—through which human beings produce an ethical self-understanding: what some scholars of his work have called "technologies of personhood."[7]

I suggest that the place of disability within the Jewish world has been shaped by recent profound changes in two key technologies that have played expanding roles over the last century in reframing contemporary personhood: biomedicine and documentary media. My work interrogates how transformations in these fields have shaped ideas about the boundaries of Jewish identity—who is in and who is out—in ways that have inspired members of this community to become "moral pioneers."[8]

In the case of biomedicine, we are living in what some have called the "second age of biology," an era dominated by new knowledge of things molecular and genetic. Its impact on daily life is felt through the routinization of prenatal genetic testing.[9] As historians of science have cautioned us, the new genetics of the late twentieth and early twenty-first centuries exists in the shadow of the last century's eugenics, haunting the present like a "ghost in the machine," to use Sander Gilman's appropriation of the phrase.[10] Gilman elaborates on this idea in an article addressing questions of Jewish genetic disease: "those who see in genetic manipulation, alteration or selection the potential for the elimination of genetically transmitted diseases are constantly forced to confront a history that they claim not to be their own."[11]

Over the last two decades assisted reproductive technologies (ARTs) have supported a growing potential for individualized "neoeugenics" in the technologically advanced West, where we find the routine use of genetic testing by individual couples and their choice to abort fetuses with genetic anomalies diagnostic of particular disabling conditions. Although U.S. genetic counselors are trained to express neutrality about the choices a pregnant woman and her partner may make around amniocentesis testing, the very existence of such a technology and the offer of such tests under the terms of consumer choice are premised on the desire for normalcy and fear of unknown abnormalities.[12] As my colleague Rayna Rapp and I have argued elsewhere, this normalizing discourse about disability, as it has emerged with the proliferation of reproductive technologies, stands in contradistinction with the one accompanying the expansive, democratizing language of civil rights that has shaped the disability rights movement in particular. As a result, almost all "modern parents" might find themselves facing the contradictions created by progress both in biomedicine—premised on selecting against certain disabling conditions—and in social movements founded on expanding democratic inclusion of all citizens, regardless of bodily condition.[13]

This is a circumstance faced more frequently by Jews of Ashkenazi descent, whether secular or religious, because of the high incidence of genetic disease in this population. For that reason Ashkenazi Jews are strongly encouraged to have carrier or fetal screening for the eleven genetic disorders for which we are considered to be particularly at risk.[14] Debates about the implications for action based on this form of knowledge run deep in this community, motivating religious innovations in the management of such knowledge. Dor Yeshorim, for example, is an ultra-orthodox Jewish genetic testing service that succeeds because of its ironclad policy of complete anonymity for its clients, whose genetic profiles are checked for compatibility even before a match is arranged, thus screening for potential genetic disease while avoiding abortion.[15] For less orthodox and even for secular Jews, the technology of genetic testing has produced a kind of collective recognition of a community at risk, a social fact given form in the emergence of organizations in the United States such as the Jewish Genetic Disease Consortium and its constituent support groups. Indeed, many who know they carry one of the mutations for these diseases see themselves as linked in a kind of "imagined community" in which the medium is not the vernacular novel or the newspaper, as Benedict Anderson discussed, but mutated DNA.[16] For example, those who know they share this mutation but who are related in no other way may refer to each other as "cousin" on Internet support groups. As Gilman notes regarding genetic disease:

> Those labeled as "ill" in complex ways accept the label and turn it into a mark of identity. For is there nothing more redolent of "identity" in the age of the human genome than our biological code? In an age of biologization, have not our genes become the ultimate definition of who we believe we are? ... In the nuclear family, the desire is to construct a world beyond the nuclear family into which the illness can be projected and given meaning.[17]

Awareness of the ghostly presence of even a single ancestral mutation that first occurred centuries ago, Gilman suggests, has particular consequences. "The phantom in the machine here is the story of the cohort [the genetic disease community] into which the family must insert itself."[18]

Media, Technologies of Personhood, and Cautionary Tales

The process of constructing that "story of the cohort" brings us to the second technology: visual media. Over the last seventy years exhilarating transformations have occurred in visual media technologies as an extension of the human capacity for witnessing, testifying, and storytelling, all forms for the production and circulation of new social facts as well as narrative invention. These changing *technai*, marked by shifts from 16 mm film to analog video to the proliferation of the digital, are identified with particular forms of evidence, historicity, narrative, and poetics.[19] Photography and film were used to document and justify eugenics projects in pre-war Europe and the United States, and they continued to play a significant role in the Nazi era (and beyond) as evidence used by the infamous Dr. Mengele, among others. Since the 1940s this visual legacy not only has been claimed and resignified as evidence of a horrific period, but also, more recently, has been appropriated by documentary makers as part of the retelling of the intimate histories of survivors for whom such footage, ironically, may be one of the few fragile forms of material connection to their former lives, even as they hope to destroy this artifact representing profound humiliation.[20] In this process of reclamation and witnessing and the subsequent creation of counternarratives, it is impossible to underestimate the impact of small-format, inexpensive, widely available media-making technologies—beginning with analog video in the 1980s and Internet and other digitally based forms that first emerged in the 1990s. These have had remarkable effects as technologies (in the Foucaultian sense) that enabled the expansion of documentary to encompass new cultural subjects whose lives previously had been stigmatized and/or rendered invisible in public space.[21]

As some have argued regarding the impact of this form of media practice, the mediated subject does not emerge out of thin air.[22] Nor does it remain singular, but rather is "subjectified" through a series of discursive regimes—religion, culture, and ethnicity being perhaps the most pronounced—that some have called attention to as the *first-person plural*.[23] In other words, the filmmaker does not simply reflect on his/her life and culture through the filmic text, but uses these media technologies as forms of cultural intervention that extend beyond the "I" to the "we" and that can reach across time and space beyond the immediacy of face-to-face interaction. These works become meaningful in new ways as they enter into social worlds in their creation, exhibition, circulation, consumption, and resignification as a constantly evolving cultural practice.

In tracing the transformative trajectory of the changing place of disability in Jewish life through documentary works, I rely on an understanding of media objects as polysemic, gaining new meanings as they follow unruly and constantly transforming paths over historical time, enter into unanticipated social and cultural domains, and take on new and different forms of authority. Once unleashed from their historical moment and original intention, media forms often promiscuously violate social and epistemological boundaries; they can move rapidly from the domain of scientific records to that of legal evidence or to the realm of personal narrative, in each case constituting new forms of visible evidence that have the potential to shape new understandings of personhood.[24]

The first set of films I want to discuss serves loosely as a collection of "cautionary tales." I borrow that term from its use in folklore studies to describe a traditional story meant to warn the audience of a danger that can be destructive to a whole community. The 2004 documentary *Gray Matter*, made by American filmmaker Joe Berlinger, cautions against the dangers of genocidal practices masquerading and documented as "science" in photography and film.[25] He also demonstrates how film and photographic archives can be powerfully reanimated in a new historical moment, serving purposes that subvert their original intention. Berlinger, who early in his voiceover of the film confesses to being "obsessed with the brutality of the Holocaust," traveled to Vienna in 2002 to witness a funeral for the human remains (mostly preserved brains) of hundreds of infants and children who had disabilities such as epilepsy, diabetes, and Down syndrome or who were orphaned or of the "wrong" religion—many of them Jewish—and who had died from brutal treatment in the 1940s after being experimented upon by forensic psychiatrist Dr. Heinrich Gross (notoriously nicknamed "the Austrian Dr. Mengele").[26] Evidence suggests that Gross oversaw their killing at the Speigelgrund Hospital in Vienna, Austria, when it served as a Nazi-era "euthanasia" clinic. Once the children were dead, Gross had their brains preserved in glass pickle jars and labeled with their names, diagnosis, and the dates of their very short life spans. Until their dignified and humane burial in 2002, they continued to be used as scientific data by Gross and others in scientific publications appearing as late as the 1990s. For Berlinger and most viewers, far more shocking than the grim story of the facts of Nazi "medicine" was the fact that these brains were considered legitimate scientific evidence for so long after the war, and that Gross continued to work in Austria as a medical expert for the court system well into the late twentieth century. As we see in the documentary, Gross—who was still alive and around ninety years old at the time of filming in 2004—was never successfully prosecuted, despite several efforts to do so, and despite the existence of definitive proof of his activities. Several Austrian historians in the film suggest that Gross had been protected by the many Nazi sympathizers who remained in the Austrian establishment despite the outcome of World War II. He lived freely in Austria and—perhaps most shockingly—was awarded the Honorary Cross for Science and Art in 1975 (although he was eventually stripped of that honor in 2003), and he collected a comfortable pension until his death in 2005. In the film, despite his best efforts, Berlinger does not succeed in meeting Gross, but he does meet survivors of Spiegelgrund whose compelling and tragic stories are far more significant in underscoring the danger at the heart of this cautionary tale than the confrontation that never happens.

This film is relevant to my argument in at least two ways. First, the opening sequence of the film shows the compelling appropriation by Austrian citizens of enlarged archival photographs of the faces of the disabled children killed by Dr. Gross: photos they hold in their arms in an effort to honor and remember these victims (see Figure 7). In ways that Gross could never have imagined, the photos are displayed not as scientific specimens, but as resignified in a context of repentance and memorialization. Removed from their original context of stigma, these images are now literally embraced in the arms of those protesting Gross's work and its link to Austria's Nazi legacy as part of the ritual accompanying the burial of the human remains in Vienna. The documentary thus captures the way the photos are sacralized in this public demonstration of kinship, insisting on their common humanity.

Second, the film generates a clear case for the power of film and photography as a technology of governmentality in the construction of "scientific" arguments that supported the Nazi project. We see not only the photos of the children, but documentary footage used in Nazi propaganda about Jews and those with disabilities used to "normalize" genocidal campaigns through medical, economic, and public health discourses that anchored these images as frightening, polluting, and dangerous. They were an essential part of the Nazi program to rid the society of genetically impure people considered *lebensunwertes Leben*, "life unworthy of life." One of the speakers at the funeral, Dr. Werner Vogt, a

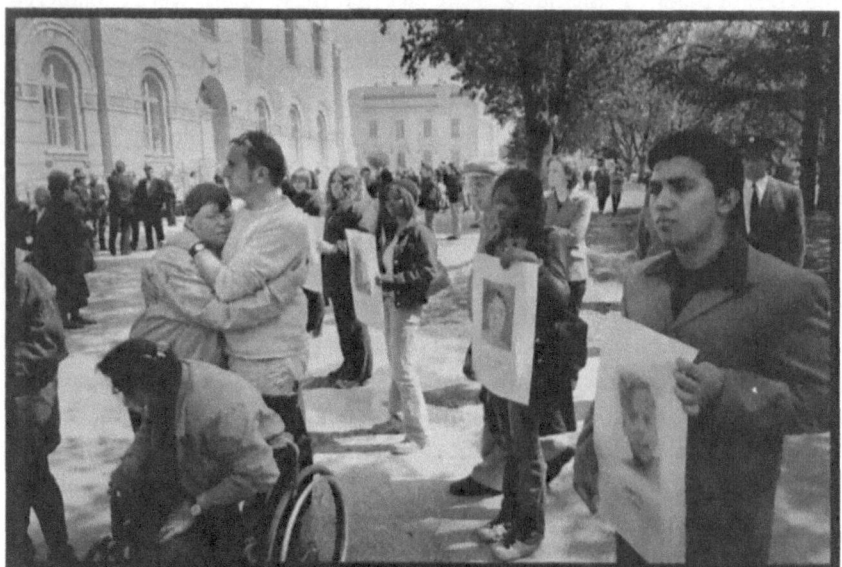

Figure 7. Austrian participants in the ceremonial reburial in 2002 of the remains of the children killed by Dr. Heinrich Gross hold enlarged photos of the victims to memorialize their lives. (Photographer: David Reinhard; photo courtesy of Milli Segal.)

physician who had gathered evidence against Gross in the 1970s, said the ceremony "destroys a secret Austrian proclamation that goes as follows: 'Let's forget the murders; let's forgive the perpetrators and thousands of silent confidants; let's defame and hide the survivors.'"[27] The cautionary tale focuses on Austria's collective denial of its own participation in such atrocities, suggesting that those who fail to come to terms with their past continue to harbor this toxic sensibility.

I now want to turn to a second documentary cautionary tale in which the resignification of genocidal "biomedicine" and archival footage—and the continued work beyond the war of Nazi scientists who had been involved in experimenting with those with disabilities—play a central role. The film *Liebe Perla* is an astonishing 1999 documentary by Israeli filmmaker Shahar Rozen, structured around the relationship between two women linked by their size and their histories.[28] Hannelore Witkofski, a short-statured German woman and disability advocate born in the post-war period, sets out on a quest to understand the fate of people like herself during the Nazi period.[29] During the process she tracks down and befriends Perla Ovitz, the only surviving member of her ten-member family. Seven of the family members were little people, and before World War II they had formed the Lilliput Troupe, performing music throughout Eastern Europe. Because of their genetic condition, her family had been of interest to Dr. Josef Mengele, who ran the infirmary at Auschwitz-Birkenau, where he carried out human experimentation on identical twins and people with genetic abnormalities. In Perla's view the Ovitz family survived Auschwitz only because Mengele chose to keep them alive for his "experiments." As she explained in a 1999 interview, "We were the only family who entered a death camp and emerged together. If I ever questioned why I was born a dwarf, my answer must be that my handicap, my deformity, was God's way of keeping me alive."[30]

At the time of filming Perla was eighty years old and living in Israel. When she tells Hannelore, her new German friend, about the humiliating experience that she and her family endured in 1944 when they were filmed naked for Mengele's research archives, Hannelore sets out on a quest: to go from archive to archive in Germany, and then to Auschwitz-Birkenau in Poland, to find this film footage and restore it to Perla, whom she regards as the rightful owner of her image.[31] As Hannelore expresses it in the film, reading aloud one of her letters to Perla, "Today is our last day in Auschwitz. We did not find the film. Often I hoped that if I do find it, as soon as I open the box, it would crumble into dust. I'm afraid that someone in some archive or other or in some attic would find it and show it. . . . The film belongs to you, and you alone."

At one archive, Chronos Films, Hannelore succeeds in finding other Mengele footage. In a remarkable moment in the film, as the archivist runs the film for her, she recognizes a face among the anonymous bodies in striped clothing, restoring personal identity and history to this dehumanizing footage. Yet she is unable to locate the footage Perla remembers. Toward the end of the film Perla receives word from Yad Vashem, the Holocaust memorial in Jerusalem, that they have found something of hers. She and Hannelore arrive there to find that it is not the missing footage; far better, it is a box containing her family's handmade musical instruments—adjusted to their small size—which they had used on their European tours.

In a meditative analysis of this film, Holocaust scholar Sara Eigen writes, "*Liebe Perla* itself manages much of the work that would be demanded of the lost film, if found; it deftly manages some creative play with archival exposure to serve history and to re-open the case against the Nazi-era and post-war German medical communities, all without exploiting the lost film's actual images as historical evidence. Hannelore's assertion of Perla's rights seem right and good; history has been served by *Liebe Perla*, and historians should return the favor by allowing the film to remain lost."[32] Hannelore's journey through the archives shapes the documentary, inviting us to witness what can happen when such documents, produced under the most racist and oppressive conditions, are taken up and transformed in a kind of ritual process of restoring the humanity of its victims.

Yet *Liebe Perla* also operates as a cautionary tale. It does not leave us with an assured sense that these problems are safely behind us, as we see some of the prejudices toward people with disabilities that Hannelore encounters in contemporary Germany. Additionally, Hannelore's archival work reveals the links between Germany's Nazi past and the present. In one scene, shot in the library at the Max-Planck-Gesellschaft in Berlin (formerly the Kaiser Wilhelm Institute), she pores over archives that make clear that Mengele and his mentor, Dr. Otmar Freiherr von Verschuer—the wartime director of the Institute for Anthropology, Human Hereditary Teaching and Genetics—had collaborated around Mengele's Auschwitz "research." After the war, rather than being punished as a war criminal, von Verschuer went on to lead the Institute for Human Genetic Research at the University of Münster. As Hannelore reads aloud from his obituary in 1969, more than twenty years after the war, she notes ironically that he was celebrated "for his contributions toward humanistic eugenic research."[33] Indeed, it was only in 2001, two years after this film was made and more than six decades after the war, that the Max Planck Institute issued an apology to the few remaining survivors of Mengele, Verschuer, and other Nazi scientists. While Hannelore hopes to bring back to Perla the film footage Mengele had shot, she also seems to be fulfilling the desire of Perla and other survivors that their stories might help prevent future atrocities. In his speech at the Max Planck Institute on the occasion of the apology, Auschwitz survivor Jona Laks made clear that revelation is not sufficient insurance against the possibility of recurrence. "It was inside our planet and a part of it, perpetrated by human beings against the lives of other human beings. It was here, amongst us. There is no guarantee that it will not return again."[34]

While *Gray Matter* and *Liebe Perla* alert us to the histories of dangers to the community—threats that may continue in new form—other films have focused their work on the troubling questions raised by the erasure of disability *within* the Jewish community during the postwar period. Susie Korda's 1999 documentary, *One of Us*, focuses not on Nazi campaigns against Jews and the disabled, but on the lack of public acknowledgment of disability in the post-war American Jewish community, bringing the cautionary tale closer to home.³⁵ Korda chronicles long-kept secrets of her troubled American Jewish family. She traces the family history and discovers a well-kept secret: an unknown sister born with Down syndrome who was sent away after her father, a Holocaust survivor, abandoned the family following the birth of this child. To make matters even more complex, her brother develops neo-Nazi obsessions, while her mother remains emotionally distant. The filmmaker eventually finds her long-lost sister living happily as a young adult in a large non-Jewish family. As other work has shown, the case of the Korda family, while distinctive, is not unique, as disabled children were routinely institutionalized during this period—a practice that was considered to be appropriate and humane well into the 1970s.³⁶ The film raises questions about where, and by whom, the boundaries of kinship and communities are drawn, while suggesting a radical generational change in attitude toward disability, as represented by the filmmaker.

Korda's parents might be considered an extreme, but exemplary case of a sociohistorical situation shaping attitudes toward disability in the postwar American Jewish Gemeinschaft. For Ashkenazi Jews, particularly after the horrendous losses suffered in Europe, beginning with the period of intense anti-Semitic pogroms in the late nineteenth and early twentieth centuries and continuing up through the Holocaust, a cultural ethos amplified the Biblical imperative to go forth and multiply. In the twentieth century, and especially the post-Holocaust era, for middle-class Jewish North Americans, having Jewish children as the foundation for rebuilding lives and communities was seen by many as an answer to the genocidal policies against Jews.

In a peculiar inversion of the eugenic policies practiced against Jewish and other populations, postwar Jewish survival was not just about having progeny. Children were needed to demonstrate the capacity of Jews not only to survive efforts to exterminate them, but also to succeed. Building on a long cultural tradition that has always valorized religious study as the highest form of accomplishment—at least for men—postwar Jewish cultural life has continued to place particularly high value on intellectual prowess, in or out of the synagogue. While certainly not written in Jewish theology, the emphasis on having children who were intelligent and high-achieving across a number of fields where brains and creativity count—such as medicine, law, science, business, scholarship, and the arts—was a built-in assumption of Jewish cultural life. "Smart genes" are imagined to be part of the inalienable cultural and genetic capital that Jews assumed they carried with them; even impoverished immigrants and refugees whose material lives had been shattered could hold on to their DNA. Children born with disabilities interfered with that narrative. Until relatively recently Jewish children with such conditions were routinely institutionalized, fostered out, or hidden from view.[37]

In ultra-orthodox communities, where arranged marriages are essential to biological and social reproduction, a "stain" on the lineage is seen as damaging to both immediate and extended kin, who will inevitably bear the stigma of being known to carry a "hereditary disease." For those unable to avoid the birth of children with genetic disease through the use of a service like Dor Yeshorim (discussed above), the question of how to care for loved ones while still keeping their status a secret can exact a serious toll. This does not mean that families would not seek the best possible medical care for sick children, even if they never told them the name of their condition for fear that they might further damage chances of marriage for themselves or other close relatives.[38]

Andrea Eisenman's *Hidden Blessings* is a documentary in progress that addresses this situation. Born with the genetic disease cystic fibrosis (CF), a life-threatening lung condition with a high incidence in the Ashkenazi population, Eisenman received a life-saving bilateral lung transplant in 1998; since then she has competed in the Transplant Olympics and is involved in organ-donor awareness through public speaking.[39] Because of her outreach work for CF, Andrea—a secular Jew—was contacted by ultra-orthodox Hasidic Jews living in Brooklyn who had been keeping their cystic fibrosis hidden from their community and loved ones (even spouses) for years, but who now recognized the need to change that circumstance. She was so astonished by their efforts that she decided to make *Hidden Blessings* to address this issue. As Eisenman explained: "There is a conflict in many closed communities, particularly the orthodox and Hasidic, between secrecy and health, privacy and disclosure. A genetic disease results in the stigmatization of an entire family in the crucial matters of matchmaking, where kinship is the primary source of cultural capital and marriage. This leads to under-reporting of illness and medical non-compliance. There is no emotional support for them in their isolation."[40]

Hidden Blessings follows the journeys of several people, including a Hasidic man, Josef. As he explains in one scene from her work in progress, "When you suffer from something like cystic fibrosis, it's painful as is. But what makes it even much harder is the secret. That you have to keep it a secret that you have CF. You can't tell anybody that you have cystic fibrosis. I know nobody understands. I know nobody understands what I'm going through, because they don't have CF." Eisenman decided to make this film as a cautionary tale, warning the audience of the physical and emotional complications caused by this culturally imposed secrecy surrounding so serious a physical condition.

Does the question of disability and its lack of cultural acceptance suggest a disturbing disconnect between the two dimensions of being Jewish discussed in the opening section of this chapter? How can we understand the tension between the restrictive Gemeinschaft of culture and kinship described by Josef in the quote above and religious concepts guided by ideas of social justice and theological injunctions for acceptance of all those rendered "in God's image"? This question was central to an essay with that title written by Rabbi Dianne Cohler-Esses, published in 2006 in *The Jewish Week*.[41] While she is not ultra-orthodox, her words eloquently describe the tensions between the realities of a particular exclusionary Jewish Gemeinschaft and the possibilities of an inclusive Jewish theology, as well as her desire to close that gap through what she calls a "search for a new story." She writes:

> I am the parent of three children, two of whom have learning disabilities. Besides Eli [my son with developmental delays], our eldest daughter Ayelet (almost eight) has language processing difficulties. . . . As a parent of children with learning disabilities I find myself resisting the powerful emphasis on educational achievement in the Jewish community and in our culture at large. What to do with those who can't live out this particular script? Are they somehow exiled from the hierarchy of Jewish communal values? Sometimes I feel like my own family members are strangers in our own land. At others, like we are a family searching for a new story. I believe it is time for us, the Jewish community, to expand this script, to create new stories where other kinds of children also become stars. And to begin by asking ourselves the following questions: Have we put so much emphasis on achievement, intellectual and otherwise, that we haven't left room for other modes of being? Other values? Are we so concerned with excelling that we've forgotten our simple humanity? Have we eclipsed, perhaps, the very fullness of the face of God? . . . Our children, those with diagnosed disabilities or those with the more typical struggles of life, are all created in the Divine image, not in the human image of mastery and perfection. . . . There is nothing at all they have to do to achieve this state of being. No fancy nursery schools, no scores on tests, and no Ivy League Schools will attest to the indisputable fact of their divine image.[42]

The Search for a New Story: Parables of Possibility

What might that new story look like? The 2007 documentary *Praying With Lior* (dir. Ilana Trachtman) is exemplary of what Cohler-Esses is seeking: what I will call "parables of possibility." In literature on folklore, parables are stories that ask us to examine our everyday assumptions about the usual order of things, "a traditional technique for coping with problematic social situations" providing "a microcosm of the life situation and a projected resolution."[43] I think of films such as *Praying With Lior* as parables because they indeed ask us to rethink our assumptions about disability, offering models of possibility rather than limits. *Praying with Lior* focuses on Lior Liebling, a Jewish boy with Down syndrome, and the way his special capacity for prayer has shaped his own life as well as those of his family and community. The documentary's director, Ilana Trachtman, was drawn to Lior's life when she first heard him pray. As she explains:

> I was not looking for a film subject, and I wasn't particularly interested in disability. I'm not sure I ever thought about disability. What I was doing had no connection to my career as a producer/director of TV documentaries. I was actually trying to pray. Searching for spiritual inspiration outside the stale synagogue experience of my childhood, I attended a retreat for the Jewish New Year. As I sat in the service, anxious, distracted, counting the pages until I'd be free, I heard Lior's unabashed, off-key, ecstatic voice. When I turned to look at the source of this sound, I was struck to see a boy with Down syndrome. And I was surprised to find myself envious of this "disabled" child, who could pray as I wished I could. Over the course of this retreat, I stalked Lior, looking for the secret to his prayer. When I heard he was having a Bar Mitzvah, I pictured the movie version. And then I realized that I could make it.[44]

The film chronicles the four months leading up to Lior's anxiously anticipated Bar Mitzvah. With intimacy and patience the film illuminates what it means to be "praying with Lior" through the eyes of the diverse community nurturing him: his father, Mordechai Liebling, who is a Reconstructionist rabbi; his stepmother, Lynne Iser; his three siblings; an embracing liberal Reconstructionist Jewish community; his late mother; and his twelve-year-old classmates at the orthodox yeshiva where he goes to school. His school peers' acceptance of him demonstrates how these young people use religious teachings to understand the value of difference. As one of the yeshiva students explains to the camera, "Let's say there are two baseball players. One could easily hit a home run and one works very hard. The person who works very hard to hit a home run, he gets more credit than the person who could easily hit a home run. Same way with Lior. It counts double."⁴⁵

The film opened at the San Francisco Jewish Film Festival in July of 2007 and has had a robust run of festival screenings since then, including a theatrical run in New York City in February 2008 at the Cinema Village Theater, with lines around the block for every screening, earning it the highest-grossing independent film that weekend. After one of the opening screenings, Lior's extraordinary, loving, and involved stepmother took questions from the audience. When asked how the film had changed her family's perspective, she answered, "While it had been fun and exciting during the making of the film, now that it is out in the world, it has changed my children. They understand they have a role to play helping other families, as activists, something they never understood before. Getting out in the world with the film has brought them a second life."⁴⁶

Similarly, Trachtman is clear that in the process of making and then circulating this film with Lior and his family, she became "an accidental activist," and the film became "the centerpiece of an ambitious outreach campaign to change the way people with disabilities are perceived and received by faith communities."⁴⁷ Despite the extraordinary way in which Lior's life had been integrated into his religious community, Trachtman points out that this is the exception rather than the rule, not only for the Jewish community, but for communities of faith more broadly:

> According to the National Organization on Disability, over 54 million Americans are disabled. Less than half of our houses of worship are handicapped accessible. This number alone speaks to the abandonment of the disabled in faith communities. In a society that literally "worships" perfection and same-ness, individuals with physical and cognitive disabilities are dismissed and discriminated against everywhere. In the place where they should receive the most welcome and derive the most comfort—their faith communities—parents of children with special needs often hear "your child shouldn't be here."⁴⁸

Praying with Lior shows how different parts of the Jewish community—broadly defined from secular to orthodox—might embrace all of its possible members. Trachtman's film, along with the others discussed above, challenges the hegemonic cultural narratives that marginalize the lives of those who have not been valued, and in this way provides a parable of possibility. All these films (and the Cohler-Esses editorial) offer chronicles of lives imagined in a new register. They provide alternative disability narratives that are foundational steps to the integration of disability, not only into everyday life in the United States, but also into their particular communities of belief and practice. Authorized by those with disabilities and/or their family members and friends, these media offer revised, phenomenologically based understandings, which at times also anchor substantial analyses of the social, cultural, and political construction of these conditions in Jewish life. Some, such as Rabbi Cohler-Esses, summon theology to underscore the ontological value of all who are rendered in God's image.

Pushing the wordplay of the title a bit (and perhaps beyond its endurance), I want to suggest that these filmmakers and activists who are interrogating the place of disability in Jewish life are acting as cultural canaries, using image-making and story-telling technologies to reframe the boundaries of acceptance as to who is in and who is out of this particular community. The cultural and social labor these kinds of media practices represent in the Jewish community are part of a modest, but growing movement that began a little over two decades ago, very much in step with the growth of both the disability rights movement and the emergence of the "New Jews," a group that more generally is identified with being flexible and inclusive, reversing the exclusionary practices of prior generations.[49] Exemplary of this trend, Yad Ha Chazakah (translation: "Hand of Strength"), the Jewish Disability Empowerment Center, was catalyzed by orthodox Jewish disability activist Sharon Shapiro in October 2005 and inaugurated in January 2008. Shapiro, who has a background in the Independent Living movement,[50] explained in an interview in *The Jewish Week*, "I wanted to know where all the Jews with disabilities are. It couldn't be that no Jews except me and a handful of people had a disability."[51]

Anita Altman, who founded the UJA's Task Force on People with Disabilities in the mid-1990s, is now turning to film as a powerful vehicle for humanizing the experience of living with disabilities, inaugurating a disability film festival, Realabilities, in 2008. Commenting on the new film work that is emerging from the community, Altman said, "I feel like we're riding the crest of a wave. This is all part and parcel of trying to change societal attitudes about people with disabilities, trying to open up not only the Jewish community but the larger community to realize people have a lot to contribute, whatever their level of ability."[52]

In God's Image: You, Me, and Everyone We Know

Before I continue, allow me to provide full disclosure about how I got into this. I am part of this story. In 1989 my daughter Samantha was born with a rare Jewish genetic disorder, one so uncommon that even

I, an anthropologist and daughter of a geneticist, had never heard of it. Familial dysautonomia (FD) is so infrequent that just over six hundred cases have ever been diagnosed; approximately half that number is alive today. Through the efforts of the parent-run Dysautonomia Foundation, for which I serve on the board of directors, the "FD gene" was discovered, and it is now routinely part of prenatal testing for Ashkenazi couples.[53] FD, which occurred because of a random mutation that probably occurred around five hundred years ago in a Jewish *shtetl* [village] near Minsk (what in genetics is called genetic drift, enhanced by generations of Jewish endogamy), accounted for a range of inexplicable and bizarre symptoms—linked, it turned out, by a dysfunctional autonomic system—that had landed us in the hospital with great frequency from the time my daughter was two weeks old. To allow her to live with a disorder that can make every basic function a struggle—swallowing, breathing, regulating blood pressure—Sam has had multiple surgeries, and manages daily life thanks to medical technologies such as feeding tubes and pumps, oxygen concentrators, and a strict regime of daily medications.

By the time she was ten, Sam had grown tired of having to explain herself to her classmates and friends and wondered why there were no others like her on the kids' shows she watched on television. A notable exception was *What Are You Staring At?*, an innovative, Emmy Award–winning special produced by Linda Ellerbee's "Nick News" in 1998 and aired repeatedly during 1999. The half-hour program featured a group of kids and teens with a range of disabilities—Down syndrome, hearing and visual impairments, cerebral palsy, polio, burn injuries—as well as "celebrity crips": journalist John Hockenberry and the actor, the late Christopher Reeve. In the summer of 1999 in New York City, Samantha surfed onto *What Are You Staring At?* and was riveted. When the final credits ended, she had come up with a solution to her problem. She announced that she wanted to talk about her disability on television. She found the website for the Make-A-Wish Foundation, a group that grants wishes to children with life-threatening diseases, and emailed them, explaining that her wish was to go on "Nick News" and talk about her life with FD.[54] Within two weeks she was working with a friend and a Make-A-Wish volunteer, making a pitch book with Polaroid photos and handwritten text about her life and disability. Sam's inventory of her life included pictures reminiscent of crime-scene photos she took of all her medical equipment, as well as photos of her dog, friends, and relatives.

By her eleventh birthday she was working with a producer from "Nick News," and by late April of 2000, the show was broadcast. Of greatest significance to Sam was that so many FD kids were able to see another child like them on television. She was deluged with email from families with FD children around the country who were thrilled to see an image and story that for once included their experience. As a result Sam has been invited to show her tape and talk to a number of groups, ranging from scientists working on medical interventions for her disorder to those interested in how synagogues can become more inclusive. Two years later Samantha took the occasion of her Bat Mitzvah to raise awareness and over $10,000 for research on FD.[55]

The media world into which Sam surfed at the cusp of the twenty-first century is evidence of a transforming public culture—religious and otherwise—in which disability is becoming a more visible presence in daily life, albeit very slowly. This anecdotal evidence—Sam's immediate sense of kinship with the disabled kids and adults she saw and heard on television and her desire to join the process of making the reality of living with a disability part of public discourse—underscores the significance of such imagery for those with disabilities who do not see themselves regularly in dominant forms of representation. Indeed, much of the early writing in disability studies focused not only on the need for changes in civil rights legislation, but also on the absence of disabled people from literature and popular media—or, where present, the negativity of their portrayal, citing the legacy of freak shows, circuses, and asylums.[56] Meanwhile, activists were working to alter the media landscape itself.[57] Their work has become increasingly evident in the growing number of photography shows and film and video festivals devoted in part or entirely to the topic of disability.[58] And, of course, the myriad websites, e-lists, blogs, and chat groups on the Internet have dramatically expanded the range of locations through which questions about disability and its public presence are being negotiated and communities of support are being formed.

The circulatory reach of electronic and digital media is a key factor in the creation of "mediated kinship," a term I coined with Rayna Rapp as a way to capture all the media practices I have been discussing. Mediated kinship can create a new sense of a Gemeinschaft among those who may be physically separated, but who share the experiences of genetic or other diseases.[59] Emerging as a neighboring—and sometimes overlapping—field in relation to the formal, institutionalized discourse of disability rights, alternative forms of mediated kinship often offer a critique of normative American family life that is embedded within everyday cultural practice. Encompassing many genres and identities, a common theme is an implicit rejection of the pressure to produce "perfect families" through the incorporation of difference under the sign of love and through intimacy in the domain of kinship relations. Mediated spaces of public intimacy such as the ones I have mentioned in Sam's case—documentaries, talk shows, online disability support groups, websites, and so on—are crucial to building a social fund of knowledge more inclusive of the fact of disability across a range of communities.[60]

An exemplary case of this within the Jewish Gemeinschaft took place in January 2007 in a series of film screenings and discussions organized by award-winning filmmaker, DES survivor, and media activist Judith Helfand, held as part of Limmud ("to learn" in Hebrew). Billed as a conference, a festival, a gathering, and "an opportunity to craft your own Jewish world," Limmud was held for four days in upstate New York. Then in its second year, it was modeled on a similar project that began in the UK twenty-five years earlier.[61] Helfand had been approached by Limmud's planning committee to program something on Jews and film, for which she chose to bring a group of innovative filmmakers and activists who are using their documentary work to reframe the question of who is a Jew in the context of disability. Pulling together this group, which included me and my daughter, was the title for the session (playing on the name of a popular independent film from 2006), *In G-d's Image: You, Me, and Everyone We Know*. The description in the Limmud program read as follows:

> This is a series of nine sessions focused on non-fiction filmmaking & story-telling about inclusion and exclusion, abilities and disabilities, family and community. Expect humor, chutzpah, a lot of hope, serious fun, voices and points-of-view you've never heard before and will want to hear from again. Our collective hope is that *In G-d's Image: You, Me, And Everyone We Know* will inspire Limmud-New York to talk openly about inclusion and exclusion. Long-term, we hope the series will be used as a resource to spark a necessary and mindful discussion within the institutions dedicated to an inclusive, human, kind and just Jewish community.[62]

A number of sessions focused specifically on independent film projects, including Trachtman's *Praying with Lior* and Eisenman's *Hidden Blessings*, both works in progress at that point. I call them projects, rather than films, because they are much more than documentary texts. Each is part of a much broader campaign of outreach, education, and intervention in multiple sites. At the first session the irrepressible Helfand looked up at the seventy or so participants gathered there—people who ran the gamut from orthodox to secular—and exclaimed, "They wanted me to program Woody Allen! Look at this! This has never happened before! When have a bunch of Jews gotten together to look at movies that can make us think about these issues? What do we do when something has never happened before to bless this occasion?" Voices called back: "The Shehechiyanu!" And, without missing a beat, the group spontaneously joined together in reciting this most basic of Jewish prayers, the blessing for all new or special experiences, traditionally said to inaugurate joyous—and novel—occasions.[63]

Getting a (Second) Life

Later that year, at a 2007 workshop about Jewish religious practice in the online world held at New York University's Center for Religion and Media, a virtual lighting of the Shabbat candles was about to take place in the Jewish section of the online world of *Second Life*.[64] The assembled group waited eagerly, watching the screen and a group of online avatars (or "javatars," as some call those virtual representatives of the self who identify as Jewish) gathered for the first set of candles to be lit (virtually) based on Israeli time, seven hours ahead of New York City. As the avatar named Namav Abramaovitch carried out the ritual, Dr. Chava Weissler (who is conducting research on Jews in *Second Life*), asked him if he would be leaving soon to go light candles in RL ["real life"].[65] To the group's astonishment, he wrote back, "No, I can't light candles in RL because I am disabled. *Second Life* is the only space where I can be a practicing Jew." Clearly Namav is not alone. In the October 2007 issue of the online Jewish magazine 2*Life*, an article described another avatar's embrace of this virtual world: "On Rosh HaShana and Yom Kippur, Serafina [the creator of the first synagogue in *There*, the Jewish section of *Second Life*], and who is homebound in RL, had an open house in the synagogue, welcoming everyone who had no other possibility to attend services, to join her in the virtual world."

These stories of Namav and Serafina are yet another kind of parable of possibility, suggesting that the virtual world of Second Life offers a second chance to participate in Jewish life for those who find RL less than accommodating.

Conclusion

It goes without saying that we are far removed from Mengele's film footage in the use of contemporary media technologies to include or exclude the disabled in the life of specific communities, whether these are national, local, or virtual. However, the deployment of media technologies—documents, documentaries, DNA karyotypes, or digital websites—is critical to the creation of a variety of Gemeinschaften in the contemporary world, whether it is the sense of relatedness that is built in online discussion groups among the dispersed Jewish families whose children share a rare mutation on chromosome 9 or the spirit of inclusion that embraces audiences who view the film *Praying with Lior*, as I have seen happen at countless screenings. The hegemonic authority of "science" and "biomedicine" buttressed the interpretive frames that gave Nazi film and photography its authority at a particular historical moment. The impossibility of tethering such media permanently to their foundational frameworks is part of their unruly productivity, as future generations refuse to let unacceptable narratives shape their interpretation, no longer allowing them to objectify and dehumanize people—in this case, those with disabilities. The passion with which archival footage is sought and repositioned through idioms of kinship and human rights is an index of the continued power of these images and the fear that, without their radical resignification, they can continue to wreak damage, like the half-life of nuclear toxins. In the hands of activists, from Hannelore and Perla, to Andrea and Josef, to Ilana and Lior, to Namav and Serafina and Samantha, these images and the people they represent can indeed have a second life.

Whereas phenotypic evidence captured on film was once used by eugenicists to make the case for an underlying pathology they imagined lurked within, the filmmakers discussed here refuse to allow such reductive interpretations of the body to separate the disabled from their social worlds. Instead they rely on what I call mediated kinship. Such forms of relatedness are not necessarily genealogical or familial. Consider the following:

1. the bond constituted between Hannelore and Perla in their shared status as little people who have suffered discrimination and join together in the search to reclaim Mengele's footage;
2. the political performance of Austrian activists who resignified photos from the scientific archive of Heinrich Gross to claim kinship with the murdered disabled children they represent;
3. the relationships created across different forms of Judaism by those with the genetic disease cystic fibrosis who share the mission to break the unwritten code of silence surrounding this and other chronic diseases in the Hasidic Jewish community;
4. the extended family and community that find themselves (in both senses) praying with the Down-syndrome teen Lior;
5. the cyber-kinship created among avatars whose lives are enriched by the virtual possibilities denied to the disabled in RL.

In any polysemic tradition there are always new ways to imagine community where exclusion once existed. The media practices considered in this chapter provide a counterdiscourse—from cautionary tales to parables of possibility—to the naturalized stratification of membership within an ethno-religious community that for so long has marginalized those disabled from birth. It is not only the acceptance of difference within families, but also the recognition of relatedness that makes these works potentially radical in their implications. As sites of information and free play of imagination, these cultural forms help to constitute new social landscapes that move embodied difference beyond the constraints of medical diagnoses. The disjunction between the aspiration for democratic inclusion and the fantasy of bodily perfectibility through technological intervention—from eugenics to ARTs—has energized much of this cultural expression in documentary media, creating a growing sense of public intimacy with experiences of disability. The resulting disability narratives offer models of lives lived against the grain of normalcy with ingenuity, courage, and joy. And in the Jewish case such narratives constitute a legacy both internal and external to a community that has too often denied the possibilities of such lives. In closing I want to return for a moment to Foucault's discussion of technologies as methods through which individuals can transform themselves and those around them "to attain a certain state of happiness, purity, wisdom." In this sense Jewish identity—as much as biomedicine or film—can be seen as a powerful technology that increasingly embraces the diversity that disability brings to this community, whether recuperating a sense of shared ancestry with Jewish kin—as Susie Korda does with simple elegance in her film's title *One of Us*—or embracing the religious imperatives that ask us to recognize that every human being is created in God's image.

(Re)Locating Religion in a Technological Age

Thinking about Melville, Religion, and Machines That Think

John Lardas Modern

Captain Ahab: How long before this leg is done?
Carpenter: Perhaps an hour, Sir.
Ahab: Bungle away at it then, and bring it to me (turns to go). Oh, Life! Here I am, proud as Greek god, and yet standing debtor to this blockhead for a bone to stand on! Cursed be that mortal inter-indebtedness which will not do away with ledgers. I would be free as air; and I'm down in the whole world's books.

—*Herman Melville, Moby-Dick; or, The Whale* (1851)

The word personality describes that which is personal, that which belongs to one human being only. To have personality means to possess . . . an original character not like that of others, but truly one's own and free from imitation. To be a personality is to be one who is distinguished and recognized among a crowd by some trait either moral, intellectual, physical, or simply practical. . . . Be the captain of your ship of destiny launched on the ocean of life.

—*Henri Laurent, Personality: How to Build It* (1916)

The Effects and Limits of Protestant Piety in the Age of Mechanical Reproducibility

"What an age," exclaimed a columnist for *Advertising and Selling* in 1927. "Photographs by radio. Machines that think . . . Vending Machines to replace salesmen. The list of modern marvels is practically endless."[1] The slippage—between mediation and immediacy, machines and humanity, advertising and selling—was as inspiring as it was unsettling.[2] With continuing innovations in the motion picture, telephone, and automobile industries, the appearance of neon signs, traffic lights, airplane travel, and lie detector devices, and most vividly, extensions of mass media into everyday life—book-of-the-month clubs, radio, the advent of modern marketing and public relations—the relationship between the self and the marvels of technology became a site of heightened religious concern, particularly among America's white Protestant majority. As "shell-shocked" veterans and amputees from World War I struggled to adjust to domestic life, their machine-induced maladies became metaphors for the experiential shocks of modernity. Articles in such popular magazines as *Ladies Home Journal* and the *Atlantic Monthly* introduced readers to the psychological minefield of Sigmund Freud—catharsis, trauma, and the uncanny—and hinted at the limitations of discerning the real from the phantasmatic on all matter of experiential fronts. In 1922 Harvard-trained psychologist Alfred B. Kuttner wrote of the strange materiality of machine-age America and the increased difficulty of maintaining a stable sense of self within it. From Kuttner's perspective, writing from within the Protestant establishment, "our society, with its kaleidoscopic changes . . . presents a problem of adjustment with which even those who are at home in America find it difficult to cope."[3]

What remains of this moment when Americans in general adjusted to the seepage of technology into everyday life? What, if anything, is religious about the affective space in which technology was passionately engaged rather than visibly seen or reasonably understood? To what degree does this space constitute what we are talking about when we are talking about modernity? Might this space of indeterminate lineage and vague contours resemble one that billions across the globe now occupy?

This chapter, inspired by such questions, explores but one node of what may be called the ever-evolving habitus of technomodernity—the way in which machines go without saying because they came without saying. Such exploration, of course, is a matter of technology and theology, which is not to say that God is a machine or machines are God. Rather, it is to broach the hazy regions in which humans are not simply human, but marked somehow, already, by the culture that contains them. This mark, among other things, signals both discipline and agency, the knowledge that accompanies free will and the ignorance associated with determinism. This mark is a contradiction. Indeed, its dense measures suggest the implosion of a static anthropology, the impossibility of an essential and unchanging nature of the human (however it may be construed). This mark, in other words, marks neither the machine nor the human, but the relationship between them.

I am particularly interested in the immensity of technology—technology as a social form, as an index of social relations, and as an organizing metaphor of human being. These are the same issues that greatly troubled post-Calvinist Protestants in the early part of the twentieth century—those who had become used to a God who had granted them capacities of agentive and social control while rarely impinging upon them. As historian Martin Marty has written, 1920s America "reeked of religion," a telling phrase that illumines the kinds of anxiety generated by the atmospheric effects of technological development.[4] Liberals, for example, pointed to the factory system as the infectious source of economic deprivation. Frederick Winslow Taylor's principles of scientific management, in addition to their potential application "to all kinds of human activities" (not just the assembly lines at the Ford Motor Company), could also pollute the voluntary ground of religious faith.[5] "In the past the man has been first," wrote Taylor in a style that was wholly apocalyptic. "In the future the system must be first."

The fires of Fundamentalism, on the other hand, were fueled by relentless attacks upon "mechanical and electrical and chemical discoveries" that "are contributing to our material prosperity [but] are more rapidly still undermining our morals."[6] On more reactionary ends of the Protestant spectrum, urban industrialism and the automobile were cited as having contributed to an increase in immigration, internal migration, and unpalatable mixings of blood and language. In the pursuit of "hundred percent Americanism," nativists fought the fight in gendered terms, erecting "virile legislation" and rallying against "the radical seeds that have entangled American ideas in their poisonous theories."[7]

Defensiveness, perhaps, was a logical response, as technological innovation and expanse threatened to dissolve the economies of origination—moral, psychological, and political—that were integral to a range of white Protestant pieties and their attending logics. In responding to what Walter Benjamin once called the machine-induced processes of "mingling and contamination," white Protestants redoubled their efforts to secure the very linchpin of their religiosity—an unencumbered act of faith made possible through conditions of epistemological clarity.[8] Such strategies owed much to the elective affinity between the spiritual rationalism of Jacob Arminius (c.1560–1609) and the empiricism of Francis Bacon (1561–1626). Arminianism had long since been the driving bass line of Protestant subjectivity, its message of spiritual autonomy spread far and wide by nineteenth-century revivalists. From the beginning of the American Republic, Scottish Common Sense philosophy—and its Baconian universe, consisting of discernible parts and governed by an aggressive and instrumental reason—achieved widespread currency through the "village Enlightenment" and industrial revolutions.[9] Both perspectives—"religious" and "scientific"—were consistent in their affirmation of individual rational faculties and the potential for perceptual transparency.[10]

By the 1920s, however, vocabularies of Arminianism and Common Sense had come to inflect and organize all manner of communication and economic networks.[11] Indeed, these vocabularies had cross-pollinated to such a degree as to become *epistemic*, at least for a Protestant majority whose power was increasing in terms of ideological diffusion, even as it decreased in other, more measurable areas. What is fascinating, then, about Protestant understandings of the self is how they generated expectations of agency even as they generated material conditions that made fulfillment of these expectations increasingly difficult. For as the grammatical blend of Arminian rationality and Common Sense empiricism continued to produce the possibilities of and conditions for technological advancement, this particular admixture was itself failing to come to terms with the world it was advancing. On the contrary, unsettling moments proliferated in which neither the self was as active nor the material environment as passive as had been promised in the instruction manuals for evangelical conversion, the social contracts of Enlightenment, capitalistic exchange, or scientific inquiry.

This chapter dwells within the failure of the explanatory franchises undergirding public Protestantism in hopes of glimpsing something about the habitus of technomodernity. In particular it assumes that cybernetic imaginings and technological developments in feedback control provide opportunities for scholars to renarrate histories of religion and to rethink what, exactly, is religious about the histories they narrate. When one takes seriously the concept of feedback in terms of both history and experience, what, then, separates the religious from the secular? What does it mean to take seriously those individuals who have taken seriously the religious, even divine, dimensions of technology? What, too, does it mean for historians to address the history that passes through them: a process aided, no doubt, by the capacity of machines to capture a moment, any moment, and to reproduce it *ad infinitum*? Indeed, what separates histories of religion from histories of a secular haunted by the effects of mechanical reproduction?

The prevalence of moving images, radio voices, telephonic messages, and automobile exhaust, for example, suggested that in the 1920s there were, in *effect* rather than *fact*, "mysterious incalculable forces" and that "all things" could not necessarily be mastered "by calculation."[12] Scholars, in other words, must entertain the seriousness with which historical actors entertained the visible effects of the invisible and the material dimensions of the immaterial. "When we learn a little more about radio it appears to be the transmission and reception of pure form, without substance," wrote W. H. Worrell in 1922. "And isn't it amazing," he added, "to think that this form, this exchange of thought, is constantly passing about us—*passing through us—from countless transmitting stations, at this very instant!*"[13] This "atmosphere of magic" defied Max Weber's contemporaneous description of the dream of disenchantment in "Science as a Vocation" (1917), not to mention the ideological prescriptions of secularism: religious belief as voluntary, morals as universal, and epistemology as optically grounded and temporally consistent.[14] According to Worrell, the atmospheric forces of technology interfered with the elective space between minds, the affective space between bodies, and the ontological space between human and machine.

Worrell's insight was not indigenous to the modernity of the 1920s. Herman Melville had already reached a similar conclusion by the time he published *Moby-Dick* in 1851. "Ineffable socialities are in me," he wrote amid the mechanization of steam power and factory floors, the spread of rail lines and telegraph wires, the extension of trade and postal routes, the accelerated production and dissemination of verbal and visual information.[15] Melville took seriously the question of humans and their devices, or rather the "springs and motives" that comprised the mechanics of human subjectivity. As Ishmael explains in the first chapter, "I think I can see a little into the springs and motives which, being cunningly presented to me under various disguises, induced me to set about performing the part I did, cajoling me into the delusion that it was a choice resulting from my own unbiased freewill and discriminating judgment."[16] According to Melville, the directives of imperial selfhood, even though they had undergirded numerous projects of American modernity—from industry and the economy, religion and philosophy, to national infrastructures and mental scaffoldings—had already begun to fail. In *Moby-Dick*, Melville explored, via Captain Ahab, how the relentless pursuit of spiritual autonomy, epistemological clarity, and ocular dominion could not only double one's submission to technology, but also result in confusion and blindness. "Here I am, proud as a Greek god," says Ahab to the carpenter who is constructing his ivory leg, "and yet standing debtor to this blockhead for a bone to stand on! Cursed be that mortal inter-indebtedness which will not do away with ledgers." Cursing his "inter-indebtedness" to technology, Ahab could also acknowledge its organic power, admitting that "the path to my fixed purpose is laid with iron rails, whereon my soul is grooved to run." He could not, however, appreciate the specters that such acknowledgment portended—first and foremost the "looming" presence of the white whale, but also the specters within himself and those generated on board the most advanced technology of its time—the self-contained industrial apparatus of the whaling ship. Indeed, by the end of the novel, the Pequod has become haunted by strange sounds, strange portents, and even "phantom" crew members. And before he is taken under by Leviathan, Ahab becomes unhinged by the "message-carrying air"—precisely those material effects that resisted his observation and calculation.[17]

By the 1920s, the air had only become more saturated with messages of various kinds. Amid Taylorized working conditions, moving pictures, and the lingering traumas of industrial warfare, Protestant understandings of spiritual autonomy and renderings of the material world as pliable and inert often failed to do explanatory justice to feelings of mechanical structuration. This chapter addresses particular responses to this charged environment, not strictly within religious institutions and groupings *per se*, but within one of the more underappreciated religious phenomenon of the time—the aptly named "Revival" of Herman Melville that revolved around his long-forgotten *Moby-Dick*. Although Melville had himself claimed that *Moby-Dick* was a new "gospel," it was not until the centenary of his birth in 1919 that his novel was fed back into the loop of popular culture.[18] With the publication of new editions of his works, critical studies, and biographies, Melville became a literary sensation and a media spectacle, capped off by *The Sea Beast* (1926), a silent-screen dramatization of *Moby-Dick* starring John Barrymore and Dolores Costello. The Melville Revival reflected, albeit from a peculiar angle, many of the anxieties and desires of white Protestant majorities across the political spectrum. *Moby-Dick*, for example, was enlisted in the service of authorizing American superiority in the geopolitical sphere as well as in the elusive sphere of culture. As the lone, solitary, masculine artist, Melville became a literary vehicle by which many revivalists expressed their own revulsion toward the sentimentalism of mass culture and the perceived threat of feminized, racialized, and ignorant masses.[19] Many (but not all) revivalists celebrated Melville and his epic in terms that mirrored American investment in the directives of possessive individualism and the essential distinction between human and machine.

The first two sections of this chapter highlight the shared anxiety coursing through American Protestantism, popular culture, and the Melville Revival. After exploring the prescient analyses of feedback technology and the fate of human organicism advanced by Lewis Mumford—a writer who participated in each of these three discourses—I offer close readings of two moments within the Melville Revival that broached issues of feedback and religiosity: Bess Meredyth's screenplay for *The Sea Beast* and the American phalanx of European Dada associated with *Broom*, the short-lived journal whose title and musings on the machine age were inspired by Ishmael's retort, "Who ain't a slave?" In their exploration of the murky ontological space between human and machine, these unorthodox readings addressed the technological environment in terms traditionally associated with religion: revelation, enchantment, mysticism, God. In the end, mine is a story about different modes of theological assessment—inquiries, one might say, into the epistemic orders of technomodernity. For what Mumford, Meredith, and contributors to *Broom* shared was an appreciation of *technologia* (from the Greek meaning systematic treatment) as itself a process worthy of theological consideration.

Feedback and the Protestant Public Sphere

In addition to "reek[ing] of religion," 1920s America also reeked of technology as principles of feedback and reproducibility emerged as central components of modern life. Telephone networks, engines powering automobiles, and movie projectors, not to mention the production of consumer desire by public relations specialists—all marked a moment in American history when technology became intensely expressive and atmospheric. By multiplying the possible selves one could inhabit, technology expanded the horizon of being human. More choices were available, more opportunities to reflect, more ways of living and dying. In their capacity for reproduction and diffusion, technologies generated the capacity for regulating both nonhuman and human systems (the ideal of machines building other machines). They were, in other words, becoming cybernetic (from the Greek *kubernetes*, meaning steersman), "recreating" the world in their own image. According to an advertisement for the advertising agency Calkins and Holden, "Your world is being recreated today by three important influences; first, the closeness of science and discovery to commercial manufacturing; second, the shortness of the link between the manufacturer and the consumer; and third, the amazing speed with which the American public makes up its mind to change its mind."[20]

As historian David Mindell argues in his history of feedback-control technology, the cybernetic ideas made popular by Norbert Wiener in the late 1940s and early 1950s were already emergent by the 1920s.[21] Feedback technologies, defined by their internal capacity to adjust themselves to the future through knowledge of past conditions, were designed by human operators to "respond" to external disturbances and maintain a secure relationship between two variables.[22] Once the human agent sets a control variable (the temperature within a room or the velocity of a turntable or projector), adjustments to external fluctuations (the temperature outside the room or the changing weight of a film reel) proceed automatically.

Feedback technology is often associated with computers and artificial intelligence. However, the capacity to transmit information in order to counter entropy and maintain equilibrium within a unified system was present in oil lamps from ancient Greece, water clocks from the Middle Ages, and temperature regulators from the early modern period.[23] The invention of the Watts steam engine (1788) and the Corliss engine (1848), the publication of James Clerk Maxwell's "On Governors" (1868), the appearance of air-conditioned factories (1902), speed governors on trucks and tractors (c. 1910), automated electric substations (1914), and the Sperry gyropilot (1920) had revolutionized the kind of material and ideological presence machines assumed within human life—no longer a wholly "artificial" other, but a "natural" component of how things fit together and moved along.

By the 1920s the fluidity between humans and machines, nature and second nature had intensified dramatically.[24] A Romantic rejection of technology was no longer as appealing as it had been in the previous century. Nor was it as practical after the massive incursion of infrastructure into everyday life that required mechanical upkeep. Self-regulating devices, automated factories, and modern office equipment were becoming so pervasive as to go *almost* unrecognized and *almost* immune to critique. Acceptance and simmering anxiety were both constitutive of the social fabric. This irresolvable tension between triumphal humanism and dread is what I am calling the habitus of technomodernity.[25] And it is precisely this lived tension that bound together white Protestants who were struggling to maintain the social, perceptual, and racial orders through which "hundred-percent Americanism" and related principles were defined. From a historical perspective, such struggles were ironic. Very little, if any, genealogical considerations were made that would have threatened core principles of Arminianism and Common Sense—in other words, no considerations that would have questioned the historicity of their shared stake in epistemic immediacy and cosmic disclosure. For even as Protestants (and those within the orbit of their public sphere) forged pure and totalizing narratives of identity, they bore other marks, other origins. Whether in retreat or optimistic embrace, the stories Protestants told themselves in order to be their natural selves had, themselves, become part of a feedback loop in which technology played a central role.

Rather than retreat from technology, liberals were inclined to see "the energy of God realizing itself in human life" through those innovations. Walter Rauschenbusch, a significant proponent of the Social Gospel, repeatedly called for progressive efforts to extend access to economic and spiritual opportunity. "The redemption of society" did not mean the abolition of the "industrial system," but the lessening of its negative impact.[26] Instead of seriously considering how technological drives and their "reality effects" might undermine projects of economic reform and self-cultivation, liberals confidently chose to direct technology in the service of a clearly defined humanity. It was a "democratic" strategy that required decisive action. For only through such action could the political and epistemological promises of Enlightenment become a religious reality. By acting upon one's God-given "instinct," the kingdom of God could be achieved and maintained on earth.[27]

In their revolt against the material incursions and ideological temptations of modernity, Fundamentalists strategically harnessed God, somewhat ironically, as guarantor of an organic version of human subjectivity.[28] The Fundamentalist defense of biblical inerrancy, for example, confirmed both the divine autonomy of the text *and* the human capacity for accurate contemplation of it. This underlying tension was resolved within the fundamentalist theory of textuality that hewed to the Common Sense dictum that seeing was, in fact, on par with authentic belief. Just as there was a transparent relationship to be had between the self and God, reader and words on the page, the promise of transparency was also fulfilled in the human act of vision more generally. God was the architect and engineer of the world. He constructed the eyes as well as the space that made visions of the world even possible. As William Jennings Bryan wrote in 1922, "I believe that God made the eyes when He made man—not only made the eyes but carved out the caverns in the skull in which they hang."[29]

With similar missionary zeal, so-called "hundred-percenters" went on the offensive and designated scapegoats for a decline in "original-stock Protestant America." The Red Scare of 1919–1920, led by Attorney General and "fighting Quaker" Mitchell Palmer, initiated campaigns of surveillance and intimidation of Socialist Party members, labor leaders, vociferous Jews and immigrants, and any others deemed politically subversive. The Johnson Act of 1921, the more restrictive Immigration Act of 1924, and the increased visibility of the Ku Klux Klan during the decade spoke to burgeoning fears over racial miscegenation.[30] At stake in these fantasies of whiteness and strategies of purification was the notion of the Anglo-self as autonomous, possessive, and immune.

In popular culture triumphant myths of individual expertise proliferated that reflected both the Protestant desire for authenticity and the limits of this desire more generally: celebration following anxiety following celebration following anxiety. And so on and so forth. Even as Americans designated signs of their essential humanity, they often came to understand these signs and themselves in and through technological terms. Babe Ruth, Henry Ford, and the business entrepreneur offered celebrity assurance of an autonomous subject who could withstand the feminizing assaults of modernity by mastering technology.[31] Advertising executive Bruce Barton (who worked for General Motors when it organized the production of automobiles around consumer orders, feedback from local dealers, and demand forecasting) introduced Jesus in his best-selling *The Man Nobody Knows* (1925) as a conflation of Ruth, Ford, and the businessman.[32] According to Barton, Jesus deftly swung his carpenter tools, created an "organization that conquered the world," and awakened to the "inner consciousness" of his "power." Barton pitched Jesus as a "mystic" and "big man" who had incorporated the technologies of business, advertising, and manufacturing into his own personality and cult thereof.[33]

As feedback technologies "neutralized" economies of origination and claims to eternal value, both Christologies and psychological narratives of restoration were mechanically inscribed.[34] In the wake of the popular *Personality: How to Build It* (1916) and the nine other titles in the "Mental Efficiency Series published by Funk and Wagnalls," self-realization was consistently equated with an engineering process of control. *Outwitting Our Nerves* (1922) affirmed "the integrity of our physical machines" as well as human "power of choice" over those machines. It was a "fact" that "we ourselves decide which of all the possible emotions we shall choose, or we decide not to press the button for any emotion at all."[35] In *Self-Mastery Through Conscious Auto-Suggestion* (1922), one of the defining books of the twentieth-century genre of "self-help," Emile Coué introduced Americans to the control panel of their inner autopilots. In *Why We Behave Like Human Beings* (1925), evolutionary anthropologist George A. Dorsey defined humans in terms of the "kinesthetic sense" and their innate capacity to enact feedback control upon themselves. He assured readers that "every human individual normal enough to live beyond the walls of an asylum lives because he has an equipment by which he can keep on making adjustments to changing conditions."[36] In *We*, Charles Lindbergh's celebrated 1927 chronicle of his trans-Atlantic flight, his airplane, "The Spirit of St. Louis," assumed its own personality even as Lindbergh became "mechanized" in the popular press.

In each of these narratives there was an insistence upon the capacity for self-control in the face of circumstances that were, at least initially, uncontrollable. For as self-assured masculinity became subject to didacticism and soft discipline, the certitude achieved could be less than satisfactory. Anxiety became inevitable, implicit in the very framing of how to avoid it—celebration following anxiety following celebration following anxiety. And so on and so forth. Yet neither time nor space for any disturbance to register its effects upon this loop.

Melville, Mysticism, and Mental Efficiency

Concerns over how to secure one's identity and maintain its coherence within a seemingly animated material world also precipitated the revival of Melville in the 1920s. As was the case with other Protestant strategies of adjustment, revivalists (predominantly white and male) embraced Melville as providing a script of American identity and self-governance. In hopes of defending themselves against the totalizing directives of technology, revivalists read Melville and his works through the lens of anti-Puritanism and the newly discovered script of Freudian psychoanalysis. Melville's celebrity increased as Elsie Clews Parson, Van Wyck Brooks, H. L. Mencken, Waldo Frank, and others accused Puritans of possessing a "repressive impulse," of denying "life and desire," and of discarding "mystical consciousness" in favor of "instrumental" reason.[37] In Melville's rejection of Puritanism's "repellant materialism," his work assumed a positively transgresssive quality.[38] Opposed to the Puritan life of "intolerable monotony," Melville was viewed as "a mystic, a treasure-seeker, a mystery-monger, a delver after hidden things spiritual and material."[39]

Raymond M. Weaver's *Herman Melville: Mariner and Mystic* (1921) set the terms of religious evaluation for the early stages of the Revival.

Weaver proclaimed that Melville, in his "escape from an inexorable and intolerable world of reality," had achieved "psychological synthesis."[40] The construction of Melville as mystic was concurrent with the discursive construction of mysticism by liberal Protestants as "ahistorical, poetic, essential, intuitive, and universal."[41] Both intellectual constructions—the latter integral to the academic study of religion in the twentieth century—sought to wrest a degree of "realness" from a world in which "the real" was felt to be increasingly susceptible to technological erasure.[42] And whereas mystically inclined Protestants denounced "secular activities" by calling for the liberation and unity of "the deep-lying powers of the inward self . . . into one conscious life" under God, revivalists called on Melville to provide them with an experiential map of that which was utterly human.[43] To be sure, such terrain was fraught with dark spaces, but only in the sense that they were there, waiting to be illuminated, ever susceptible to the demands of human reason. Melville's romanticism—unlike the enchanted pantheism depicted in a chapter like "The Mast-Head"—was sufficiently scientific. Indeed, it was heady, focused, and efficient. As Henry A. Murray flatly announced, "Melville discovered the Unconscious and commenced to explore it."[44] As a model for authenticity and self-governance, Melville was both analyst and analysand—"a gentleman adventurer in the barbarous outposts of human experience," not a "staged dip into studio savagery." Melville had penetrated the depths of his own psyche, no doubt aided by his strategic mingling among South Sea islanders, as detailed in his first two novels, *Typee* (1846) and *Omoo* (1847).[45]

Whereas Weaver expressed nostalgia for a simpler, less commercial, and more fully "real" existence, another Melville biographer, Lewis Mumford, depicted Melville as a visionary: someone who possessed a prescient understanding of the affective dimension of technology and the complex simulations ushered in by a market economy. Mixing cultural criticism, history, and theological speculation, Mumford was a keen observer of the technological revolutions in feedback control. In his most memorable and encyclopedic work, *Technics and Civilization* (1934), he claimed that in the seventeenth century mechanics had become "the new religion, and [it] gave to the world a new Messiah: the machine." In dramatizing the extent to which technology had shaped and continued to shape human consciousness, Mumford explored in exacting and illustrated detail the history and material conditions that were allowing "tools and utensils" to assume "an independent existence." This "neotechnic phase" had begun in the early part of the nineteenth century and was marked by efficiency, flexibility, "complete automatism," and synthetic materials—a "mutation" that was rapidly integrating "the machine and the world of life."[46]

Such integration signaled a restoration of the human, but was not without its dangers. "With the invention of the telegraph," wrote Mumford, "a series of inventions began to bridge the gap in time between communication and response despite the handicaps of space: first the telegraph, then the telephone, and finally television. As a result, communication is now on the point of returning, with the aid of mechanical devices, to that instantaneous reaction of person to person with which it began." The sympathetic relations between family and friends could now be replicated on an unprecedented scale through telepathic technologies—giving rise to "[immense] possibilities for good and evil." The building of a personality was no longer a "local" affair. On the contrary, when "mass-reactions" were "mobilized and hastened," the needs and interests of the human became those of the machine. As Mumford suggested, technology was becoming a "creative force, carried on by its own momentum" and "producing a third estate midway between nature and the humane arts." The drive to overcome distance—between individuals as well as between self and world—had created unprecedented, immaterial, and ungraspable forms of mediation. "*In projecting one side of the human personality into the concrete forms of the machine*," wrote Mumford, "*we have created an independent environment that has reacted upon every other side of the personality.*"[47]

According to Mumford, such technological interference had been of intense and abiding concern for Melville.[48] In *Herman Melville* (1929), Mumford had chided fellow revivalists for exaggerating Melville's retreat into mystical idealism. "Melville was a realist," countered Mumford, "in the sense that the great religious teachers are realists." Furthermore, Melville had witnessed the "volcanic intrusion" of "industrialism [as] a value in itself."[49] But things had become much more complicated since the mid-nineteenth century—for, whereas Melville beheld "the servile routine of the factory system," Mumford was now witnessing the birth of "the machine system . . . the network of relationships that have followed the financial exploitation of machinery." The difference, in other words, was the full-scale emergence of self-governing technologies: "handicraft devoted to mechanical reproduction and machinery that is set to reproduce endless simulacra." For Mumford, this "machine ritual," this "endless" loop of "mechanical reproduction," threatened to efface "the human arts of seeing, feeling, and living."[50] Technology, from his perspective, had achieved the capacity for feedback on two different, but related levels: first, in material devices that could copy both nature and themselves; and second, in humans that governed themselves according to the latest control variables set by the machine. As Mumford argued, the totalizing power of feedback technologies resulted not simply from designs, motors, or even material outputs, but through their economically driven expansion of "the very domain of the symbol itself."[51]

Mumford's insights take on more ominous implications when one considers the rise of the American public relations industry during this period.[52] Public relations consultants such as Edward Bernays and advertisers such as Bruce Barton actively sought to shape and change the beliefs of individuals in the service of larger economic agendas. It was no accident, Bernays wrote in 1923, that a "man belongs to one church rather than another or to any church at all." It was no accident that "Boston women prefer brown eggs and New York women white eggs." Because the judgments of individuals were not arrived at through "research and logical deduction," but were "dogmatic expressions accepted on the authority of his parents, his teachers, his church, and of his social, his economic and other leaders," a "public relations counsel" must do the work of reauthorization.[53] Through the strategic "saturation" of images, text, and workplace incentives, an entire professional class sought to provide the terms for and effectively monitor the conditions of self-realization.[54]

What, then, did Melville have to offer those living within "the machine system" of the 1920s? Mumford and other mainstream revivalists championed *Moby-Dick* as a blueprint for living within an increasingly mechanical, routinized, and bureaucratic world. And despite different emphases, these revivalists depicted Melville as a representative human, the last best hope for fending off the incursions of modernity. In this vein many revivalists also heaped admiration upon Captain Ahab, an odd choice given the outcome of *Moby-Dick*. Contrary to those who would later read Ahab's technologically enhanced demagoguery against the political backdrops of Italian Fascism and National Socialism, Ahab's madness in the 1920s could be considered "active and courageous," as well as a sign of "genius"—"the very pinnacle of human self-assertion."[55] Such readings conflated the white whale with the power of technology. They framed Ahab as defiantly affirming the principle of free will and defending the boundary between human and material worlds. Mumford, for example, wrote of Ahab as the "spirit of man" who stood in opposition to "the brute energies of existence, blind, fatal, overpowering." Ahab was self-directive and "purposive," and he pitted his "puniness against this might and [his] purpose against the blank senselessness of power." So even though Ahab's "methods are ill-chosen," wrote Mumford, his "defiance is noble."[56]

Errant readings of Melville's essential humanity, although not central to the story of Melville's canonization, did, however, exist. Within the Melville Revival—an almost clichéd instance of modernism's vogue for the solitary genius—seeds of post-Cartesian doubt were being sown and the enchanting dimensions of technology reconsidered in light of Melville's own musings. Because Melville "was spell-bound by the strange slidings and collidings of Matter," his work, in the eyes of less sentimental critics, exposed the enchanting conditions of the machine age. "It is the material elements he really has to do with," wrote D. H. Lawrence in 1923. "His drama is with them. He was a futurist long before futurism found paint."[57] And to these futurist leanings we now turn—errant readings of Melville that extended Mumford's line of inquiry to its (theo)logical conclusion, accounting for, among other things, the excessive power of machine-enhanced publicity.

People Who Portray Themselves, or Ahab on the Subject of Ahab

Film projectors, in addition to utilizing concepts of feedback internally, generate external feedback loops between humans and machines, nature and artifice. Such loops arguably constitute the "society of the spectacle," Guy Debord's term for the image-saturated environment that arose in the 1920s with the confluence of sound film and the perfection of propaganda techniques. As one of the more grim assessments of an image-based postmodernity, Debord defined the "spectacle" in terms of negative feedback: "It is the omnipresent celebration of a choice *already made* in the sphere of production, and the consummate result of that choice. In form as in content the spectacle serves as total justification for the conditions and aims of the existing system. It further ensures the *permanent presence* of that justification, for it governs almost all time spent outside the production process itself."[58] In America Debordian paranoia was rampant as Victorian fears over the exploitation of pleasure were morphing into general anxieties concerning voyeurism and cinematic determinism. "The spectacle of mechanical progress has made so deep an impression," argued Walter Lippmann in 1922, "that it has suffused the whole moral code." What disturbed Lippmann and other public figures was the specter of circular causality and the quiet "insertion between man and his environment of a pseudo-environment" composed mainly of images.[59] Unbeknownst to them, Americans were in danger of becoming automated by images and trapped within what Debord would later call "an uninterrupted monologue of self-praise."[60] Their perpetual affirmation of self, however, was wholly cybernetic, given the fact that they were oblivious to the fact that "on the screen the whole process of observing, describing, reporting, and then imagining, has been accomplished for you."[61] These Americans, in other words, were inter-indebted to the machines that perpetually affirmed their inviolability through story, image, and song.

In a strange twist that Melville might have enjoyed, the most compelling representation of *Moby-Dick* and portrayal of Captain Ahab may have occurred via the technology of the moving picture.[62] The 1926 silent film *The Sea Beast*, adapted for the screen by Bess Meredyth and starring John Barrymore as Captain Ahab, was compelling precisely because it dramatized the feedback dimensions of film and its capacity to regulate the human personality. *The Sea Beast*, I argue, challenged more able-bodied academic interpretations by reveling in its status as a technological reproduction. *The Sea Beast*, with its odd juxtapositions, visceral jump cuts, and perverse attention to Ahab's stump and artificial limb, rather than affirming the desire for self-transparency, suggested that the equipment-free reality of the self was, quite literally, an enabling fiction. What Americans lacked, according to Meredyth's scenario, was the tragic recognition of themselves as always regulated and already enhanced by technology. What they lacked, in other words, was a genealogical perspective, unable and/or unwilling to broach the technical contingencies that had given them their human certainties.

In 1925, at age forty-three, John Barrymore was one of Hollywood's most bankable actors (part of the "star system" promoted by Edward Bernays, who for his part clearly saw the potential for cross-marketing between entertainment, business, and political campaigns). Barrymore easily convinced Warner Brothers to turn *Moby-Dick*, one of his favorite novels, into a movie and to cast him in the role of Captain Ahab. Having played Hamlet in the 1922–1923 Broadway season, Barrymore had developed a keen interest in psychoanalysis and, in particular, Freud's account of Hamlet in *Interpretation of Dreams* (1913).[63] The role of Captain Ahab, like that of Hamlet, allowed Barrymore to reach a larger audience with his newly emotive acting style. As Captain Ahab he could also remind his audience of his depth and manly credentials. He was tired, in his words, of playing "scented, bepuffed, bewigged and ringletted characters."[64] Promotional pamphlets for *The Sea Beast* seemed to reinforce Barrymore's gendered strategy, featuring a picture of Barrymore in a business suit puffing contemplatively on a pipe. "John Barrymore is more than a name," declared the advertising copy, "more than a personality; he is a world institution."[65]

The opening credits to *The Sea Beast* begin imprecisely with a close-up of the film's nonexistent textual referent, *Moby Dick, or the White Whale*. This simulated text begins not with "Extracts" or even "Call me Ishmael," but with the following words: "There never was, nor ever will be, a braver life than the life of the whaler. Compared to the game they hunted the mightiest land beast was but a poodle dog." Adapted to the screen by Bess Meredyth, former actress turned writer, *The Sea Beast* is noteworthy as one of the earliest, if not the first, public appropriations of Melville's novel by a woman. By 1926 Meredyth had become a Hollywood regular, having written the scenarios or continuities for *Ben Hur* (1925), *Don Juan* (1926), and at least seventy other films. "There is no woman writing today," read the promotional copy of *The Sea Beast*, "who has contributed so much to genuine screen values as Bess Meredyth."[66] The "genuine" sense Meredyth made of Melville's epic is significant in its relentless focus on the self as a technological construct. In Meredyth's scenario one literally glimpses the spirit of Melville's critique of the contemplative, insular, and hyper-masculinized self of mid-nineteenth-century religion and science. In its plot and perverse attention to Ahab's stump, *The Sea Beast* suggests that nothing will, or even can, make up for the loss Ahab suffers.

After the opening credits the audience is introduced to a healthy Captain Ahab atop the masthead. He looks out over the sea and down on his crew hard at work, his feet tapping to the beat of the sea shanty "Hanging Johnny." Nostalgia and the logic of substitution are both broached in the opening scenes—not in terms of idealism, but in ways that hint at their subsequent negation. As Ahab reads a letter from his beloved, Esther Harper, the daughter of a Christian missionary played by the nineteen year-old Dolores Costello, Ahab looks longingly at her name tattooed on his arm. His mind drifts back to their last embrace. Following a long close-up of his legs, Ahab descends from the masthead, the camera sliding down the rope in real time and, from Ahab's point of view, his legs leading the way. The experience of vertigo engendered by the shot suggests that Ahab's identity is already unstable, already marked by a palpable lack of ground. This shot, however, is quickly offset by numerous scenes that depict the fullness of Ahab's vigor, particularly in relation to his healthy pair of legs. He jumps, he hops, he runs around.

When Ahab's ship docks in the bay of Mauritius, the audience is introduced to Esther as well as to Derek, Ahab's scheming half-brother. It is here that one is reminded of the words from the 1925 promotional publication of *Moby-Dick*, accompanied by scenes from *The Sea Beast*: "the screen version of 'Moby Dick' exceeds the book. The discrepancy between the two must not be considered as a profanely wanton alteration." To portray the "psychological study" of Captain Ahab, "the camera has resorted to means of its own. A mental state, therefore, particularly an involved condition of mind, must be expressed by means of the incidents which produced it; each tortuous thought composing Ahab's madness must be traced to the event which engendered it."[67] The most obvious incident referred to here was the loss of Ahab's leg. But the film compounds this sense of material loss by turning Melville's tale into one of endlessly deferred desires—from the love triangle between Ahab, Derek, and Esther to the triangulation of reality, fiction, and the mechanics of representation.

On shore, Ahab and Esther declare their love to each other. But after a few days Ahab sails from Mauritius and scans the shore with his telescope. He spies Esther's window. She comes to the window and returns Ahab's gaze through her own telescope. Technology has literally become the lens through which they see each other, through which each declares commitment. They wave and blow kisses until they are both out of range. At sea, Ahab is betrayed by Derek, who, unbeknownst to Ahab, pushes him overboard into the waiting jaws of Moby Dick. After losing his leg, Ahab is distraught. Derek then taunts Ahab and suggests that his symbolic castration is too much for any relationship to bear. As Derek reminds him, "Esther was always crazy about your bein' so strong and perfect." Having been fitted with his ivory stump, Ahab arrives back at Mauritius. Derek then shames Ahab even further by telling him that he and Esther are in love and that Esther cannot bring herself to tell Ahab of the deceit. Derek then goes to Esther to convince her that Ahab has abandoned her. When Ahab arrives at Esther's house to confirm Derek's story, he sees their shadows, cast by the light of spermaceti candles, and mistakenly believes that Esther has indeed left him for Derek. It is here that Ahab descends into his infamous monomania.

Ahab goes on to slay Moby Dick, but not before uncovering his half-brother's double betrayal. In a dramatic confrontation, Derek pulls a knife on Ahab and is about to get the best of our hero. But wait! Ahab wedges his ivory stump into the deck, leveraging himself in order to fend off Derek. Ahab then casts Derek overboard and into the sea. An ivory technology marking the absence of Ahab's leg has been transformed into a salvific presence (the stump having regulated Ahab, making him complete and free to pace the deck). Or so it seems when the audience is treated to the restoration of order upon the Pequod's return to port, and Ahab's reunion with Esther is consummated in their tearful embrace. Having staged and seemingly resolved the crisis of masculine identity (the *raison d'être* of melodrama being that the resolution is already present in the staging), *The Sea Beast* did anything but restore the full presence of Ahab's self. The film suggested through both content and form that whatever reality the self possesses, whether it be the character of Ahab or the spectator in the theater, was neither fully resolvable nor equipment-free.

Ahab achieves a kind of liberation on screen by recognizing that he is always already a figment of an imagination that is not his own. After the tearful reunion between Ahab and Esther, the screen goes black. The audience is then given a glimpse behind the scenes, as it were: a scene of the director, Millard Webb, in his chair issuing directions to Ahab and Esther in Esther's living room. A man in a business suit plays the violin in the background. As Ahab and Esther look longingly into each other's eyes, Ahab slips a ring onto Esther's finger and they embrace once again. Or is it Barrymore and Costello? It is unclear, particularly in light of the rumors of an off-screen tryst between the middle-aged Barrymore and his nineteen-year old co-star (they would later marry). The loving embrace is seemingly real, an ambiguity reaffirmed by the fact that after Webb yells "cut!" he has to step between the couple and remind them that they are on film! Webb then turns to the camera and smiles as the screen abruptly cuts to black once again.

The ending of *The Sea Beast*—playful, uncanny, vaguely ominous—suggests that Ahab's journey toward reconciliation did not end with self-exposure, but that it could never really begin. Rather than achieve restoration of nature in and through a cultural construction, Ahab's artificial leg points to a previously "excluded and illegible domain that haunts the former domain as the specter of its own impossibility, the very limit of intelligibility, its constitutive outside."[68] The ending harkens back to the sea shanty "Hanging Johnny," Ahab's introductory descent from the masthead, and his telescopic flirtation with Esther, both of which constituted vertiginous slides into the unfathomable layers of mediated perception that signal the "execution" of possessive individualism. Rather than erase the sign of Ahab's trauma—his ivory leg—the ending of *The Sea Beast* suggests that Ahab and Barrymore are two sides of the same character vacillating within the loop of continuous performativity. One is reminded here of Walter Benjamin's insight into the traumatized subject in the age of technological reproducibility. As Benjamin argues, the trauma can be understood as a shift from the stage to the screen, in which the actor performs for a "piece of equipment" rather than for an audience.

Citing the Italian playwright Luigi Pirandello, Benjamin suggests that the modern subject is

> exiled not only from the stage but from his own person. With a vague unease, he senses an inexplicable void, stemming from the fact that his body has lost its substance, that he has been volatilized, stripped of his reality, his life, his voice, the noises he makes when moving about, and has been turned into a mute image that flickers for a moment on the screen, then vanishes into silence.[69]

Pirandello's borrowed words speak directly to Meredyth's reconfiguration of Melville's text. Whereas Melville's Ahab tried and failed to conquer the very source of visual illumination—the spermaceti oil that allowed antebellum Americans to see in the dark—Barrymore's Ahab revels in the technologically enhanced gaze of his audience. When the lights come up, the selves of Ahab, Barrymore, and the audience have been renarrativized as cybernetic—that is, as permanently divided and fundamentally transient. In affirming the really real off-screen relationship between Barrymore and Costello, the penultimate gesture of *The Sea Beast* supported a notion of selfhood as always already mediated. Or better yet, the film insisted on the necessity of experience to be mediated in order for it to become real, or maybe even the necessity of acknowledging that the reality of the self is really made up. Taking "*pleasure* in the confusion of boundaries" and "*responsibility* in their construction," *The Sea Beast*, in the borrowed words of Donna Haraway, made "an argument for the cyborg as a fiction mapping our social and bodily reality and as an imaginative resource suggesting some very fruitful couplings."[70]

Barrymore's self-conscious performance, inspired by his reading of Freud and designed to overcome middle-class mores, did not so much penetrate the inner depths of his character as it did the emotional life and perceptual apparatus of his audience. *The Sea Beast* does not dramatize the individual conquest of nature as much as it dramatizes visual technology's seduction of the individual. *The Sea Beast*, in its staging of a cybernetic reality, interrupted the narrative closure on which self-presence depended. Neither Ahab nor Barrymore nor the audience is ever alone, even in solitude. They are all haunted, not simply by the unconscious, but by the specters generated in and through technologies of reproduction. They are, in Benjamin's apt phrase, "people who portray *themselves*."[71]

For Benjamin photography and cinema were technologies of religious revelation, for better or for worse, in that they both exposed various feedback loops that constituted one's identity. Both technologies, in other words, denied the epistemological purity and ontological totality portended by "one hundred percent" Americanism. On one level Benjamin argued that the category of originality had been challenged by visual technologies that put copies "of the original in situations which the original itself cannot attain."[72] On another level the decay of the "aura" of authenticity and the blurring of original and reproduction enabled individuals to recognize the fact that they were implicated in the perceptual field and no longer insulated from what they saw or heard. "Reception in distraction," wrote Benjamin, "which is increasing noticeably in all areas of art and is a symptom of profound changes in apperception—finds in film its true training ground."[73] Influenced by Johann Wolfgang von Goethe's notion of "after-images" in *Theory of Colours* (the same text that informed Melville's "The Whiteness of the Whale"), Benjamin announced the birth of the "optical unconscious."[74] According to Benjamin, images had become *the* currency of consciousness, structuring thought and determining the range of possible actions. Mechanical means of reproduction had liberated the perceptual capacities of humanity. They had also ushered in the prospect of mass deception and control. Either way, they had resulted in a "massive upheaval in the domain of objects" and a "shattering of tradition."[75]

The Theological Musings of American Dada

In broaching the aporias of modernity, Lewis Mumford praised Melville for having given the lie to Weberian diagnoses of disenchantment. The capacity to effectively turn night into day, Mumford suggested, the experience of a subway car rumbling past, the solid structures of a skyscraper vanishing into the air, the peering into a microscope, and the observation of a "row of bottles, each of identical size, shape, color, stretching away for a quarter of a mile" were enough to induce a particular kind of vertigo. "The special visual effect of repeating pattern[s]" occurred *simultaneously* with the experience "of the unique and the non-repeatable."[76] The experience of intense systematicity—precisely what feedback technologies were designed to induce—could be positively disorienting when the infinitely calculable assumed the "special quality" of the "incalculable."[77] According to Mumford, when technology no longer made imperfect copies of nature but perfect copies of itself, the very notion of "natural" could become radically suspect. With the "liquidation" of the solid bookends of authenticity and artifice came the prospect that the spectrum itself was socially constructed, for better or for worse.[78]

For Mumford, Melville had not simply dramatized the incursion of machines—a traditional Romantic trope. He had also come to recognize those parts of the world and himself that had already been produced by machines, insisting that the plasticity of self was something with which Americans had to struggle and, to their spiritual detriment, repress. Having torn aside the veil that "man has thrown between his own experience and the blank reality of the universe," Melville neither succumbed to the temptation of nihilism nor retreated into his own private morality. On the contrary, he urged his contemporaries to own up to the constructedness of any and all cultural forms and, more importantly, to the fragility of the faith commitments that undergirded them. "As soon as you say *Me, a God, a Nature*," wrote Melville, "so soon you jump off from your stool and hang from the beam."[79] Or as Mumford wrote, "to appreciate the reality of the White Whale is to see more deeply into the expedience of all our immediate institutions, all the spiritual shelters man puts between himself and the uncertain cosmic weather. Meaning, significance, attends only that little part of the universe man has built up and settled."[80]

Whereas Mumford assessed the religious dimensions of technological "progress" in a tragic key, others tended toward the comic, as was the case with a group of experimental artists associated with *Broom: An International Magazine of the Arts Published by Americans in Italy*, published between 1921 and 1924.[81] *Broom*'s coeditor, the poet Alfred Kreyemborg (who from 1927 to 1931 would later coedit with Lewis Mumford the yearly anthology of American literature *The American Caravan*), had adapted a passage from *Moby-Dick* for its title, logo, and statement of purpose, which appeared on the back cover:

> What of it, asks Ishmael, if some old hunks of a seacaptain orders me to get a broom and sweep down the decks? What does that indignity amount to, weighed, I mean, in the scales of the New Testament? Do you think the Archangel Gabriel thinks any less of me, because I promptly and respectfully obey that old hunks that particular instance? Who ain't a slave?[82]

The first issue of *Broom* included poems addressing Albert Einstein's theory of relativity as well as Emmy Veronica Sanders' declaration that "the American Machine" was "transforming itself, with all its attributes and characteristics, into American Mind." "America," she continued, initially "made of the Puritan, by the Puritan, for the Puritan," was now being "remade of the Machine, by the Machine, for the Machine."[83] Following

Sanders' piece was David O'Neil's hymn of supplication to the new gods of the machine:

> When you are sweeping us
> With Your cosmic broom
> Sweeping us out of mouldy ruts
> Sweeping us clean and sweet—
> Remember
> When we're quivering—
> Sensitive— bare—
> We shall be grateful
> For just a few shadows. . . .[84]

Broom took Ishmael's retort quite seriously, addressing the revolutionary dimensions of technological artifice and the shadows cast within the realm of technological illumination.

O'Neil's insistence on enchantment, for example, was a longing for machines to become theologically significant rather than divine in and of themselves. His was a radical invocation of *technologia* as disruptive, a treatment of the human that, in casting its shadows, negated the service the possibility of a totalizing systematicity.

Unlike Futurism, *Broom* did not celebrate the beauty of war. It did, however, come to express the "dreamed-of metallization of the human body" and the playful cybernetic fantasies of Dadaists such as Man Ray and Francis Picabia.[85] After some initial hesitation, *Broom* began to embrace Dada's perspective on the liberatory dimensions of the human-machine interface. "Everything is artificial," gasped *Broom* contributor Blaise Cendrars. "The eyes, the hand . . . the sexual frenzy of the factory. The wheel which turns. The wing which flies. The voice which travels far, on a wire. Your ear in a trumpet. Your sense of direction. Your rhythm. You melt the world in the mould of your skull. Your brain is hollow. . . . Like a religion, a mysterious pill hastens your digestion."[86] Jean Epstein, from a slightly different angle, argued that technology had "become part of ourselves" and had democratized human perception—"man has not one memory of [the] landscape; he [now] has a thousand different ones, which may or may not resemble each other. Everything possesses hundreds of apparent diameters which never superimpose exactly."[87]

Broom was soon translating less inflammatory Futurist manifestos such as Enrico Prampolini's "The Aesthetic of the Machine and Mechanical Introspection in Art," in which he declared, "Is not the machine today the most exuberant symbol of the mystery of human creation? Is it not the new mythical deity which weaves the legends and histories of the contemporary human drama? *The Machine* in its practical and material function comes to have today in human concepts and thoughts the significance of an ideal and spiritual inspiration." The kind of worship that ensued was that of the cyborg, neither reverent nor memorializing of cosmic law.[88] (See Figure 8.) Or, as Prampolini wrote, "Our experience has convinced us of the truth of certain of our plastic truths and has allowed us to perceive the errors that lie in others."[89]

One important piece of American Dada captured precisely this point: *God* (c. 1917), designed by Baroness Elsa von Freytag-Loringhoven and photographed by Morton Schamberg (see Figure 9). The inverted cast-iron plumbing trap atop a carpenter's miter box was emblematic of the Melvillean appreciation for technological enchantment. Indeed, the pipe is part of an indoor plumbing apparatus, a modern convenience whose history dates back to some of the earliest feedback technologies on record—the water clocks and float regulators of ancient Greece.[90] *God* resembled the mechanical

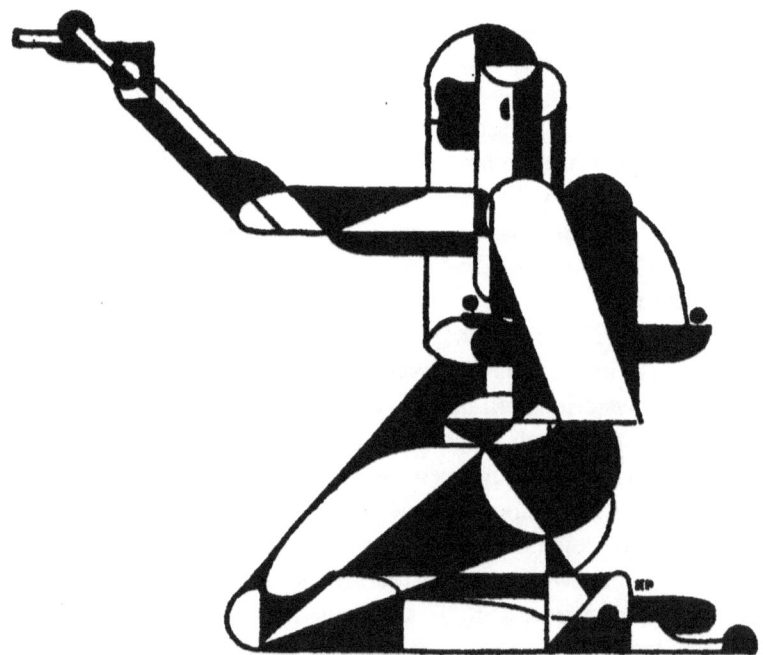

Figure 8. "Robot-Worship." Illustration accompanying Enrico Prampolini's text in *Broom* (October 1922).

Melville, Religion, and Machines That Think   207

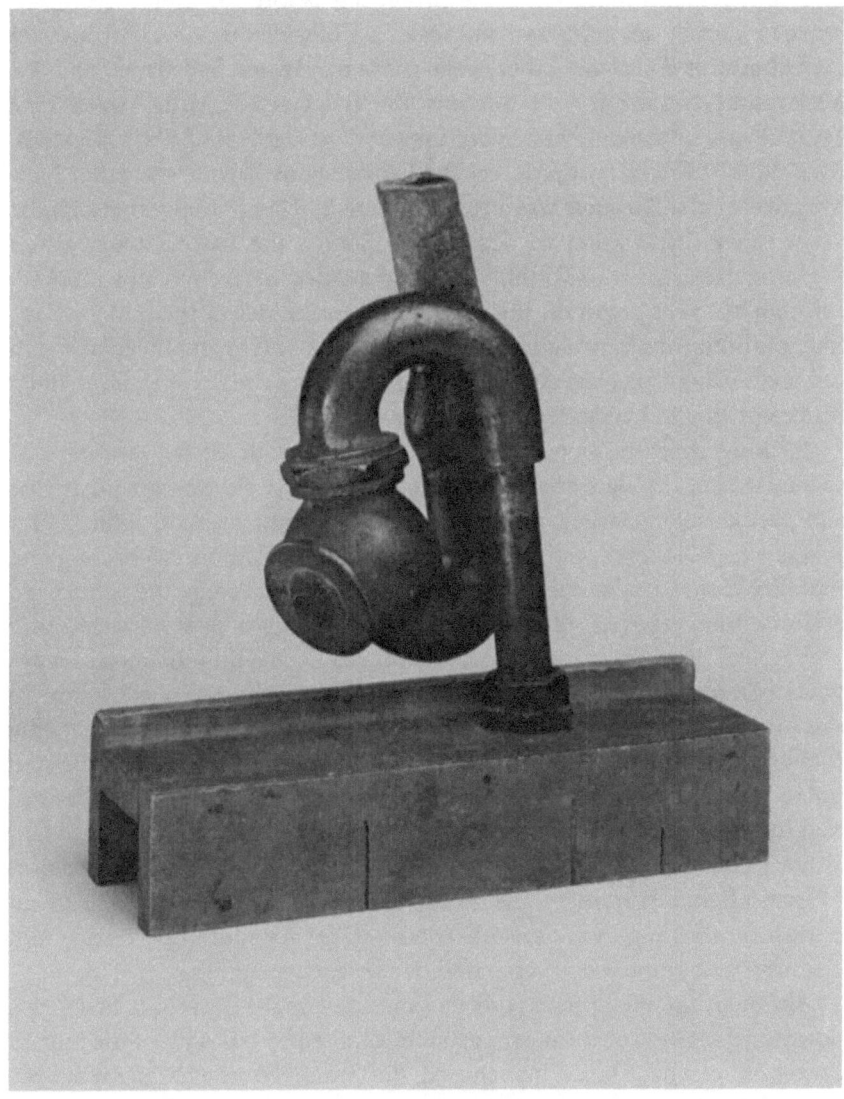

Figure 9. "God" (1917), by Elsa von Freytag-Loringhoven and Morton Schamberg. (Reproduced with permission of the Philadelphia Museum of Art.)

abstractions Schamberg had been producing before his premature death in 1918 during an influenza outbreak in Philadelphia. The Baroness, a contributor to *Broom* and other avant-garde magazines, had arrived in New York from Germany in 1913. She was "the first American dada," wrote Jane Heap in 1922, "the only one living anywhere who dresses dada, loves dada, lives dada."[91] Friends with Marcel Duchamp, Djuna Barnes, and other New York artists, the Baroness was a central figure in a burgeoning, transatlantic avant-garde. In addition to her art and poetry, the Baroness was also a performance artist who skillfully inverted gender hierarchies and attacked, through her very presence, the traditional sensibilities of the middle-class. She was notorious for walking around the streets of Greenwich Village with her shaved head painted purple, postage stamps pasted to her face, and a bird cage around her neck housing a live canary.[92]

In what must be considered a prescient assault on all manners of logocentrism, the Baroness also carried with her a plaster-cast penis that she periodically revealed to passersby for maximum shock value.[93] But it was the Baroness's sculpture *God* that, in addition to celebrating the mobility and reproducibility of that which was supposedly the most fixed and essential, repossessed the power of technology as ever imperfect and incomplete. As a companion piece of sorts to Duchamp's infamous ready-made, *Fountain*—an inverted urinal displayed in the 1917 exhibition of the American Society of Independent Artists—*God* invited more expressly theological speculation about the limits of singularity. First of all, it insisted on supplementing the three traditional symbolic centers of Western religious reflection—God, humanity, nature—with the machine. And although it has since been viewed by critics as "sacrilegious" and an instance of "antireligious scatology," the transgressive dimensions to *God* also affirm a shadowy opening to radical otherness—in the form of imperfection and chance—within the loops generated by feedback technology.[94]

Although the metal pipe ends up pointing toward heaven, it first loops downward in a nod to its human ground. Limited by the skills of the human carpenter on whose box it is anchored, the contorted pipe narrativizes both the pitfalls and prospects of the machine age. Shit eventually flows up in the case of *God*, not down, suggesting that even the most lofty and noble ideals of the imagination maintain their human rank. Rather than assume the power of divinity classically construed, *God* staged divinity as nothing more, and nothing less, than that which made life livable—that which kept the smell of human waste artificially at bay or, more ominously, managed the flow of things through feedback control. But even more literally, *God* called attention to the human work in the making of artifice and celebrated the biological possibility for the endless unmaking (and remaking) of self. Feedback technology was not really God, but it was, for all practical purposes. Or as the Baroness wrote in a 1927 letter to Peggy Guggenheim, God had much to learn from Henry Ford, for he was "clumsily subtle—densely—intelligent—inefficiently—immense—(Lord not Ford—of course)."[95] God, the Baroness playfully warned, had "better hotfoot it toward progress—modernize—use his own omnipotence intelligently—smart or we'll all expire in tangle. Well Lord knows—(Does he?)."[96]

Conclusion: Deus in Machina Movet

As Protestant majorities struggled to adjust themselves and their theological inheritance to new technological conditions, theologies of the machine age, both compelling and disturbing, emerged from outside the precincts of traditional religious discourse. For in addition to being inspired by the ghost of Herman Melville, the Melville Revival was quite literally haunted by the power of feedback technologies—specters that were affective rather than concrete, strangely resistant to rational contemplation, yet recognized through anxious admixtures of thought and feeling. On one hand, the Revival reflected the spectrum of Protestant fears over technological miscegenation. The capacity of machines to redraw the boundaries of race and gender disturbed Protestant leaders and revivalists alike. On the other hand, subversive elements within the Melville Revival offered what must be considered a theological critique of how Protestants understood themselves and their God in relation to technological materials. In other words, the range of Protestant sensibility had refused to come to terms with phenomena that called into question the terms that had already provided for the relationship between God, human, nature. Grant Overton, for example, saw in *Moby-Dick* a deep appreciation for how technological developments had come to undermine—quite literally haunt—the epistemological and ontological assumptions that made them possible. "No longer able to instance the *deus ex machina*," wrote Overton, Melville was "unforgetful that *deus in machina movet*, and while most of mankind [has] become unable to see the god for the machine, [he] can scarcely perceive the machine for the god agitating it. ... [His] reports of the machine are somehow unrecognizable, [his] realism is confronted by Reality."[97]

Both Bess Meredyth's reimagining of *Moby-Dick* and Baroness Elsa von Freytag-Loringhoven's *God* also explored the otherness that technology engenders within the modern subject, a trace that lingers despite all attempts to extinguish it. Their errant readings challenged contemporaries to reimagine their relationship to technology from an enchanted perspective. Moreover, these readings subverted the soteriological and epistemic directives of American individualism. Resisting the advertisements of both Arminianism and Baconianism, these readings insisted that there was something else—something wholly other—occurring *within* the technological workings of secular modernity. Excess, or that which unsettled the boundaries between body and machine, masculine and feminine, had resulted in a modernity defined more by its fears than by any rational and/or instrumental ambitions. The prospect that either machines or women had begun to think for themselves, or at least possess a kind of agency once attributed to the enlightened male subject, now seemed as likely as a whale vengefully turning against a whaleship.[98] As Melvillean riffs on the deferred project of religious identity, *The Sea Beast* and *God* marked the space between human creation and technological determination, consent, and compulsion, and therefore hinted at the prospect that belief was not an individual state, but an embodied activity. Consistent with Lewis Mumford's assessment of the symbolic and material powers of feedback technology, these works raise numerous questions concerning the relationship between religion and what Thomas Carlson calls a "networked" subjectivity.[99] Indeed, the material practices of automation could streamline definitions of human nature—that is, make humans in their own image. But they could also disrupt, radically so, making and remaking humanity so as to reveal the universality of inconsistency. Either way, the subject is inter-indebted to the machines that surround it.

It is one thing to note the limitations of agency—as both a concept and experiential phenomenon. But how might a relentless focus on power and the porousness of subjectivity change how one views matters of religion within history? How might a greater attention to the aesthetic conditions that mediate any and all beliefs challenge the ways in which we distinguish the religious from the secular? How do technologies and vested interests realize themselves through the discourses of agency, choice, and mobility? What, in other words, are the conditions of possibility that allow a historical actor (rather than a Hollywood actor) to make a particular faith commitment or, for that matter, have any faith at all? In what language do historical actors dream about themselves and divinity, and how does that language change over time? And finally, to what degree is faith itself a technology?[100]

Such questions shift the scholarly emphasis from explicit expressions of religious belief and practice to the space between those beliefs and practices and the world at-large. Individuals within American religious history, for example, have often been depicted as fully formed agents making choices between various faith commitments and ever-combining religious idioms in order to suit their specific needs and circumstances.[101] No doubt this is true. But there is another side to this story of radical religious pluralism—one that, if accounted for, suggests new directions on the study of religious history. Although the "lived religion" perspective has done much to overcome the distinction between "dabblers" and "true believers," the question of power still lingers.[102] Religious beliefs and practices are not essential things; nor do they reveal themselves to the scholar *in toto*.[103] Such a position does not replicate the either/or discussion regarding the agency of historical actors. On the contrary, it suggests that agency is a looping effect of intent and instinct, immediate response and mediated principle, knowing and unknowing.[104]

N. Katherine Hayles has argued that the principle of feedback, or "reflexivity," must be appreciated if one is to begin to grasp the rich and complex history of modernity.[105] Such appreciation of feedback shifts scholarly focus from religion-as-ideology to the way in which ideas become living convictions—self-perpetuating rather than essentially misguided. From the perspective of traditional mechanics, ideological regulation amounts to sustained repetition of a single sequence. From the perspective of feedback, however, such repetition is responsive to the point of becoming a metasequence, "or a sequence for determining other sequences, in which a goal is compared to some outcome and action is then taken to bring the next outcome closer to the goal."[106] To account for the principle of feedback, then, in addition to the machines that embody it, is to begin to see religion differently. It is to view religion not as something primarily ideological—that is, about ideas, beliefs, creeds; not as some lived extension or revision of such ideas, beliefs, and creeds; not as something that can be seen at all. To look the other way, then, is to encounter the aporias of discourse and to appreciate the mechanical reproduction of power/knowledge as the ever-receding object of theological inquiry.[107]

It is with a hint of irony, then, that one may return to the promotional pamphlet of *The Sea Beast* that celebrates the "conquest" of Ahab and the invisible, wafting presence of screenwriter Bess Meredyth: "There is no woman writing today who has contributed so much to *genuine* screen values as Bess Meredyth." Indeed, her son, John Meredyth Lucas, born in 1919, continued down his mother's unsettling path as a successful television screenwriter and director. His credits included episodes of "Star Trek," "Logan's Run," and that other story of "hundred percent" Americanism, "The Six Million Dollar Man."

Amazing Stories

How Science Fiction Sacralizes the Secular

Peter Pels

Cyberpunk science fiction has been an important empirical base of the critique of modernist conceptions of science and technology and their relationship to magic and religion. Novelists such as William Gibson, Vernor Vinge, and Neal Stephenson have helped to create a popular imagination in which digital technology erases the distinctions between religion, magic, and science and/or technology. They picture, respectively, "space cowboys" confronting godlike or voodoo artificial intelligences in cyberspace; electronic identification tags as magical "true names"; and a computer virus as a language as well as a religion.[1] By thus encouraging a conception of travel in cyberspace that identifies the virtual and the spiritual and the realist fiction that the latter can penetrate the physical world through the former, they have helped to persuade scholars and hackers that, in postmodern society, the relationship between religion and technology has decisively changed. Some argue that cyberspace has produced an alternative realm akin to Dante's heaven and hell;[2] others that digital technology has kick-started a mode of gnostic thinking implicitly inherent to technology in the first place;[3] yet others that the cyborg phase of human endeavor heralds a posthuman society.[4] The "countercultural" hacker imagination is even more radical. It sees a new magic or a "digital polytheism" emerging from this technological breakthrough.[5]

This volume shows, among other things, that, while the "modern constitution" (as Latour called it) usually pretends to maintain a radical distinction between religion and technology, the salvationist expectations of technology are not really new, at least as far as modern society is concerned.[6] An interrogation into such fusions of religion and technology is needed in order to go beyond the simple dichotomy that lies at the base of the modernist ideology—namely, that the spread of technology equals the spread of rationality, which in turn equals the demise of religion.[7] Cyberpunk science fiction seemed to bring these realms together because it also appeared to draw on a different technology. Instead of space rockets, atomic engines, the Hoover Dam, or the Empire State Building, its technology seemed to be closer to us, more intimate—usually inside our minds and under our skins.[8] Yet such interpretations of cyberpunk science fiction are, just like closely related assessments of postmodernism, often too modernist in assuming a clean break with modernity. While there is much reason to argue that the cybernetic subject (or "cyborg") heralds a posthuman mode of being, this chapter interrogates science fiction in general to raise serious doubts about the extent to which such current fusions of technology and religion really go "beyond" modernity.[9] As is shown by nineteenth-century Spiritualism, fusions of religion and technology have always been part of modern culture, even if only in its less dominant, plebeian guises.[10]

This chapter formulates its doubts about the presumed break of cyberpunk with earlier modernist science fiction on the basis of three theses. First, it proposes that science fiction (SF)—the literary genre most insistently associated with technology in the twentieth century—has *always* been preoccupied with religion, even if only as its antagonist. Second, it argues that modern SF sacralized secular space as well as the technological means to overcome it, but by means of narratives that often seemed to obscure their religious provenance. And third, it provides a *sociocultural* analysis of SF by indicating how, in the translation from literary genre to science-fictionalized everyday life, the sacralizations of space and technology of SF have reinvented "religion" to fit the secular experiences of modern people.

These reinvented and secular forms of religion call for a rethinking of religion in modern society. Many students of religion pay, I feel, far too little attention to the cultural forms of the nonreligious institutions in which modern religious traditions are being reproduced—not just individually, but in the public sphere, as well. In the course of this chapter

I will mostly dwell on SF as a literary genre, but some cinematic and sociocultural diversions from the texts that I target will be needed for my analysis. The result is, I hope, an argument that clarifies certain specific aspects of the cultural features of modernity without claiming to be an exhaustive analysis of SF, modernity, or religion in general.

This chapter focuses mostly, therefore, on experiments with science, technology, and religion during the heydays of modernism as epitomized by the pulp and Golden Age periods of SF publishing (roughly from the 1920s until the early 1960s), in which SF was dominated by writers and editors from the United States.[11] This will serve to show that the cyberpunk SF of the 1980s, while different from its predecessors, is not novel because of its fusion of religion and technology (that had already happened much earlier), but because its acceptance of religious repertoires is much less agonistic. More importantly, the rediscovery of religion at the heart of modernist SF shows that we need a different attitude toward religion in order to understand its salience in modern societies: an attitude that recognizes the paradoxical fusions of science and religion, or of reason and faith, that make up modern consciousness—fusions that are sometimes gnostic, but in any case refuse to be reduced to either one of the polar oppositions.[12]

Quant Suff! Quant Suff!

In the October 1956 issue of *Galaxy Science Fiction*, one of the most acclaimed SF novels of the twentieth century saw the light: Alfred Bester's *The Stars My Destination* told the story of Gulliver Foyle's revenge against the spaceship *Vorga*, which had left him behind in outer space when his own ship, the *Nomad*, was wrecked. In that novel Foyle is rescued by the Scientific People: the remains of a scientific expedition, stranded in a remote corner of the solar system, and forgotten by the rest of it. Its descendants live off space debris and have developed their own ritualized version of science. As they carried the semi-conscious Gulliver Foyle into their junkyard asteroid,

> [A] crowd around the litter was howling triumphantly. "Quant Suff!" they shouted. A woman's chorus began an excited bleating:
>
> "Ammonium bromide .... gr. 1½
> Potassium bromide .... gr. 3
> Sodium bromide.................. gr. 2
> Citric acid .... quant. suff."

"Quant Suff!" The Scientific People roared. "Quant Suff!" Foyle fainted.[13]

In this scene the Scientific People ritually incorporate Gully Foyle, couple him to a young woman by "Natural Selection" and "genetic choice," and tattoo his face with his new name (N♂mad), so that Foyle appears as tigerish outwardly as his desire for revenge on *Vorga* makes him feel inside.

More about the novel below. For now, I want to use this vignette to reflect on the relationship between SF, technology, and religion. "Quant Suff!" is, of course, the banal technology of calculation turned into a religious mantra. "Machines and technology are," indeed, "what we most associate with SF."[14] The "science" in "science fiction" is often taken to imply that the genre deals with how people cope with new worlds generated by new machines—that it deals with a future defined by the rational extrapolation from (as-yet not realized) technoscientific advancements.[15] From a modernist framework—which says the spread of technology equals the spread of rationality equals the demise of religion—this rationality would seem to exclude religion.[16] From the nineteenth century onward, classical liberalism predominantly defined religion in one of two forms: that of the church as an unquestioning acceptance of authority, or that of belief as an irrational or metaphysical conviction. In the 1950s modernization theory transmuted this liberalism into the theory that religion is supposed to disappear or become privatized; pushed out of the way by the spread throughout society of positive scientific knowledge, materialized in technology. Since (like most of us moderns) many SF writers have their positivist moments and desires, they frequently have recourse to this scenario for their plots. Indeed, a large number of SF writers, critics, and readers would agree that SF as a genre is about rational, liberal, and techno-savvy protagonists who pit their enlightened expertise against superstitious or religiously tyrannical adversaries (whether human or extraterrestrial). In *The Stars My Destination*, Gully Foyle faints when he realizes that he is being taken up into a world of people who have gone crazy with ritual: people who have, in fact, lost their understanding of what real (technological) life is like outside the isolation of their space station. Plots that set a secular hero against an adversary who is either gullibly superstitious or who cynically advertises his (rarely her) metaphysical status seem to sell well (and I hope to show that this is not a trivial observation about SF plots or about SF markets). Thus a minimal observation about SF and religion would be that SF is one of the social spaces in which modern people reflect on religion outside the world of church and belief, even if this reflection is antagonistic and secularist, and thus *against* whatever many SF writers and readers think religion stands for. Even the most atheist and technologically boosted SF writer needs some kind of religion to argue against, if only because heroes usually must have their villains.

However, "Quant Suff!" reminds us that things are more complicated than that. The ritual confuses the modernization scenario by showing that "facts"—positive knowledge—are dependent on social and cultural situations. The Scientific People demonstrate that any rational and technoscientific idea can be turned into its opposite—into religion and ritual, given certain conditions (such as social and cultural isolation). The Scientific People show us, therefore, a second, reversed version of the relationship between SF and religion: an inclination to experiment with the ways in which modern people can undo the disenchantments of technology and rationalization, thus (re)sacralizing the secular. Such modern people may, paradoxically, be backward even in a future society— as is conclusively shown by the elaborate nostalgia of the Touareg-type desert society portrayed in Frank Herbert's famous SF novel, *Dune*.[17] A second observation would therefore be that SF is one of those discourses by which modern people can criticize a unilinear association of technology with progress and use religious repertoires to set out alternatives to the modernist trajectory.

However, at the core of its plot, there is a third relationship between religion and technology hidden in Bester's story, one that I will try to show to be representative of much of the Golden Age of SF writing in the 1940s and 1950s. Bester's plot turns around Gully Foyle's desire for revenge, which pushes him (at first unconsciously) to turn *jaunting*—a form of earthbound mental teleportation common in this future society—into a mode of space and time travel. In more strictly speaking religious contexts, only gods, angels, or shamans can "jaunte"— that is, abolish the limitations of space and time by a purely psychic exercise (as I shall discuss below). While Bester's narrative continually portrays religion as degeneration or a sin (not just because the Scientific People are backward, but also because Christian worship is depicted as an underground, pornographic, and punishable act), teleportation both in space and time—rather than the physical transportation by spaceship technology—turns out to be the salvation of both Gully Foyle and his society. Near the end of the novel Foyle learns that his desire for revenge on the spaceship *Vorga* is less important than what he has learned as a human being. If he is to space jaunte and even to time jaunte, he has to have "faith" and to "believe" in something, it does not matter in what. "'Faith in faith,' he answered himself. 'It isn't necessary to have something to believe in. It's only necessary to believe that somewhere there's something worthy of belief.'"[18]

These statements bring 1950s SF remarkably close to earlier ideas of nineteenth-century occultism, as well as to 1970s "New Age" discourse. In all these discourses, technoscientific contents were routinely coupled with modernized repertoires of religious belief on the basis of expectations about esoteric psychic transformations that owe much to late-nineteenth-century popular renderings of psychology, evolutionism, and the comparative anthropology of religion.[19] There is, therefore, another history of the ways in which SF was connected to religion: a genealogy that is still being discovered and that traces this connection back to modern religious repertoires invented in the second half of the nineteenth century. This genealogy shows that the New Age conceptions of personal salvation in terms of ufology, posthumanism, and/or supernatural mental powers, even when they only emerge into the mainstream from the counterculture of the 1960s, 1970s, and 1980s, can boast a much longer modernist heritage. Mystery fiction—of which SF is a twentieth-century offspring—was one of the main transmitters of this heritage during the era of high modernism. My final and most important proposition in this chapter is therefore that SF provides one of the most important social spaces in which modern people experiment with undoing disenchantment and sacralizing the secular. To understand such secular salvation—an intellectually necessary oxymoron—we have to be prepared to recognize religion outside religious contexts. An outline of the latter will precede my sketch of how SF sacralized secular space and prepared modern people for the expectations of posthumanism that we associate with cyberpunk today.

On Religion Outside Religious Contexts

What is the social context for the foregoing propositions about the religious importance of SF? It hinges on the idea that SF transmits "religion" in nonreligious contexts. These nonreligious contexts lie, by definition, off the beaten track of religious studies. Religious studies have, for example, long ignored the more feminized domestic realms in which religious repertoires of healing, ghostly visitations, and communications with the deceased continued to flourish. Now that studies of the combinations of this heritage with exotic ethnographic knowledge and marginalized forms of Western esotericism are proliferating, they help us to understand why offshoots of mesmerism, phrenology, and Spiritualism were so often characterized by female leadership.[20]

In this chapter I am more interested in another, closely related institutionalization of religious discourses outside religion proper: the one that, in religious studies, Lawrence Moore pioneered with his *Selling God* and that, for the purposes of this discussion, one could gloss with Benedict Anderson's term "print capitalism."[21] Elsewhere I have argued that Anderson reproduced modernist ideology when he portrayed secular nationalism as replacing religion via the medium of print capitalism, but that he failed to see that print capitalism includes (as Talal Asad has also argued) "the simultaneous growth of serialized novels published in periodicals and the enormous expansion in the market for imaginative 'literature.'"[22] The mystery fiction market turned out its first bestsellers—including the earliest SF—by the end of the nineteenth century and flirted extensively with both science and modern occultism. Occultism, therefore, resembles nationalism in being a specifically modern cultural form institutionalized in—among other places—the networks of commerce.[23]

From the nineteenth century onward, mystery fiction has often (but not exclusively) focused on the masculine realms of fantastic voyages and adventures, celebrations of brainpower, and sacralizations of science. Such works first figured intrepid explorers, then mechanical engineers and scientists, while both have been succeeded by the "techies" or nerds of today's cyberpunk SF. Although the term "scientifiction" was first coined during the launch of the journal *Amazing Stories* by editor Hugo Gernsback in 1926, we should not forget that the first science to be fictionalized in the bestselling world of mystery fiction was geography: Jules Verne's *Journey to the Centre of the Earth* was, for example, shortly followed by Edward Bulwer Lytton's similar "hollow-earth" story, *The Coming Race*, the mentally enhanced race of which directly influenced the construction of Madame Blavatsky's Theosophy.[24] The two first bestsellers in the English publishing market, *King Solomon's Mines* (1885) and *She* (1887), both penned by H. Rider Haggard, are based on similar "fantastic voyages." Together with books such as Arthur Conan Doyle's *The Lost World* (1912), such works turned contemporary field scientists—archaeologists, anthropologists, geographers—into adventure heroes long before the torch of fictionalizing science was handed over to physicists, engineers, or computer hackers.[25] Additionally, such works provided the first popular presentations of telepathy, time travel, and the technological sublime.[26]

I therefore want to suggest that, starting in the late nineteenth century, print capitalism provided another, usually more masculinized trajectory of popular religious modernity, paralleling and contributing to the feminized domestic spheres of spiritualism and occultism. If, in contrast with the overwhelmingly female readership and attendance of New Age texts and events, many of the utopias and salvations imagined in contemporary cyberculture are a kind of "New Age for men," then SF seems to have played a central role in its construction, most of all by providing an alternative nonreligious institution of transmitting religious messages in modern society.[27]

But what exactly is nonreligious about SF as a form of print capitalism? As Talal Asad has shown, we should never take the secular for granted. Instead we must subject it and its ideological reconstruction, secularism, to cultural analysis.[28] Following from this we might ask, What does it mean to package religion in mystery novels and sell it through commercial institutions? A sociocultural analysis can answer this question in three ways: first, by identifying how the culture of commerce determines religious contents; second, by researching how SF works translate into the lives of people—both in terms of power relationships and of modes of identification and expectation—as sociocultural capital in the broadest sense; and third, by recognizing the specific ways religion is located in a field that is not specifically religious—that is to say, a field that is already shaped as secular.

Institutionalizing religious content in commercial networks implies that religious contents become subject to relations implying forms of contract and voluntary choice. It also implies that religious differences can be made subject to measures of abstract equivalence and that religious contents can be turned, through commodification, into a private possession. In SF texts, as in modern occultism, one therefore often finds the corresponding arguments that one can (or must) decide for oneself what religious message to accept; that all religions can be treated as equal; and that merchandising and proselytizing are essentially similar and obstruct free individual choice. These arguments indicate a consciousness of the secular conditions of individual transaction that inhere in this form of transmitting religious content. As such they are a symptom of the contradictions and paradoxes that characterize a world where spirituality is necessarily mediated by commercial materialism. Yet, while these observations seem to be true at the level of ideology or hegemony, they are based on the original abstraction of a market model: individual person-to-person transactions from actual social relationships.[29]

In order to study such abstractions of hegemonic notions in social practice, social theorists such as Theodor Adorno often fell back on the idea of overarching commercial powers that are said to contextualize the consumer's use of religious contents, making his or her choice subject to a "culture industry." Indeed, it may not be an exaggeration to say that SF and occultism are together responsible for a large part of consumer society's bestselling industries. This can lead, on the one hand, to the neofunctionalist perspective that says such religious contents can only be forms of false consciousness, self-deception, or misrecognition of the powers that wield instrumental rationality.[30] On the other hand, the popularity of SF and occult literature might also indicate a situation in which their mystical assets are used as tactical counters to the powers-that-be, whose secularist interests dominate the commercial world.[31] Again, the contradictions of mediating spirituality through materialism lie at the core of these lines of thinking. But how do such contradictions manifest themselves? How do SF works translate into SF lives?

An ethnographic perspective—one that not only notes the modern shape of dominant ideals, but also asks how these ideals are being put to work in everyday life and popular culture—may turn out to be indispensable, but, in the case of the study of SF, it is unfortunately rare. Two of these rare examples are Christopher Roth's study of ufologists and Tom Wolfe's much older journalistic account of the "techie" side of the emerging counterculture.[32] They support the conclusion one can draw from another critical account of SF popular culture: Vivian Sobchak's seminal study of early SF film.[33] I interpret Sobchak as highlighting what happens once one studies SF as popular culture rather than as literature. She shows that the initial attitude toward SF film by writers as well as critics was based in revulsion toward its vulgarity and its perceived association with superstition and horror or a fear of technology.[34] As I hope to show below, this revulsion mirrors the attitude of Golden Age SF writers toward contemporary popular renderings of the UFO visits and forms of telepathy that they themselves wrote about and that present-day critics are still loath to abandon, precisely because popularized SF seems to violate the distinction between utopian design, history, and technology on the one hand and religion and magic on the other.[35] Instead of maintaining such a distinction, Sobchak argues that "we need a definition of science fiction which gladly recognizes these hybrid forms as part of a spectrum which moves—on a sliding scale—from the sacred to the profane."[36] This is necessary because this sliding scale is itself the social context. It determines how and when people position themselves in social practice vis-à-vis the ideals authorized by the culture industry, among other things, through its most influential writers and critics.

I partly employ Sobchak's perspective of acknowledging—à la Malinowski—the universal presence of religion, magic, and science in all societies.[37] However, I want to add one more line of thought. If commerce is the institution through which SF's preoccupation with religion manifests itself, we should also acknowledge that commerce itself is a symptom of a society in which secular relationships have become self-evident to the extent of being often unquestioned. Even if Sobchak recognizes that modern people live their everyday lives in social contexts that are partly determined by a sliding scale from the sacred to the profane, this does not deny that modernist conceptualizations of the secular have irrevocably changed the scale itself. While acknowledging that religion and magic do indeed figure universally, it is equally important to ask what specific shape they acquire in societies that have gone through different and sometimes even contradictory secularization processes. If I succeed in showing that SF has distinct ways of resacralizing what Asad has identified as the main categories of the secular—nature, history, and the human—I am also on the way to showing that there is good reason to regard SF as a religious force *even in nonreligious contexts* such as modern commercial transactions. In turn this insight allows us to grasp what is specific about modern religion (or modern magic) and, moreover, helps to explain why modern religious repertoires—in SF, but also in New Age contexts—often exert their force by strenuously denying that they are religious.[38]

SF exerts its religious force at least partly by conveying a "sense of wonder"—the "amazing" and "astounding" stories of the title of this chapter—that generates awe for the secular and transsecular powers its imagination conjures up. Awe, Robert Marrett argued, is at the core of religious emotion even before it gets articulated in clear-cut conceptions (such as "ghost" or "spirit"). Awe brings humans into a personal emotional relationship with "superior powers" even before any conception of those powers has been formulated.[39] Awe (or the "amazing") is something "not so much thought out as danced out": only when it is moralized (as good or bad, or *mana* or *tabu*), can it "become [religion's] essence."[40] The sense of wonder evoked in countless SF novels is the "raw material" of religious emotion. The choreography of amazing and astounding powers pirouetting around moral feelings takes place, for example, when SF sacralizes space.[41]

What Is "Amazing"? On Sacralizing Secular Space

What does SF present as amazing, astounding, or wonderful? On the surface of SF image and text, we often see awesome technology, the proverbial bug-eyed monster, or artificially reproduced human life. These sources of wonder have been abstractly defined as technological, mental, racial, or environmental novelties (or "nova") that effect cognitive estrangement discussed in a discourse of possibility ("what if. . . .").[42] In relation to religious discourse, horror, or fantasy, however, the SF genre's potential to *transform or transgress* the limits of secular nature, history, or humanity seems particularly distinctive. SF seems to be based on a *double* articulation of awe and wonder: awe for the powers of the secular (the limits that nature, history, or human capacity impose on the future) is coupled with wonder at those supernatural, suprahistorical, or superhuman powers that, for better or worse, threaten to overcome the human protagonists of these stories.

This fundamental relationship between SF and the secular (and therefore the religious) was brought home to me by an unusually religious and somewhat marginal SF novel—C. S. Lewis's *Out of the Silent Planet*.[43] This novel is remarkable neither for its plot nor for its nova: it recounts the abduction of a philologist from Earth by the spaceship of two fellow Earthmen in order to surrender him to the unknown designs of an alien race on Mars. Its somewhat heavy-handed Christian message, however, makes it unusual. While the chief character (the abductee) initially fears the *horror vacui* of space, he later experiences his trip to Mars as a form of bliss: as an immersion into a life-giving radiance. On Mars he finds out that Earth is the only planet no longer ruled by the disembodied, omnipresent, faster-than-light intelligence that makes sure every other planet's races cohabit in harmony. This is because Earth's secular technoscience has turned it into a "silent" planet, one that no longer speaks to the other spirits filling the universe. With a trick of realism common to many mystery stories, a postscript reveals that the main character has conspired with the writer, C. S. Lewis, to attempt "to effect" in its readers "a change-over from the conception of Space to the conception of Heaven."[44] Precisely because it stands out as unusually explicit in its attempt to communicate a religious message, Lewis's book therefore throws into sharp relief the fact that most SF writers live in a post-Newtonian world of secularized, empty space, dotted only sparsely by matter and force.

While Lewis's 1946 attempt to reconvert SF readers to a belief in "Heaven" can hardly be judged successful, his unusual critique of the conception of secular space highlights some of the fundamental features of space as it rules early-twentieth-century SF. The Newtonian billiard-ball universe is perhaps the most powerful and certainly one of the most successful conceptions of "nature" to ground the discourse of science as it emerged in the Enlightenment. Secular nature in the form of "outer space" presupposes almost infinite distances across a silent emptiness, imposing fundamental limits to movement, velocity, and communication. Lewis's book also indicates the two most important ways by which SF overcomes these limitations: either by the physical motion of the spaceship or by the faster-than-light or immediate psychic communication of telepathy. Even more, in the final sentences of the book, Lewis suggests that, in the absence of space travel, it is only time travel (in this case, through the traditional literary practice of rediscovering the truth about the "heavens" in "the old books"—that is, the Bible) that will teach us about the planets.[45] Thus, Lewis's book displays, in a nutshell, what I think are the most crucial features of science fiction literature: the attempt to overcome the secular limits of nature, the human mind, and history, the three basic categories of the secular identified by Asad. SF plays with the various forms of near-instantaneous communication— mechanical velocities faster than light, telepathy, teleportation, or time travel—that promise to overcome these secular limits. At the same time, Lewis makes clear that these options are situated on what Sobchak called a "sliding scale": some being closer to religion than others, even to such an extent that Lewis's own assumptions about planetary intelligences seem to have crossed a border into religious fantasy.

Lewis also shows that these means of overcoming the limits of the secular are by no means unequivocally positive. In the novel the scientist who built the spaceship did so only to allow humans to destructively colonize outer space, thus portraying the scientific conquest of space as inherently dangerous to the harmonious life of the radiant beings that populate "the heavens."[46] Since Jules Verne's fantastic voyage to the moon, SF literature has more often than not portrayed the scientific overcoming of the secular limits of nature, history, and humanity in terms of human advancement. Yet H. G. Wells' 1898 story of the attack by Martians in *The War of the Worlds* shows that these same technologies can also spell the near-demise of humanity.[47] In this respect these late-nineteenth-century novels resemble the ufology of the 1950s, which also juxtaposes benevolent extraterrestrial visitors with evil invaders and abductors; or, subsequently, to present-day cyberpunk juxtapositions of optimistic disembodiment, as in the case of Rudy Rucker's *White Light*, with dehumanizing dystopias, such as the one depicted in the film *The Matrix*.[48] SF constructs its own "heavens" by overcoming secular space, but it simultaneously produces corresponding "hells."

This serves to show that SF sacralizes the secular in a number of ways—if, that is, we are ready to adopt Emile Durkheim's insight that the sacred is opposed to the profane rather than the secular.[49] The secular, in fact, becomes a *condition* of such sacralization because the awesomeness of the forbidding physical, temporal, or mental limits that secular space offers can only be overcome by an even more forbidding or miraculous intervention. Even if SF is a "discourse of possibility" (as Darko Suvin had it),[50] its question "what if. . . ?" cannot but build on the extraordinary *limitations* (the impossibilities) that characterize secular nature, history, and humanity. It turns these everyday limits of the secular from profane fact into a kind of hell (or *tabu*) or heaven (or *mana*)—a *moralized* realm—without losing the awesomeness of their secular nature. It is only on the basis of the secular that SF can produce new representations of salvation and perdition—a sacralization that occurs regardless of whether these representations remain mere commodities of an entertainment industry or become everyday forms of modern belief and ritual. The sacralizations of SF are impossible without a dialectic of secularization and sacralization.[51]

Arthur C. Clarke's *Childhood's End* clearly shows this principle; it is the story of the coming to Earth of the Overlords, who end global wars and poverty, and who herald "a completely secular age."[52] Moreover, by means of a kind of (time travel) television that shows the past from as far back as five thousand years ago, the Overlords use positive historical knowledge to finally convince humanity that its heritage of religious truths was mostly fantasy without empirical foundation. As it turns out, this miraculous extraterrestrial intervention—by a race that initially hides its appearance to humans because it looks like the devil—is meant to transform humanity into a new, collective telepathic race: one that can conquer space without being limited by physical travel and thus can join the "Overmind," a cosmic intelligence that directed the Overlords' intervention in the first place.

The positivism of Clarke's novel makes it far more representative of SF writing than Lewis's *Out of the Silent Planet*. Yet it also sacralizes space: it not only uses modernization theory to define a new fall (by religion) but also defines a new state of grace. It requires the spiritual transformation of humanity into a new—posthuman—race *in addition to* secular enlightenment. As such the narrative resonates heavily with late-nineteenth-century Theosophy (as I shall elaborate below). The secular salvations of SF, therefore, take place in a dialectic of secularization and sacralization *even* when—paradoxically—religion spells original sin and disbelief spells redemption.

The examples discussed so far—of Bester, Lewis, and Clarke—indicate two of the main SF tropes by which the secular is sacralized: outer-space technology and the psychic powers of telepathy, telekinesis, and teleportation. I shall discuss these tropes in the next two sections.

The Aesthetics of Scale: Future History and the Technological Sublime

One of the most obvious sacralizations that SF exerts on our conceptions of the secular is a transformation of the sense of awe rendered by the "technological sublime." Globalized to a considerable extent by the typically North American structure of feeling of "the machine in the garden," the image of awesome technology juxtaposed with primitive or rural nature drew upon colonial tropes of impressing the native by superior technology or neo-Luddite visions of a technologically driven apocalypse.[53] But while writers like Thoreau and Melville geared the awesome powers of technology to overcome secular limits to the changes that technology was actually making in the historical landscape, the SF version of the technological sublime was placed in the future.[54] Its optimism about technological advancement, now redirected to "hard science," is most graphically represented by both the pulp and the Golden Age phases of SF magazine publishing and by the "space opera" in particular.[55]

Space opera featured vast spaceships that hurtle through infinity to bring their hero-engineers to their destiny.[56] This "approximation of Miltonic sublimity" was defined by the man often regarded as its originator, E. E. "Doc" Smith, in terms of an "aesthetics of scale."[57] The range of literary and imaginative consequences of space opera's scalar dramatization of vastness and infinity is perhaps best conveyed by the opening passage of Smith's first novel, *The Skylark of Space*, even when its point of departure is not outer space, but the much more banal scientific laboratory:

> *Petrified with astonishment*, Richard Seaton stared after the copper steambath upon which, a moment before, he had been electrolyzing his solution of "X," the unknown metal. As soon as he had removed the beaker with its precious contents, the heavy bath had jumped endwise from under his hand *as though it were alive*. It had flown with *terrific* speed over the table, smashing a dozen reagent-bottles on its way, and straight out through the open window. Hastily setting the beaker down, he seized his binoculars and focused them upon the flying bath, which now, to the unaided vision, was *merely a speck in the distance*. Through the glass he saw that it did not fall to the ground, but continued on in a straight line, its *rapidly diminishing size* alone showing the *enormous velocity* at which it was moving. It grew smaller and smaller. In a few seconds it disappeared.[58]

The emphases added convey how this representation of a technical discovery (aided by a mysterious metal) of a power capable of propelling a spaceship away from earth at incredible velocities relies on the aesthetics of scale and sublimity. This is replicated in the description of the Skylark, the spaceship that results from Seaton's initial experiment: "Six *tremendous* fabricated columns radiated outward; branching in *maximum-strength* design out into the hull. The floor was *heavily upholstered*."[59] The story subsequently turns to the abduction of Seaton's beloved by an adversary engineer, leading him to chase them both into outer space and subsequently encountering a different race. Although in this part of the story some of the (female) protagonists are "awed by the immensity of the universe" itself, the general message is nevertheless clear: it is the overwhelming power of the new machine, engineered by men, that does the hyperbolic job in the narrative.[60]

Space opera is a genre analogous to (and, as a term, derived from) "soap opera," and this signposts the fact that the genre is often regarded as a literarily inferior, "machines-over-people" formula.[61] As with soap opera, the pulp fiction provenance of the space opera genre does not make it any less popular.[62] Whatever space opera's genealogy, it should not distract us from the fact that some of the genre's major features—the future technological sublime in particular—have become basic to SF in general. Perhaps the most celebrated series of novels from the Golden Age of SF, Isaac Asimov's *Foundation* sequence (originally published from 1942 onward in serial form in *Astounding Science Fiction*), displays a set of tropes characteristic of the space opera genre. For instance, Asimov's narrative opens with a description of the moment of arrival of a young scholar from a distant rural planet at Trantor, the planet at the center of the Galactic Empire:

> This was Trantor! The air seemed a little thicker here, the gravity a bit greater, than on his home planet of Synnax, but he would get used to that. He wondered if he could get used to its *immensity*. Debarkation Building was *tremendous*. The roof was almost *lost in the heights*. He could see no opposite wall; just men and desks and converging floor till it *faded out in haze*.[63]

The immensity of space travel—impossible, as I argued in the previous section, without the Newtonian secularization of space—is an absolute (in the sense of "universal") backdrop of space opera, even when this immensity is relocated in imaginary places like Trantor. Writers such as Asimov and Clarke, however, developed an alternative way to exploit this sense of awe. They not only fell back on metaphors of "tremendous" scale, but also employed narrative sequences that focused first on individual human protagonists, only to dwarf them by jumping in the next story or chapter to a development centuries later and light-years away, in which the original hero of the story has already been forgotten or historically stereotyped.[64] The shifts from one protagonist to the other signal a kind of desubjectivation of the narrative—the characters become, in effect, pawns or patients (rather than heroic agents) of a larger evolutionary ("future-history") sequence. In later space operas the narrative device of dispersing action along differently placed protagonists indicates that the desubjectivation implicit in the aesthetics of the large scale of space runs into limits once faced with the literary need to produce identifiable protagonists.[65]

However, while Asimov's *Foundation* and *Galactic Empire* novels certainly were "space opera on a grand scale," the technological sublime (which I take here as the initial twentieth-century mode by which SF sacralized the space of nature through [near-] instantaneous communication) was not always the most important narrative feature of SF's Golden Age in the 1940s and 1950s—that is, if we understand "technological" to be restricted to machines and ships.[66] *Foundation* starts out predominantly as a modernization narrative in the typical SF style of future nostalgia: the story of how a typically modern, technological society established itself at the edge of the galaxy to avoid being swallowed up in the demise of the (increasingly religiously retarded) Galactic Empire. But the rest of the narrative of the first *Foundation* sequence is about the surpassing of natural space (and the limits of the human body) by extraordinary *mental* powers.[67] At first Asimov concentrates on the mathematical predictions of "psychohistory": a kind of social engineering supported by quantified measurement that predicts the downfall of the Galactic Empire. The subsequent stories move into an account of how the leaders of the "Second Foundation" (whose mathematical insight has turned them into psychic manipulators) must combat the disruption of the mathematical model of the future of psychohistory by an unexpected mental mutant, "The Mule." As such Asimov's early *Foundation* sequence heralded a second form of the sacralization of secular space: a sacralization precipitated by the extraordinary powers of telepathy.[68] This relation of "technological" SF to the "soft" imagination of psychic powers was, as we shall see, complex. While it often tried to deny its provenance in forms of popular religion by its emphasis on "hard" mathematics and experimental psychology— and hence, profane technology—it nevertheless remained thoroughly implicated in occultist and proto-New Age conceptions.

Posthumanism in the 1950s: The Golden Age of Scientific Telepathy

When he introduces "jaunting" at the start of *The Stars My Destination*, Alfred Bester specifies that someone who wants to learn to use this innate human capacity requires, first, the development of the faculties of visualization and concentration, but above all, "faith": "the slightest doubt would block the mind-thrust necessary for teleportation."[69] Anyone who has read a description of the average New Age ritual directed at unleashing "the hidden potential of the self" will recognize these three requirements: visualization, concentration, and faith are basic to a majority of Western esoteric ways of imagining a release from existing conventions in order to realize the "true self."[70] What is really interesting is that these requirements were written in 1956 in an SF novel at least twenty years before they came into everyday use in New Age circles. Did SF prefigure New Age discourse? Or, put differently, has SF helped to transmit the contents of the nineteenth-century reinvention of Western esotericism to its 1980s New Age descendant?[71] I think the answer is affirmative, provided we recognize that, unlike in the 1880s or 1980s, the transmission of occultist ideas in the 1950s took a peculiarly positivist form.

A brief list of some of the major novels of the Golden Age of SF can give some idea of the prominence of the theme of extraordinary mental powers in SF: telepathy, mind-reading, teleportation, and telekinesis. I already mentioned the central narrative importance of telepathy and mind-control at a distance in the work of Isaac Asimov (the *Foundation* sequence, but also *Pebble in the Sky*).[72] Likewise, we have noted the evolution toward a posthuman collective mind that travels intergalactically in Clarke's *Childhood's End*, as well as in Alfred Bester's descriptions of a telepathic police force (in *The Demolished Man*) and teleportation (in *The Stars My Destination*).[73] In addition, we find the theme of extraordinary mental powers heralding a new breed of humans in James Blish's *ESPer* as well as in A. E. van Vogt's *SLAN* and *The World of Null-A*.[74] Both Blish and van Vogt refer to the popularity during the 1940s of Alfred Korzybski's ideas about a new "non-Aristotelian" (or in van Vogt's terms, "null-A") way of using the human brain and its superhuman capacities, making telepathy and teleportation plausible through a "scientific" mode of reasoning.[75] This was "posthumanism" long before it became a currently fashionable topic of discussion among present-day intellectuals.[76]

Korzybski's thought was only one of the channels through which, at the time, a "hard SF" type of reasoning could be employed to give new credence to telepathy and teleportation and thus create a new kind of posthuman subject. Asimov, for his part, initially presupposed a mathematicization of psychology and sociology to make "psychohistory" possible, even if he went from psychohistory to mind-reading and mind-modifying at a distance in the rest of the Foundation trilogy. In *Pebble in the Sky*, it is an as-yet experimental machine (in a future laboratory) that produces the mental change that generates mind-bending powers at a distance. Clarke's *Childhood's End* achieved a similar effect, but did so by describing an inevitable process of evolution (guided by the extraterrestrial intelligence of the "Overmind"). The posthumanism of the 1950s generates the plausibility of occult psychic powers, therefore, by applying "hard science"—i.e., the "facts" of mathematics or evolutionary biology—to psychology, sociology, and other "soft" topics.[77] The positivism of popular science is, in these works, generally opposed to the fraudulence of religion (as Clarke's *Childhood's End* and Asimov's *Foundation* amply illustrate). Contrary to the "hands-on" engineers of earlier pulp fiction technophilia or the adventurer-scientists of the late-nineteenth-century "fantastic voyages" genre, the esoteric scientist is the hero of the 1940s and 1950s SF imagination.

Interestingly, many contemporary SF stories display this positivism by an overt disdain for the publicly known manifestations of the heritage of Western esotericism and modern occultism. James Blish tells of an upcoming new breed of "ESPers" who fight against a group of "super-minds" who have been trying to keep people ignorant of their innate telepathic and teleportation capacities through the dissemination of "mumbo-jumbo" (that is, faked religion). In his quest to discover his real (liberating) mental capacities, the protagonist of the story runs up against "astrology, hollow-earth notions, Lemuria, pyramidology, phrenology, Vedanta, black magic, Koresanity, Theosophy, Rosicrucianism, crystalline atoms, lunar farming, Atlantis, and a long list of similar asininities."[78] Similarly, in another story, an almost too skeptical journalist and a seemingly occultist professor encounter the former owner of an esoteric bookshop who presents them with "an amazing compost of lost-continentism, the Ten Tribes, anti-fluoridation, vegetarianism, homeopathic medicine, organic farming, astrology, flying saucers, and the prose-poems of Khalil Gibran."[79] The supreme SF positivist, Arthur C. Clarke, caps this attitude of disdain toward the genealogy of New Age by dismissing flying saucers. In *A Fall of Moondust*, he argues that earth people might have believed, out of uncertainty, that their planet would be destroyed during the nuclear age unless some Flying Saucer civilization intervened to make things right. But the "dawn of the space age" dispelled all these irrational visions and—apart from a "lunatic fringe" that persisted in believing in flying saucers and interventions from outer space—restored humanity's faith in its limitless possibility to expand into the space beyond.[80]

Yet, if Clarke dismissed the lunacy of flying saucers in this 1961 novel, he made extraterrestrial invasion necessary to posthuman life in *Childhood's End*. There, science and séance merge: before the coming of the Overlords, psychic experimentation by humans was premature. To prevent human occultist practices from disturbing the evolution of humanity toward its mature transgalactic form, the Overmind sent in the Overlords as guides. Thus Clarke ridiculed the flying saucers cult in one book, while providing a closely related posthuman evolutionist vision in another.

The one SF writer known more for his contribution to New Age than for his science fiction—L. Ron Hubbard, the father of Dianetics and Scientology—does not seem to mention his New Age experiments in his science fiction stories. But this may be because he regarded "spiritualism, mythology, magic, divination, the supernatural, and many other fields of that type" as belonging to the sphere of fantasy rather than "real SF."[81] The fact that A. E. van Vogt became a committed Dianetics follower suggests that van Vogt's own "hard SF" version of telepathy was in fact quite compatible with Hubbard's Scientology, and indeed Scientology can at least partly be seen as a kind of positivism turned into religion.[82] However, this did not prevent an author like James Blish to include Dianetics in the list of proto–New Age follies mentioned above.[83]

The clue to the Golden Age SF writers' paradoxical attitude toward religion and telepathy—based on their desire to turn the "soft" social relationship of narrative into "hard" mathematical or evolutionary fact—can be found in this contradiction between, on the one hand, the limits of the awesome powers of nature, history, and the human, and on the other, the imagination required to go beyond these limits. But there is only a finite stock of imaginative resources by which to transgress the boundaries of secular power, especially when such resources should appeal to a more public or popular sphere. It seems no coincidence, therefore, that shortly after the group of Golden Age SF authors came into print capitalism's limelight (via John W. Campbell's journal *Astounding Science Fiction*), a new editor of *Amazing Stories*, Raymond Palmer, "co-founded much of UFO lore" in 1943 on the basis of the "paranoid"—and very Theosophical—"delusions" of Richard Shaver.[84] Modeling "stim rays" on the basis of Bulwer Lytton's and Blavatsky's *vril*, Palmer and Shaver's *I Remember Lemuria* transposed Theosophy's conception of sequences of (mentally) superior races to the idea of extraterrestrials fertilizing a series of Earth races with its superior intelligence (culminating in the most famous account of all, von Däniken's *Chariots of the Gods*).[85] Palmer and Shaver are the immediate sources and predecessors, not only of the binge of "contactee" extraterrestrial stories associated with George Adamski and the amateur anthropologist George Hunt Williamson between 1953 and 1959, but also in the "abductee" stories of alien races experimenting on humans that would later come to dominate a peculiar (and large) section of New Age fantasies. Christopher Roth's first attempt at a historical ethnography of such visitations underlines, most of all, that we are here dealing with the reinvention of humanism along Theosophical racialist and evolutionist lines. In the words of one of the extraterrestrials, "We are men [sic] like yourselves. We are only far ahead of you in progression."[86]

The "antinomian agnosticism" of ufology is, at least in its *social* spirit, close to the antinomian "cybergnosis" we identified elsewhere.[87] What is more important, however, is that the lists of "asininities" ridiculed by Blish and Kornbluth above—which include astrology, hollow-earth notions, Lemuria, phrenology, Vedanta, pyramidology, Theosophy, lost-continentism, the Ten Tribes, vegetarianism, organic farming, and Atlantis, to name just the most prominent—perfectly replicate the spiritual heritage of late-nineteenth-century occultism. While the hard science of early, technologically sublime SF seemed to distance itself from such pseudo-science, occultism was once more taken up by ufology from the mid-1940s onward. *Amazing Stories*, therefore, seems to have presented itself, starting around 1943, as a somewhat subaltern transmitter of spiritual or modern religious content in comparison to the—I would say alternatively religious—boost of telepathy by the Golden Age SF authors of the rival journal *Astounding Science Fiction*. The latter—Blish, Kornbluth and Clarke, among others—ridiculed Theosophy and the flying saucer cult (at the same time that these were popularized by Adamski, Williamson, and others). Yet Blish, Kornbluth, and Clarke also established their own transgressions and transformations of secular power, as if they wanted to counter the rival positivisms of Theosophical and proto–New Age posthumanist evolutionism. But if so, were they successful? This requires us to look at New Age, the emerging counterculture, and its relation to cyberpunk SF.

The First Subway to Heaven

It is tempting to date a shift toward a "softer" approach to hard science in SF with the publication of its most quintessentially proto–New Age novel, Robert Heinlein's *Stranger in a Strange Land*.[88] The story of Valentine Michael Smith, a human child raised by Martians and therefore possessing the Martian capacity for telepathy and teleportation, not only marks the revival of interest in sciences (such as [linguistic] anthropology) that had lost popularity among SF writers since the early twentieth century, it also inaugurated a feminization of the genre exemplified by Mike Smith as an unusually meek hero. Mike Smith preaches a Martian creed of peace, free love, tolerance, and astounding mental powers: a combination that would give the novel a cult status in the 1960s and 1970s. Its central (proto–New Age) message that all religions are true, and that "Thou art God," emerges from a prolonged discussion about religion that takes places throughout the book.[89] Mike's martyrdom at the end of the book gives it a Christian taste, and Heinlein, usually more martially inclined, cannot resist taking a swipe at astrologists (associating them with stage magicians). But the reception of the book alone allows it to be interpreted as a turning point from "hard telepathy" to soft New Age.

I base this retrospective judgment on one of the most interesting ethnographies of the way in which secular salvation was sought (and, at least to some extent, found) in mid-modernity. Tom Wolfe's *The Electric Kool-Aid Acid Test* recounts how, in the mid 1960s, a small group of visionaries (the Merry Pranksters) led by novelist Ken Kesey achieved a consciousness of a substitute god ("Cosmo," "The Management," or the "Overmind") on the basis of drug-induced experiences, mainly with LSD.[90] In one of his first efforts at "new journalism"—that is, "to re-create the mental atmosphere or subjective reality" of the Pranksters—Wolfe dotted his account with the word "grok(king)," signifying a deep experiential understanding of a reality beyond words, that was shared by the Pranksters as well as, at a remove, the whole "flower power," electric-guitar, countercultural scene that was to follow from the Pranksters' first initiatives.[91] To *grok* is the single word from Martian to be explored in depth in Heinlein's *Stranger in a Strange Land*.[92] Wolfe explicitly refers to Heinlein's novel only once, but by saying that the book's "vibrations" emanated from the Pranksters' own bookshelf, binding Mike Smith and the Pranksters "by some inexplicable acausal connecting bond."[93]

The Merry Pranksters were, indeed, devoutly SF: Clarke's *Childhood's End* also figured prominently on their bookshelf, and they often defined their LSD-induced ecstasy in terms of participation in the "Overmind." Ken Kesey's attempts to shock the world out of lethargy and toward liberation, in addition to being inspired by Heinlein's "grokking" and Clarke's "Overmind," talked of being "on other planets," "on a spaceship," in another "time-warp," of sailing the "intergalactic" seas, or embodying a "Space Man."[94] This shows an often forgotten part of the genealogy of modern New Age religion: the fact that the Merry Pranksters were not your usual New Age Buddhists "returning to nature," but a spiritual movement for whom salvation was very much *technologically* enhanced—both chemically (with LSD and other drugs and Day-Glo paint) and electrically (guitars, amplifiers, and much more). Yet Wolfe argues that, in the end (by 1966), the technological "summer of love" initiated by the Pranksters succumbed largely to the Buddhist-inspired, nature-loving conservatism of New Age guru Timothy Leary and his followers.[95] This techno-savvy, SF-induced New Age religion missed, in Kesey's words, "the first subway to heaven."[96]

Is Cyberpunk Really Different?

Ken Kesey and the Merry Pranksters, and their roots in earlier SF literature, serve as a reminder of the fact—referred to in the introduction to this chapter—that the fusion of religion and technology often attributed to cyberpunk SF does not mark a clean break with earlier modern cultural forms. It is, therefore, useful to distinguish some ways in which cyberpunk SF does or does not emulate the sacralization of the secular characteristic of earlier SF. In much cyberpunk SF, technology often seems to lose its sublimity and become banal, even profane at times. Often cyberpunk does not exalt technology, but on the contrary, unmasks the technological amazement once produced by the SF authors of the 1940s and 1950s as "technolatry."[97] If we take our cue from the final scene of cyberpunk writer John Shirley's *Eclipse*—when guerrillas confront an evil Fascist mercenary corporation on top of the Arc de Triomphe—sublime technology is the enemy, resisted by a subversive rock-guitar warrior.[98] Here established secular powers are confronted by a countercultural (rock-'n'-drugs) prank, similar to the kind performed by Kesey and the Merry Pranksters.

Indeed, cyberpunk has clear affinities with the Pranksters' electrically amplified reinvention of religious fervor.[99] Cyberpunk, however, is much more "noir" than the style invented by the Bay Area technophile hippies. This can be at least partly attributed to the influence of "New Wave" SF in the 1960s and 1970s on cyberpunk and its tendency to depict a post-apocalyptic world destroyed by awesome technology. New Wave SF objectified the countercultural suspicion of technologically enhanced salvation, whether in the post-nuclear urban hell of Samuel Delany's *Dahlgren*, the technological alienation of Philip K. Dick's *Do Androids Dream of Electric Sheep?* or the impending environmental apocalypse in John Brunner's *Stand on Zanzibar*.[100] The dreams of technological advancement that inspired the Golden Age writers gave way, in much of this 1960s and 1970s wave of SF, to the destruction of nature and the human. The reemergence of some measure of positive appreciation of technological salvation in SF mostly had to await the neo-liberal 1980s and the emergence of cyberpunk—although cyberpunk has always maintained a strong tendency toward the "noir" and the interpretation of cyberspace as an "underworld."[101]

If cyberpunk is much less naïve about technology than the SF of the 1930s or the 1950s, it also seems to be more casual about religion than was the case with SF's high-modernist predecessors. Rather than opposing organized religion as something inimical to technoscientific salvation, cyberpunk is interested in the coping strategies of a *"street* religion" such as voodoo or in the seamless connection between a virus, a language, religion, the afterlife, and advertising.[102] In fact, cyberpunk SF's most significant contribution to reinventions of our religious repertoire is caused by the translation of the cyberpunk novels into a new popular culture of hacking, especially through the notion of "uploading" consciousness to the realm for which William Gibson coined the term "cyberspace." As is well known, Gibson's "space cowboy" hero Case became a role model for a majority of hackers after the publication of *Neuromancer* in 1984, even if the book's general message about computer technology was far more pessimistic and *noir* than most of the utopias cherished by hacktivists.[103]

Yet the genealogy of twentieth-century SF should make us skeptical about claims to the novelty of cyberpunk fiction. Gibson's accounts of cyberspace in *Neuromancer* and other books still tend to describe a "colourless void" across which unfold "lattices of logic," an "endless beach," "towers," or, I think most commonly, data stacked like "one big neon city," despite Gibson's invocation of cyberspace as a "space that wasn't space."[104] In *True Names*, the "datasphere" is a straightforward copy of the castles and swamps of Ursula Le Guin's *Wizard of Earthsea*, a fantasy novel that inspired Vinge to write the story.[105] In other words, by visualizing an alternative space for their readers, cyberpunk writers rarely fell back on anything but a Newtonian conception of a natural emptiness filled with objects and forces, with the significant difference that their "space" was usually urban. But the superhuman "space cowboys" of cyberpunk SF flitted across space instantaneously, much in the same way that Gully Foyle and the other telepaths did in earlier SF novels. And of course, just as it is impossible to find a visual image of telepathy or teleportation on an SF book cover, it seems impossible to visually represent cyberspace except two-dimensionally, which, in our current imagination, is not "natural" (that is, three-dimensional) enough.[106] Many cyberpunk writers (such as Bruce Sterling or Vernor Vinge) have recourse to the classical scale of outer space found in the space opera genre: Newton's vast emptiness, through which tiny specks of matter move, whether digitally enhanced or not.[107] In this sense cyberpunk SF does not have, to use Mark Dery's words, the "escape velocity" to break out of the orbit of the modern secular world any more than other cyber-technological fantasies do.[108]

Conclusion: SF, Religion, and Technology

What does this partial genealogy tell us about the relationship between science fiction and religion and, more broadly, about the relationship between science and technology and religion in the modern world? First, the least we can say is that it confirms Vivian Sobchak's conclusion that SF is one of those cultural realms in which modern people discuss the relationship between science and technology on the one hand and magic and religion on the other, and where they reinvent these categories in order to fit their own experiences. Contrary to the expectations of the theory of modernization, this does not lead to a straightforward demise of religion and magic for the greater glory of science and technology. Instead, the rise of a popular scientific consciousness implies reinventions of religion and magic that are sometimes made to contradict and sometimes made to support existing notions of magic and religion, and in other instances even to introduce novel forms of magic and religion closely akin to those of modern occultism and New Age. Moreover, once one shifts one's attention from the "high" literary canon of SF to include films and other popular cultural forms (such as ufologists' cult activity or "hippiedom"), the scientistic aura of SF turns out to have transmitted a large number of those new forms of religion through the decidedly nonreligious carriers of print capitalism. While they may be less "public" than established science and official religion, these religions outside religious contexts are nevertheless public, at least in the sense that their mode of publicity takes the form of a bestselling publishing market.

Second, we need to reflect on the nature of these religious repertoires. Modern occultism was fed by the fictionalization of sciences and technologies belonging to geography, anthropology, and archaeology—modes of scientific travel, new and comparative ethnographic knowledge—and this in itself showed how modern modes of communication and travel helped to reinvent religious repertoires. This reinvention of religion was reinforced by new technologies promising to radically reduce physical and imagined distances (such as the telegraph and the photograph).[109] The emergence of the technological sublime, and especially its popularization through pulp fiction SF, was therefore continuous with an earlier form of time-space compression epitomized in this chapter by the space opera's overcoming of secular space through instantaneous communication. The words that could shape this overcoming of secular space in popular consciousness had to come from religious repertoires, for modern humans had little else with which to conceive of such new experiences. At the same time, in modern societies, the new fusions of religion and technology achieved by SF (and other discursive genres) could not but be based on the secular—both in terms of their awe for the secular limits of nature and also for the technological means to overcome them. Secularization in this sociocultural field does not mean that religion is marginalized vis-à-vis technological rationality, but that religious repertoires are based on and incorporate secular reasoning.

Finally, we should take into account the fact that this incorporation of the secular into modern religious repertoires takes a number of different forms that, I feel, have not been sufficiently studied. In this chapter I have ignored at least two main forms of sacralizing the secular in SF: robotics and the computer, and time travel and its related issues of alternative histories. Both are important, among other things, for the interpretation of cyberpunk SF (in the sense that cyberpunk cannot be understood without the question of nonhuman intelligence or of computerized total recall). This is perhaps the most important lesson we can draw from the conclusion in the previous section: that cyberpunk SF is not as novel and distinct from previous fictionalizations of science and technology as originally expected. Futurism—the expectation that things will be radically different from then/now on, on the basis of some sort of decisive change or intervention—is itself a particularly modern religious form: it can be traced to late medieval monastic imaginaries of religious utopia brought by human technological prowess and came to its full flowering when Europe started to measure "others" by means of its superior technological capacity. Futurism, therefore, derives from the Enlightenment idea that the future is malleable, but also from the model of such malleability: the invention and intervention of new technologies—a model that became particularly ubiquitous in the nineteenth century.[110] Futurism's insistence on the malleability of the future by human hands implies the secularization of history, and it is against this background that we should interpret the dialectics between the "techno-noir" of many cyberpunk SF texts and the technological optimism that characterizes its popular reinterpretation by countercultural hackers, as well as by leaders of the IT industry. It is the *sine qua non* of both policy-makers and SF writers that the future is open to fabrication and therefore open to their own interpretations of secular salvation.

SF, however, is characterized by a greater secular liberty: it can commercially explore and cultivate the possibility of taking the personal predicaments of its protagonists (the Gully Foyles, denied their place in society by the powers that be) more seriously than is the case with the big salvationist schemes of secular policy-making and governance. This, finally, connects the desire for telepathy of Golden Age SF with the optimism of those inspired by the instantaneous communications promised by cyberpunk. Both share a common desire to overcome the limits, not just of secular space, but of secular social powers, as well. However, we need a sociocultural, ethnographic analysis of SF (and thus of the modern relationship between religion and technology) to understand why religious repertoires are so important in modern, technologized societies—why amazing stories need to be told in order to make sense of these societies and to gauge their impact on people's lives.

Virtual Vodou, Actual Practice
Transfiguring the Technological
Alexandra Boutros

Haitian Vodou has a long history as a secret religion. In the French colony of Saint Domingue—until 1804, when it became the independent nation of Haiti—Vodou was practiced covertly by slaves of African origin who hid their rituals to avoid penalty under Louis XIV's *Code Noir*, which sanctioned brutal corporal punishment for the practice of any religion other than Roman Catholicism. The religion continued to be practiced largely in secret even after Haitian independence, in part because its practitioners continued to be persecuted. The "anti-superstition" campaigns waged until the 1940s by the politically influential Catholic Church are just one example of a protracted history of persecution Vodou has faced.[1]

The secrecy of Vodou has also traveled with its practitioners. As Haitians emigrated from Haiti, often fleeing political and religious persecution, they brought Haitian Vodou to North America. While Haitian migration to North America has existed at least since the advent of the Haitian nation, it has more recently come in waves that have shaped the Haitian diaspora in Canada and the United States. The first major wave of contemporary Haitian migration happened in the 1950s and 1960s and consisted of mainly upper-class urban Haitians opposed to the government of François Duvalier (1957–1971). Duvalier's dictatorship, followed by that of his son, Jean-Claude Duvalier (1971–1986), made life in Haiti increasingly difficult and untenable, compelling Haitians from the lower classes to seek refuge in North America, many arriving by boat in perilous journeys from Haiti in the period between the early 1970s and early 1980s. Race relations in the United States and Canada, combined with a particular anti-immigration attitude toward Haitian "boat people," meant that many Haitians were reticent about publicly displaying their Haitian-ness. Not surprisingly, Vodou, always closely associated with Haiti, remained an underground religion in North America.

After a long history of persecution and secrecy, Vodou has gradually become more publically visible in both Haiti and North America. The recent recognition of Vodou as an official religion in Haiti has had an impact on its public presence in that nation. At the same time media technologies have introduced this once intensely secretive religion to a global public sphere. In North America the dissemination of Haitian popular music, the production of large-scale cultural and aesthetic events such as the traveling exhibit *The Sacred Arts of Haitian Vodou* (1995) and film festival screenings of *Des Hommes et Dieux* (*Of Men and Gods*, 2002), and a growing online presence have all contributed to the public visibility of Haitian Vodou.[2] Practitioners themselves mobilize media and technology in order to educate people about Vodou, to work toward religious tolerance, and even to seek new members.

All of this public visibility brings what Wade Clark Roof has called "religious seekers" to Vodou.[3] These individuals have no genealogical or geographic connection to Haiti, the cosmological center of Vodou, and they often "find" Vodou not initially through direct contact with Vodou practitioners, but through mediated representations that instigate a desire to seek out more information. This chapter explores the intersection of digital technologies and the public visibility of Vodou. It examines not only how digital technologies are used and understood by practitioners (including newcomers to the religion), but also how the affordances of digital technologies—the possibilities and limits generated by the interaction between technology and technology use—shape manifestations of Vodou in the digital public sphere.

While Vodou may have only recently gained official public recognition, the religion has long been visible, albeit problematically, in the realm of popular culture where Vodou—or as it is more colloquially known, Voodoo—has a ubiquitous presence in films, television, kitsch, and popular music. Such images seem completely divorced from the more authentic practices, representations, and discourses of Haitian Vodou. But instances of pop Voodoo need to be critically explored in order to understand the cultural work they are performing. Many popular representations of Voodoo encode a host of disenfranchising meanings—from racist and colonialist histories to more contemporary Western anxieties about Haiti. Some representations also contain recognizable traces of Haitian Vodou. Such representations are sometimes incorporated into the spiritual journeys of newcomers to Vodou, acting as catalysts that inspire a search for more information about the religion. Negotiations of pop culture Voodoo by practitioners of the religion are thus characteristic of the constitution of Vodou in the digital public sphere.

Many religions negotiate images of themselves in popular culture. The Catholic Church, for example, used a variety of official and unofficial venues to address and manage negative representations of the church found in Dan Brown's popular novels *The Da Vinci Code* and *Angels and Demons* (as well as the subsequent blockbuster movies based on those novels).[4] Vodou, however, is not an institutionalized religion with a defining central text, nor does it possess a centralized religious institution from which official or authoritative discourses can be promulgated. Vodou is a fluid and orthopraxic religion in which multiple voices from multiple geographic centers can potentially address the constitution and the constituents of the religion. This multi-vocality maps itself onto the workings of new media, where social networking and software publishing practices seem to create an all-access public sphere. Yet any analysis of Vodou and digital technology must be attentive to not only who literally has (and who does not have) access to the digital public sphere, but also to the limits and possibilities that constitute that sphere itself. What information or representation circulates and thrives in online forums and platforms, and what disappears in the detritus of dead links and defunct web pages? More critically, what does it mean for a religion such as Vodou—already occupying a unique place in North American popular imagination—to become visible in the cybersphere?

Thinking through the intersection of religion and technology requires not only an exploration of technology use by religious groups, but also an examination of the multiple ways in which religious and technological narratives interconnect. As discussed in the introduction to this volume, the intersection of religion and technology is often negatively framed. Perennial questions that pepper North American media about whether religion can "withstand technology" belie an assumption that the two are incommensurate.[5] Scholars of technology have argued that religion and technology represent two separate and opposing worldviews.[6] Such theories align not only with post-Enlightenment assurances of the triumph of secularization over religion, but also with a modernist narrative of technological progress: the belief that new developments in science and technology will inevitably bring about social change or, more specifically, social betterment.[7] These discourses of progress and modernity collide with deeply embedded assumptions about Vodou. Haitian Vodou is imbricated in colonialist discourses that paint it as premodern—a relic of a precolonial African past that survived in the New World. Such an archaic image of Vodou seems to conflict with the hypermodern narratives of technological progress.

At the same time Vodou is inevitably intertwined with assumptions about race and technology. The "digital divide"—referencing the ways in which access to computers and the Internet are limited by social or economic factors—is an important area of investigation in places like North America, where computer literacy seems increasingly important. However, the digital divide risks becoming an easy shorthand for assumptions that black users (often cited as some of those most affected by the digital divide) must always play "catch-up" when it comes to digital technology practices. These assumptions run the risk of obscuring the actual uses of digital technologies by black populations, as well as those populations' contributions to technological innovation. As Anna Everett explains, discourses of the digital divide are rife with "the often overlooked or unacknowledged fact of historical and contemporary black technolust and early technology adoption and mastery."[8] Running underneath much discussion of the digital divide is a still-pervasive utopic view of new media, which sees them as liberating technologies that free us from the constraints of social identity positions such as gender or race. The famous mid-1990s "Declaration of the Independence of Cyberspace" by John Percy Barlow is indicative of a foundational conceptualization of cyberspace as a raceless place: "Ours is a world that is both everywhere and nowhere, but it is not where bodies live. We are creating a world that all may enter without privilege or prejudice accorded by race, economic power, military force, or station of birth."[9] However, as Alondra Nelson points out, such discourse tends to figure race as a liability; in the rhetoric surrounding digital culture, "racial identity, and blackness in particular, is the antiavatar of digital life. Blackness gets constructed as always oppositional to technologically driven chronicles of progress."[10] Implicit in Barlow's manifesto, as in much of the utopic discussion around the Internet that emerged in the 1990s, is the belief that social differences (such as class, race, or gender) will disappear in virtual spaces, where identity is mutable and the signifiers of difference can be masked. While this utopic image of cyberspace may stem from a desire to overcome prejudice and marginalization based on social difference, it perpetuates perhaps less obvious, but equally problematic conceptualizations of social difference. The myth of technological progress is a deterministic one that narrates social change as the inevitable conclusion of technological innovation. Yet technophilic iterations of this myth harbor longstanding cultural precepts about what constitutes social betterment.

As part of my investigation into online Vodou, I interviewed Samuel, a Haitian man in his late twenties who immigrated to Montreal in his early teens. Involved in digital cultural production—from digital art to digital media—and often producing work about Haitian nationalism, Samuel got angry at the suggestion that, as a black man and a Haitian, he was bucking the assumed trends of the digital divide. "I had access to computers in school. My parents bought me a computer so I could do my homework, like everyone else in my CÉGEP.[11] And there are computers in Haiti too, you know. There is Internet and everything." "Yes, sure. But not everyone in Haiti has access to computer and Internet technology," I argued. "Not everyone has access to it here," he retorted angrily. "I know what you are going to say," he continued, forestalling my response, "that more people have access here. That's true. But what I hate is the idea that if we [Haitians] get to a computer, we won't know what to do with it; we'll just stand there and stare at it, or dance around it, sacrifice a chicken to it, or something." In this exchange, Samuel gives voice to obvious frustrations with what he sees as some of the problematic assumptions underlying discourses of the digital divide. He also succinctly articulates the potential racisms that can surface when issues of access are reduced to the assumption that Haitians in particular or blacks in general are inherently less capable of understanding computer technology than other races. Anna Everett argues that, despite the "unanticipated dramatic upsurge in black participation on the Internet from 1995 onwards, the overwhelming characterizations of the brave new world of cyberspace as primarily a racialized sphere of whiteness inhere in popular constructions of high-tech and low-tech spheres that too often consign black bodies to the latter."[12] While discussions about the digital divide are vital to understanding how access to digital technology is shaped by social factors such as race, gender, and class, they risk overlooking existing links between practices of digital technology and religious and cultural identities. Because conceptualizations of Vodou as "primitive" and assumptions about the digital divide coalesce, instances of technologized Vodou are often left unexamined. Understanding how Vodou circulates within narratives of technology and, correspondingly, how technology circulates within narratives of the religion is a necessary step for teasing apart the web of cultural discourses that enmesh Vodou.

In part such an analysis requires examining those moments when Vodou and technology intersect, not only in religious practice, but also in the popular imagination. Interestingly, Vodou/Voodoo appears in some of the founding narratives of cyberspace. It plays a significant role in William Gibson's influential *Sprawl Trilogy* (*Neuromancer*, 1984; *Count Zero*, 1986; *Mona Lisa Overdrive*, 1988) and it appears again in an article by the journalist Julian Dibble published in *The Village Voice* in 1993, at the height of early discussions of cyberspace, virtual reality, and the consequences of our actions in this seemingly new technologized terrain.[13] Dibble's article, "A Rape in Cyberspace, or How an Evil Clown, a Haitian Trickster Spirit, Two Wizards, and a Cast of Dozens Turned a Database into a Society," is foundational for early cyberculture studies in part because it was one of the first texts to provide an ethnographic account of an online community, allowing those unfamiliar with the "new world" of cyberspace insight into some of the activities that constituted it in the early 1990s.[14] A few years before Dibble's text, William Gibson was credited with coining the word *cyberspace*. Although it first appeared in his short story "Burning Chrome" (1982), the word was not popularized until the publication of *Neuromancer* in 1984. In Gibson's novels, where the organic form is fused with technology, cyberspace is not simply a "virtual world" mediated by cybernetic technology. Instead, for Gibson cyberspace is "a consensual hallucination," the entire condition of being wired, networked, fused with, and addicted to a technologizing reality. It is into this highly influential understanding of cyberspace that Gibson introduced Voodoo. While some pop culture images of Voodoo are so bastardized as to be unrecognizable, Gibson's representation depicts identifiable gods and goddesses (or *lwa*) from the pantheon of Vodou. Gibson's work thus stands out from many popular representations of Voodoo because it merges signifiers of the religion—so often assumed to be premodern—with images of a futuristic and highly technologized world. In *Count Zero* (volume 2 of the *Sprawl* trilogy), for example, Gibson introduces a cybernetic, viral image of the *lwa* Erzulie,[15] who appears to the main character, hacker Bobby Newmark. Similarly, the *lwa* Legba is Gibson's "lord of communication."[16]

Gibson's amalgamation of cybernetic technology and signifiers of religion may represent an unusual iteration of Vodou, but his work also encodes sometimes-familiar iterations of race, sexuality, and nationality. Cyberpunk in general and Gibson's work in particular almost always depict a futuristic (although dystopic) world that is inherently transnational. This transnationalism is represented by the iconic figure of the cyberpunk cyborg, who is not simply a hybrid of human and machine, but also of different races and ethnicities. As Emily Apter puts it, "the cyborg's transracial, transnational body conjures forth an identity no longer split between First and Third World, between metropole and native home, but rather, a body so fragmented that its morphology is a diaspora."[17] Although this image is futuristic, it also encodes the past. The cyborg embodies "postcolonial conceptions of nation and race as part of the politically charged relationship between the diaspora and transnationalism, pigmentation and desire, and, most controversially, hybridity and miscegenation."[18] Voodoo/Vodou has long been encoded in colonial discourse as a contaminant and the visceral fear often associated with the religion has functioned as a warning against miscegenation, or the dilution of the purity of the colonial race.[19] The fragmented morphology outlined by Apter and fears of miscegenation that can be found in Gibson's fictional world—where gender, race, and technology collide with the signifiers of Vodou in depictions of the Vodou ritual of possession—are explained through the metaphor of hacking. For instance, the possession of Jackie, a female character, by Danbala, a god (or *lwa*), is described in the hacker's vernacular: "Think of Jackie as a deck, Bobby, a cyberspace deck, a very pretty one with nice ankles.... Think of Danbala, who some people call the snake, as a program. Say as an icebreaker. Danbala slots into Jackie's deck, Jackie cuts ice. That's all."[20]

This sexualized passage is more than a simple explanation of possession or even a counter-explanation of hacking. It is also an acknowledgment that, in cyberspace, humans are always potentially penetrated by technology: always at risk of contamination. Such sexualized imagery inevitably echoes a fear of miscegenation, or the viral spread of racial impurity. The translation of a fear of viral contamination into the technologized, cybernetic world of science fiction perpetuates colonialist conceptions of race and religion. Representations such as Gibson's provide a node in a "figural strand" that, as Barbara Browning has observed, links "voodoo, sex, and viruses," in which everyone is concurrently at risk of both hybridization and contamination.[21]

Although problematic, Gibson's representation of Voodoo is significant in that, like other forms of pop Voodoo, it makes visible a particular iteration of the religion. Gibson's work had enormous impact on the collective consciousness of those people deeply involved in the developing digitalized and networked world of new media technologies. Allucquère Rosanne Stone explains:

> *Neuromancer* reached the hackers . . . and it reached the technologically literate and socially disaffected who were searching for social forms that could transform the fragmented anomie that characterized life in Silicon Valley and all electronic industrial ghettos. In a single stroke, Gibson's powerful vision provided for them the imaginal public sphere and refigured discursive community that established the grounding for the possibility of a new kind of social interaction. . . . *Neuromancer* . . . is a massive intertextual presence not only in other literary productions of the 1980s, but in technical publications, conference topics, hardware design, and scientific and technological discourses in the large.[22]

Similarly, in "Space for Rent in the Last Suburb," Scott McQuire suggests that Gibson's work is significant because of the "itineraries of desire it cathected."[23] McQuire reads Gibson's popular success and critical influence as "symptomatic of a complex of social changes and cultural anxieties" taking place around the birth of digital networked communications.[24] But Gibson's work has reached beyond the early architects of the Internet to generations of "spiritual seekers" who turn to such easily accessible representations, not only for metaphors of the wired world, but also for information about Voodoo. Gibson's depiction of Voodoo is cool, highly technologized, subversive, underground, and, above all, efficacious. In *Neuromancer* a character by the name of Beauvoir explains:

> "Voodoo" isn't concerned with notions of salvation and transcendence. What it's about is getting things done. You follow me? In our system, there are many gods, spirits. Part of one big family, with all the virtues, all the vices. . . . Voodoo says there's God, sure, Gran Met, but he's big, too big, and too far away to worry himself if your ass is poor, or you can't get laid. . . . Voodoo's like the street.[25]

When exploring Gibson's work in conjunction with cybernetic representations of Vodou, the "itineraries of desire" in Gibson's work take on a particular tenor as they function as catalysts that sometimes send readers on a journey for more information. For instance, the creator of one website on "magic and the occult" describes how Gibson's depiction of Vodou as a "practical religion" sparked his own interest:

How did I come to find out about Voodoo? Well, it's very silly. To this day, I still find it silly and even ridiculous. However, it's how I came to be interested in Voodoo. It happened when I was reading William Gibson's "Sprawl" series of novels—specifically *Count Zero* and *Mona Lisa Overdrive*. Gibson makes heavy use of Voodoo in both books, and in *Count Zero*, there is this dialog, where Bobby (*Count Zero*) is talking to Beauvoir about Voodoo, and Bobby doesn't understand why anyone would be into Voodoo.... "It isn't concerned with notions of salvation and transcendence. What it's about is getting things done." So anyway, I became very interested in Voodoo after reading this, because I too am interested in getting things done. I didn't figure Gibson made any of it up.... It just didn't sound made up. But information on Voodoo is quite hard to find, due to the fact that most people have a very serious misunderstanding of what it's all about.[26]

Gibson's novel acts as a starting point for a search for information on Voodoo, in this instance because his depiction of the religion seems "real" and "authentic"—not something "made up." As we will see, concerns about authenticity (around what constitutes "real" Vodou) haunt discussions about Vodou in the cybersphere. The presence of Vodou/Voodoo in some of the foundational cyberculture literature may seem merely coincidental, or it may point to a deeper connection between the historicity of Vodou/Voodoo in the North American popular imagination and in the origin narratives of cyberspace.

While popular culture makes the intersection of religion and technology visible, users of new media, digital technology, and networked communication also contribute to the visibility of Vodou. In the realms of cyberspace, where everyday citizens produce as well as consume online content, there is vast, varied, and ever-changing information about Vodou. This online visibility provides a host of people—many of whom have no genealogical or geographic connections with Haitian Vodou—with portals to the religion in the form of informational and educational websites, listservs, chat rooms, and e-commerce. This same online environment facilitates the continued circulation of pop Voodoo. Voodoo and Vodou are constantly juxtaposed with one another in the cybersphere. Many websites on Vodou are specifically geared toward those unfamiliar with the religion. They not only impart rudimentary information, but also spend time dispelling common misconceptions. For example, one of the most prominent online practitioners of Vodou, Mambo Racine, provides "Vodou Lessons" on her website that promise to "teach you about Vodou, how the religion is structured, it's [*sic*] history, it's [*sic*] spiritual entities, and what it means to Vodou believers."²⁷ At the same time she is careful to distinguish Vodou from what she calls "Hollywood Voodoo—a malevolent mishmash of magic conjured up by movie producers and bearing little or no resemblance to anything else on earth!" Even the Wikipedia entry on Haitian Vodou contains a subsection on "Myths and Misconceptions" that addresses not only popular stereotypes—such as Voodoo dolls—but also misrepresentations within popular culture productions (citing the 1973 epic James Bond film *Live and Let Die*).²⁸ This practice of distinguishing "real" Vodou from its popular counterpart in the online environment reveals an acute awareness of how frequently Vodou/Voodoo conjures up pop culture stereotypes for web surfers. This speaks to both colloquial and academic understandings of the Internet as a vast, searchable compendium of information. What does the seemingly ubiquitous impulse to search this compendium do to a religion like Vodou? If Vodou is becoming more visible or more accessible via digital technologies, it is within a context in which it is closely juxtaposed with pop-culture Voodoo: so much so that the most popular search engine, Google, will ask, "Do you mean Vodou?" when you type in Voodoo and vice versa.²⁹ Software and hardware technologies don't determine how religion is made visible in the cybersphere, but they do generate conditions that circumscribe that visibility. While the technological affordances of cyberspace may collapse the distance between Vodou and Voodoo, users continually address the differences between the two.

The visibility of online Vodou—a visibility that always negotiates the specter of pop Voodoo—brings up particular concerns about authenticity, authority, cultural appropriation, and cultural belonging. Not infrequently authenticity and cultural appropriation are tackled head-on. The creator of one website (*gede.org*), for example, gives voice to her own misgivings about the proliferation of websites representing Vodou online, many of which, she argues, are created by newcomers to the religion:

> The majority of Vodou web sites are written by people who have converted. Converting to a religion isn't, in and of itself, a bad thing. I, myself, have done so. But I can't argue that my experience of [Vodou is the same as] someone who grew up in a household where the spirits were served regularly. . . . My problem with a lot of these sites . . . is that there is very little acknowledgement of that difference. Sometimes that difference can be opportune. I remember some of the things that I didn't understand about the spirits, and that makes it easier for me to explain things to people like me: North American new-age-types who did not grow up in a culture that served the spirits. But it's important to be honest about difference and ignorance.³⁰

This passage speaks to the unease some feel not only about how and by whom Vodou is being represented in cyberspace, but also about the place of newcomers in the religion. Issues of ownership—of who gets to represent (or even what it means to represent) Vodou—are magnified in cyberspace, where it is easy to lose track of who is speaking for what. Vodou's online visibility is congruent with the rise of user-generated media that can (although they do not have to be used in this way) blur and even hide the identity of the user behind the keyboard.[31] The tension between the growing online visibility of Vodou and the ways in which online producers of Vodou websites can potentially obscure and construct identity and authority is not lost on the creator of *gede.org*, who laments, "I wish more sites would be clear about their sources, because I'm not sure that they are really speaking about the religion that they learned from their *maman kanzo* or *papa kanzo* or if they're just telling me what they read in a book somewhere."[32] Concerns about the difference between religious experiences grounded in a Haitian cultural heritage and the experiences of those who are, in the words of this webmistress, "North American new-age types,"[33] is indicative of larger issues surrounding the difficulties both of authenticating web sources and of deciding what (and maybe even who) counts as "authentic" in an orthopraxic religion.

Some argue that problems of authenticity and identity in cyberspace are indigenous to the realm itself: part and parcel of how cyberspace promotes anonymity and unmoors individuals from their accountability to others.[34] In the early 1990s "cyberspace" was often conceptualized as a world apart from reality, and the beings born within it epitomized a postmodern concept of identity as fluid and fragmented. Although the term has fallen out of favor with some Internet researchers (frustrated by its lack of specificity), cyberspace is still part of colloquial language use and popular imagination. Online religious practitioners often amend the term to talk about cyberrituals and cyberspiritualities, and more mundane concepts such as cybertalk and cybermalls pepper everyday speech. This vocabulary points to a hybridized conception of cyberspace as a terrain that blends the virtual and the actual, making durable links to tangible geographies and undercutting the notion that cyber-identities are free-floating entities with no connection to "real life." N. Katherine Hayles, among others, has called for a resuscitation and redefinition of the term, suggesting that the early construction of cyberspace as "an immaterial place where mind reigned supreme" is giving way to a more nuanced understanding of a "seamless mixing of virtual and real spaces."[35] This mix is evident when websites and forums on Vodou not only disseminate information about the religion, but also attract a host of "spiritual seekers" who, not always satisfied with exclusively online experiences, seek out actual Vodou communities and rituals via online portals.

Large-scale ceremonies centered around possession, a central ritual of Vodou, involve dancing, drumming, and the preparation of ceremonial food as well as the participation of multiple practitioners. These communal rituals are seldom (if ever) replicated online. What does manifest in the realm of cyberspace, however, are the smaller-scale interpersonal transactions that occur between ritual specialists and practitioners as part of everyday practice. In Vodou it is common to seek out a ritual specialist (*houngan* or *mambo*) for help with problems. These transactions have both ritual and economic elements. Vodou priests and priestesses will help members of their congregation by preparing rituals and ritual objects designed to ameliorate a variety of hardships, from illness to romantic troubles to difficulties finding employment or even problems with neighbors. It is expected that these individualized ritual services will be paid for. This economic exchange, even when nominal, ensures that the pantheon of Vodou gods and goddesses looks upon the ritual transactions favorably. While large-scale ceremonies may be inaccessible to online seekers, this latter aspect of Vodou practice is readily found in the online environment, where e-commerce thrives. Many *mambo* and *houngan* have set up websites that function as online stores, making available both ritual supplies and ritual objects. When the spiritual marketplace of Vodou is transcribed onto the cybersphere, the interpersonal relationships that constitute the social world of Vodou become spread out. The priestess who may work closely with members of her immediate or actual congregation to create rituals and ritual objects must, in the online environment, adapt her practices to work with individuals she may never meet face-to-face. Similarly, Vodou practitioners who may have direct recourse to their local priest or priestess, should the rituals and objects they commission fail in their efficacy, have to take much more on trust in the online environment. Like other forms of e-commerce (such as eBay.com and Etsy.com), online transactions around small-scale Vodou rituals are very much about building trust and reputation for the vendor and managing risk for the buyer.[36] While other e-commerce sites that facilitate relatively direct interaction between seller and buyer must generate a system of trust around the transaction itself, the trade in Vodou rituals and supplies must additionally assure buyers of the efficacy and authenticity of the practices behind the computer screen. For instance, the *Legba's Crossroads* website, which provides "supplies for practitioners of Haitian Vodou," assures purchasers of the sacred nature of the supplies:

"All items are worked on the altars of Mambo Chita Tann ("Mambo T") before shipment. Additionally all products, with the exception of media, saints, and some jewelry items, are handcrafted for each client, blessed and assembled in the mambo's *badji* (altar room)."[37] Like other e-commerce sites, online sellers of Vodou rituals and supplies build their reputation through buyer feedback. However, this feedback is often presented so as to reinforce trust not necessarily in the economics of the exchange (whether the exchange was honored, for example), but in the authenticity of the practices behind the product or service. Feedback for the "Legba Store" (the store affiliated with the "Legba's Crossroads" website), for example, speaks not about the ease of the economic transaction, nor even the efficacy of the items themselves, but rather about the authenticity of the ritual specialist who prepared them: "I wanted to thank you for being real about your items. You are the REAL DEAL and you know your stuff."[38] Once again, issues of authenticity are brought to the fore in cyberspace, where assuring visitors to online stores that the ritual services and supplies are prepared by "real" ritual specialists is of paramount importance. Concerns about authenticity, authority, and belonging drive the production of online Vodou in both representative and participatory ways.

While the differentiation between pop Voodoo and Haitian Vodou made on many websites is one manifestation of the tension around how Vodou is being defined online, other concerns about belonging and about the authenticity of online Vodou (as both information and practice) can be found in the attestations (or suspicions) of the "realness" of online specialists and in online discussions around initiations. Vodou is a hierarchically organized religion with several levels of initiation, ranging from the lowest, or *hounsi kanzo*, to the highest, which involves one's initiation as a priest or priestess (*houngan* or *mambo*). Although the creator of *gede.org* (discussed above) speaks of conversion to Vodou, there is no formal conversion mechanism, and it is not necessary to either convert or to become an initiate in order to practice the religion. In fact, in some Vodou congregations, non-initiates outnumber initiates. Despite this, initiation is a prevalent topic of discussion in the online world of Vodou. In part this prevalence is indicative of ontological concerns. Non-Haitians who discover the religion from outside Haiti and the Haitian diaspora often find themselves in various states of becoming. Unlike Haitian practitioners, who are immersed in a culture in which Vodou (although never an easy identity) is a heritage and birthright that forms a part of everyday life, non-Haitians inevitably wrestle with how to identify with a religion so closely tied to the history and culture of Haiti. Initiation is one way for non-Haitians to authorize their own belonging to Vodou. But discussions about initiation, particularly of non-Haitians, are contentious in the online sphere.

One concern much discussed online is the possibility that newcomers to the religion are easy prey for ritual specialists with uncertain credentials or shady intent who seek to profit from these potentially naïve individuals. This concern is augmented by the financial exchanges that are an intrinsic part of Vodou ritual practice. Since it is conventional to pay for ritual services such as initiation in Vodou, the fear expressed by many is that unscrupulous individuals will take money from those newly interested in Vodou without providing the "authentic" rituals or services. Houngan Kay Aboudja, a notable figure in the online world of Vodou (and himself a non-Haitian initiate), observes on one website that "many non-Haitians now adhere to the faith and have taken Vodou initiation at one grade or another," but he laments the existence of "charlatans" who fool these gullible newcomers with shoddy, false, and needlessly expensive rituals.[39] Moreover, because Vodou initiation must take place on Haitian soil—the home of the ancestors and the gateway to *Ginen*, the residence of the pantheon of *lwa* (the gods and goddesses of Vodou)—initiates depend on specialists who will conduct the rituals of initiation and who also ensure their safe passage when in Haiti, a place portrayed as dangerous.[40] Indeed, the cost of a guide and accommodation is often added to the initiation fee. When newcomers to Vodou apply for initiation online, they are implicated in a complex set of social and economic relationships between established Haitian practitioners and non-Haitian newcomers, local residents and visitors (or tourists), "First" and "Third" World citizens, insiders and outsiders, and not infrequently, black and white.

Haitian identity is, of course, tied to discourses of race. However, "race" signifies differently in different cultural locations. In the Haitian context, for instance, race has to be understood not only in terms of the country's specific legacies of slavery and colonialism, but also in terms of the Haitian Revolution and the struggle for Haitian sovereignty. For instance, in an effort to reverse the entrenched, racialized division of the population that had existed under French colonialism:

> The first constitution of Haiti proclaimed that all Haitians no matter what their shade of skin were to be called "black"; this included even those German and Polish groups in Saint Dominique who had fought with the liberation movement and had become citizens. . . . Furthermore, the constitution stated that no white man, whatever his nationality, should

set foot in Haiti as a master or property owner, and that he was unable to acquire property in the future.... Just as colonial Saint Domingue had been based upon a system of white superiority, so Haiti became a symbol of black power.[41]

It is into this complex and culturally specific understanding of blackness that newcomers to Haitian Vodou step. Race becomes another site of contention when it comes to authorizing oneself as a Vodou practitioner online. Online practitioner Mambo Racine, for instance, admits that "[t]here is an unspoken understanding among some unscrupulous Houngans and Mambos that they will never reveal the 'secrets' of Vodou . . . to a person who is not both black and Haitian." Nonetheless, she maintains that "in Vodou, racial, ethnic, or national origin is no bar to participation."[42] Despite this declared openness of Vodou to non-Haitian participants, black and Haitian identities inevitably signify a certain proximity to notions of authentic Vodou in both Haitian and North American contexts. Non-Haitian producers of online content about Vodou must inevitably negotiate the ways race is signified when defining the religion in the online context. This negotiation sometimes brings certain aspects of the intersection of Haitian Vodou, Haitian identity, and race to the forefront while submerging others. For instance, Racine's webpage "Race in Vodou" makes no mention of the cultural specificity of blackness in the Haitian context (namely, the constitutional redefinition of all Haitians, regardless of race or ethnicity, as "black" citizens), but it does make mention of those *lwa* (gods and goddesses) of Vodou who have "white," "mulatto," or "English" characteristics.[43]

Internet and computer-mediated communication practices are often conceptualized as inherently "disembedding" (to use Anthony Giddens' term): lifting individuals out of social relationships and removing them from social consequences. For new practitioners to Vodou, the online experience clearly *can* be a means of getting to actual community and ritual practice. The communication and (virtual) mobility made possible by the Internet affect practitioners' experience of what Giddens has called "time-space distantiation": the stretching out of social relationships that were once defined by proximity and are now defined by the pull between presence and absence.[44] Although the Internet arguably allows for geographically dispersed social relationships, it can also make geographical distance (particularly when geographic distance is coupled with cultural notions of First and Third World, or of safe and unsafe destinations) appear less distant. Haiti—a sacred site and pilgrimage destination for many new Vodou practitioners—no longer "feels" very far away to those who can now book travel, accommodation, and "native" tour guides and even arrange for a ritual initiation online.[45] While the Internet is not alone in (re)shaping time-space distantiation, experiences of proximity, presence, and absence may be reconfigured in cyberspace. The potential of online visibility to bring an influx of newcomers to Vodou is a site of contention for those who might worry that the authenticity of Vodou may be lost when traditional ritual roles are passed on to those who have no active memory of Haiti or kinship ties.

Negotiations of authenticity and authority in the online world of Vodou are further complicated by the fact that those *houngans* and *mambos* (priests and priestesses) who have had the longest-lasting and most visible presence online—and who thus most easily attract the attention of "spiritual seekers"—are often themselves non-Haitian. These non-Haitian ritual specialists have to create online identities that affirm their authority as Vodou ritual specialists, which may involve displaying images or videos of themselves conducting Vodou ceremonies in Haiti, making references to their own initiations in Haiti, or invoking the Haitian-born *houngans* and *mambos* with whom they work. Just as often these online ritual experts insist on their authority and authenticity by warning visitors against following other online priests or priestesses. For example, Houngan Hector—who uses his website to provide information about Vodou as well as to advertise and sell his services as a ritual expert—counsels newcomers thinking about Vodou initiation: "If you ever decide to become *kanzo* [an initiate], you will be invariably excited. Along with the excitement, you need to approach things with caution. There are many people out there running scams."[46] He goes on to sound a note of caution aimed specifically at those whose encounter with Vodou is strictly online: "There is one widely known *mambo* online, who has a large online presence, and who charges her initiates five hundred dollars for 'advanced training!'"[47] By denouncing other online practitioners allegedly "running scams," Hector positions himself as an authority on authentic Vodou ritual practice. But, as has already been observed, it can be difficult to discern authenticity in the online environment, and those who reach Vodou via cyberspace may find themselves witness to sometimes raucous arguments about the veracity of rituals and the intent of ritual experts.

In 2004 concerns already swirling around issues of authenticity and initiation in a loosely networked online Vodou community boiled over into a controversial feud between two individuals: Mambo Racine, a well-known online *mambo*, and Ross Heaven, author of numerous books on shamanism and spirituality. Racine, an American-born woman, is the creator of an extensive website on Vodou (*www.rootswithoutend.org*), the moderator of one of the largest Vodou online forums (*Vodou Arts*), the founder of a charitable organization directed toward helping the disadvantaged in Haiti (*Vodou Aid*),[48] the proprietor of the *Vodou Emporium* (an online store that sells, among other things, supplies for use in Vodou rituals), and the orchestrator of an online portal that allows individuals to book travel for initiations in Haiti.[49] Ross Heaven is a non-Haitian British citizen who runs a website that offers workshops in shamanistic practices and an online store with links to his books. Heaven is also an active discussant in multiple online forums dedicated to Vodou. The feud between Heaven and Racine became visible after the publication in 2003 of Heaven's book *Vodou Shaman: The Haitian Way of Healing and Power*, in which Heaven discusses Vodou in general and chronicles his own initiation conducted in Haiti by Racine in January of 2000. Soon after publication Racine accused Heaven of revealing initiatory secrets in his book. Heaven countered that claim, in part, by suggesting that Racine's practice was "inauthentic" and that her credentials as a ritual specialist were suspect. Heaven argued publicly that he could not have revealed any initiatory secrets because Racine's practices "probably bear no resemblance to what goes on in a real *mambo's* house."[50] Racine, for her part, made her displeasure with Heaven known in multiple online forums, including, interestingly, the Customer Reviews section of the *Amazon.com* website, where she posted the following response to Heaven's book:

> Hello! I am Mambo Racine Sans Bout, the same Mambo Racine about whom Ross Heaven has so many nice things to say in his book, "Vodou Shaman." It is with some regret that I must warn the prospective reader that most of what is in this book never actually happened—Ross is willing to say anything for a buck, apparently. He never let me see what he was writing until the book was published, and I never imagined he would make up so many stories! Now that I have refused to support his activities he is very angry with me, but the fact remains that this book is 99% BUNK.[51]

In a 2004 interview with *Metro* (a free daily newspaper based in the United Kingdom), Heaven was forthcoming about his feud with Racine and denied any unethical behavior, but he further fueled the controversy with the suggestion that he was the victim of what some sensationally labeled a "Vodou fatwa."[52] "There is an ongoing war at the moment between Racine and myself. I have been threatened with violence. I've asked her on a number of forums on the Internet what the secrets are that

I'm supposed to have revealed and she can't say."⁵³ Racine was quick to counter the claims by Heaven and others that she (or her supporters) had threatened Heaven with harm. An article about the controversy quotes Racine as saying, "It's a bit idiotic of Ross to enter an ancient tradition which requires secrecy, reveal these secrets and then go screaming across cyberspace complaining that people are angry with him. I have been very disappointed in Ross, in his shameful behavior and in his bizarre statements on a variety of Internet forums. Despite all this, I personally do not seek to do him any harm, as I have repeatedly made clear to him in private emails and public statements."⁵⁴

In this long-lasting and bitter feud, both Racine and Heaven insisted that each "knew best" what constitutes and defines authentic Vodou practice. Because of the nature of the forum—the easily archivable content of online blogs, websites, and Internet forums—this feud has been woven into the information about Vodou found on the Internet and, as such, plays a part in the way that Vodou has become visible online. As this feud crossed cyberspace (the phrase used by Racine, "screaming across cyberspace," is apt), social and participatory media allowed interested cyber-citizens to not only view statements made by those involved, but to comment on them, adding their voices to the discussions of veracity in Vodou, the place of newcomers in the religion, and concerns over online (and offline) representations of the religion.

While the feud was ostensibly about initiatory secrets and the veracity of initiations performed for newcomers to the religion, the controversy has clear implications for ongoing concerns about definitions of Haitian Vodou found in cyberspace. Racine and Heaven's very public argument about what constitutes "real" Vodou practice has itself become part of the searchable compendium of online Vodou. It has also been attached to cyber-promotion of cultural commodities (such as books) disseminated in the offline world. By constituting part of the available information on Haitian Vodou found online, the feud has also created a forum for two (by their own definition) non-Haitians to contribute not insignificantly to the representation of Haitian Vodou in cyberspace. The greater ease of access to everything from web design software to stable Internet connections in the West may account for the greater visibility of Western Vodou practitioners and specialists on the Web. But it would be overly simplistic to attribute this visibility solely to the inequities engendered by issues of access.

Although non-Haitian practitioners are highly visible online, the importance of Haitian identity and Haitian culture for constructions of "authentic" Vodou remains. Haitian Vodou is closely tied to the cultural and geographic specificity of Haiti. For instance, sacred spaces located in Haiti are the sites of important pilgrimages, Haitian Kreyol is the language used in ritual celebrations, and initiations must take place on Haitian soil. In addition, the *lwa* (or the gods and goddesses) of Haitian Vodou are closely tied to the history of Haiti. Stories told about the *lwa* often give them roles in historical events such as the Haitian Revolution, and during large-scale Vodou rituals *lwa* who are identified with important figures in Haitian history often appear through possession. While it has always been possible for non-Haitians to participate fully in the religion by becoming initiates, even rising to the level of a *mambo* or *houngan* (priestess or priest), Haitian identity and genealogy signify a tangible connection to the complex historical and cultural specificity of Haitian Vodou. The intersection of Haitian identity with claims of authenticity and authority in ritual practice may be of concern in offline Vodou communities, particularly in the diaspora, where practitioners are more likely to be second- or third-generation Haitians and where non-Haitians may also participate in diasporic Haitian Vodou communities. But the stakes around authenticity and identity are different in the online context. Identity online is tied to negotiating who is authorized to speak for (or represent) the Vodou religion as well as to build a reputation for being an effective Internet ritual specialist, despite conditions of limited interpersonal contact. For this reason, genealogies and kinship lines are sometimes used to attest that online practitioners have connections to Haiti, the spiritual and cultural home of Haitian Vodou. When these genealogical connections are absent, as they are for newcomers to the religion, connections to Haiti are sometimes mapped out by proxy.

One mambo (or priestess) who provides online Vodou services, for instance, does not outline her own genealogical lineage, but is careful to outline those of the ritual experts who initiated her into the religion. Mambo Chita Tann (or Mambo T), whose website, *Legba's Crossing*, provides ritual Vodou supplies for purchase, advertises her credentials as an online Haitian priestess by publicizing her initiation into a particular Haitian Vodou *peristyle* (temple): "Mambo T was re-initiated as mambo *asogwe* in a second *kanzo* in January 2006 at Sosyete Sipote Ki Di, a historical Port-au-Prince *peristyle* jointly administered by Mambo Marie Carmel and Mambo Ya Sezi. At her baptism Mambo T was honored with the public name *Chita Tann*, a name passed down through several mambos in the house's lineage."[55] In addition, Mambo T is careful to point out the lineage of the *mambo* (Marie Carmel) who had initiated her: "Mambo Marie Carmel is a well-known Mambo both inside and outside of Haiti. She maintains residences in New York and Haiti and has more than 25 years' experience in Vodou, having taken the *asson*[56] at age 18 from Mambo Jacqueline Anne-Marie Lubin, herself an initiate of the famous Kintonmin Bon Mambo of Bel-Air (Mambo Felicia Louis-Romain), the chief priestess of Haiti's first *asson* lineage in Port-au-Prince in the 1920s."[57] This history of Mambo T's initiation and the genealogy of those who initiated her serve to reassure visitors to *Legba's Crossing* that they will be dealing with an established and authentic Vodou priestess. While reputation matters in the offline environment, online transactions necessitate the building and maintenance of reputation that attest to identification with Haiti in particular ways. Haiti often circulates just below the surface in online representations and practices of Vodou. Haitian identity may not be a determining factor for participation in (online or offline) Vodou communities or practices, but it can be used in the online environment to authenticate certain practitioners and practices.

Online Vodou has undoubtedly raised the public profile of Vodou, making certain aspects of the religion more easily accessible to a population that may not have a direct or unmediated experience with this oft-misunderstood religion. Online Vodou includes representational practices that not only inform interested web surfers about the Haitian Vodou tradition, but also dedicate web space to dispelling misconceptions about the religion. In addition, practitioners of online Vodou must negotiate issues of identity in the building (and tearing down) of reputation in the online environment. Race and Haitian identity can circulate in the online environment as signifiers of authenticity and authority for those trying to generate spiritual businesses online. At the same time issues of race and cultural proximity to Haiti become an uneasy (but still visible) subtext for newcomers to Haitian Vodou, who can now access the religion via mechanisms such as booking online initiations or purchasing online ritual services. While the matrix of technologies that intersect to support online Vodou does not determine the shape Vodou takes in the digital public sphere, the technological affordances of computer-mediated representation and communication intersect with both the cultural precepts of Vodou (or Voodoo) in the North American popular imagination and the cultural specificity of Haitian Vodou to give shape to a particular form of virtual Vodou.

Both colloquial and academic discussions about the promise of digital media and technology rely heavily on Habermasian notions of participatory democracy, arguing that the proliferation of individual citizen voices online can only enrich the public sphere by providing equal access to all. In some sense, this is true. A cursory glance via the workings of a search engine, for instance, demonstrates a multitude of voices contributing to the knowledge base of any one topic. Certainly this is the case with online Vodou. But attentiveness to the specificity of online Vodou demonstrates how the conversation can be circumscribed—how certain stories and representations recirculate with great frequency, while others never get told at all. Whether it is about dispelling misconceptions of the religion born in the Western popular imagination, negotiating the ontological status of non-Haitian practitioners who find their way to the religion via digital portals, or affirming the reputation of online practitioners and ritual specialists, online Vodou is very much about drawing and redrawing the borders of the religion. This is not unprecedented, nor is it a result of digital technologies themselves. But the digital public sphere—which functions as both a searchable compendium and a site for user-led cultural production—situates Vodou in a context where ongoing dialogue about authenticity and authority becomes central.

TV St. Claire
Maria José A. de Abreu

"A monastery of the Poor Claires in Canção Nova?" I asked, doubting my ears. The initial procession had just entered the alley by the left rear part of the building. The priest leading the procession walked down the aisle, raising the holy monstrance. "That's right!" said the woman I had befriended, adding, "They came here because of a moment like now, a Thursday, just like today, when Canção Nova was offering contemplation to the Holy Eucharist." This information brought in me a mix of perplexity and excitement. Could it be that Canção Nova, a multimedia campus located in São Paulo, Brazil, that belonged to the Catholic Charismatic Renewal (CCR) movement, shared its physical space with a Franciscan female monastery?

The Canção Nova media campus traces its origin back to February 1978, when its founder, Padre Jonas Abib, whom many considered a prophet, was speaking to an audience of young Catholics. The event took place in the vast green region of the Paraiba Valley, in the state of São Paulo, a place well known for its many mystical happenings and nowadays a privileged site for eco-religious tourism. The story goes that on a February morning of that year, Padre Jonas Abib asked who among those present would be willing to leave everything behind in order to fulfill a wish God had placed in his heart.[1] That the source of Padre Jonas's words would be regarded by many Catholic Charismatics in Brazil as divine was attested to not so much by the cryptic nature of his request than by the fact that as he spoke, precisely twelve people volunteered ("as though moved by an incredible force") to join the priest in establishing this "new worldwide media apostolic community."[2] Modeling themselves on the lifestyle of the first Christian community as "fishermen," these "new media apostles" promptly followed their leader in conflating and exploring metaphors and analogies associated with the "Net."[3] The "nets of the apostles" (*as redes dos apóstolos*) and their "art of fishing" (*arte de pescar*) found the emerging terrain of new technologies of communication in the Brazil of the 1970s and '80s to be a particularly rich environment for them to widen and expand. But while juxtapositions between the fishing net (an object with profound spiritual connotations) and the new vocabulary sprouting out of the technological—in its capacity to diffuse, reproduce and interconnect—were being aptly explored by this community of twelve, a readaptation of concepts concerning the specific theological status of the CCR was also taking place. Not only were religious terms and ideas informing the reception and accommodation of new communication technologies, but also the reverse was occurring: new technologies also came to recontextualize the use of religious vocabularies. The liquid environment associated with the sea into which the apostles launched their nets—just as with the contemporary association of the cybernetic as a nautical space[4]—was emphatically explored in daily interchanges of the "apostolic community" of the Paraiba Valley. In addressing the link between theology and technology, liquid terms began, as it were, to evanesce. This elemental readjustment responded to an aesthetic fad as much as to a conceptual necessity to have the theological principle of *pneuma*—the Greek word for breath, air, or spirit—rendered existentially compatible with the aerial/electrical nature of media such as radio, television, and the Internet. By stressing the ontological as well as the linguistic compatibilities between the aerial substance of the Spirit as *pneuma* and the airborne nature of electronic technologies, it became possible to juxtapose and interconnect religion and technology, two spheres kept apart by the more disenchanted theories of modernity.

That a medieval-inspired mystical order, the Poor Claires, would set themselves up within a global media campus belonging to the Charismatic Renewal of Brazil provides us with a striking example of interconnection between the religious and the technological. It is also an instance where interconnectivity itself is the event. The apparent incongruence between, on the one hand, the silent, introverted, and monastic existence of the Poor Claires and, on the other, the boisterous and highly mediatized Catholic Charismatic Renewal in Brazil comments, among other things, on the ability of technology to link parallel—even competitive—events: to update, synchronize, and reticulate apparently unrelated information or phenomena onto a single plane. This possibility, moreover, is not reducible to the message. Rather, it encompasses the very medium through which such messages are communicated, such that two extrinsic media—such as the Holy Eucharist and television—may emerge, as we will see, as citations of one another.

Whereas classical theories have tended to associate "contemplation" with a higher state of purity and authenticity, there is increasing historical and ethnographic evidence to support just the opposite view.[5] An expanding literature on the intersections between religion and media has been particularly helpful in demonstrating how the most spontaneous and uncalled-for of our actions are likely—if not primarily—reliant on techniques.[6] Such a focus does not stem from a sheer need to expose the social fabrication of things. Rather, its prime aim is to evaluate the constitutive role of technology and technique in the production and modulation of religious dispositions and embodied practices, such that neither religion nor technology could be said to exist before the other. In the present account such an interconnection will be made by tracing the (aerial) circuit that links the world of St. Claire in her medieval monastic cell to the TV screen of Canção Nova in contemporary Brazil. Contrary to modern European conceptions of vision, predicated on the existence of an active subject observing a passive object, this chapter calls for a redefinition of modern perspectival vision and of the distrust of materiality upon which such vision is based. It does so by engaging with three main arguments. The first entails revising our conception of "the air" as a substance rather than as a dimension. The second relates to how the perception of air as both material and dynamic affects our inherited conceptions of the singularity of the modern subject and the contemplated object. The third deals with the conceptions of time and historicity and their relation to our definitions of tradition and modernity. Whereas often the old and the new are articulated in terms of a break or opposition, the possibility of rethinking that relation through the medium of breath exposes how interruption and difference are not so much opposed as integral to the notions of continuity and tradition. In an attempt to question some of these assumptions, Walter Benjamin's notion of the aura will be reassessed as something not so much "seen" as "breathed."

Clairvoyance

Named after St. Claire (1194–1253 CE), a contemporary of St. Francis of Assisi, the Poor Claires are recognized for their rigorous discipline organized around the Liturgy of the Hours. In addition to their vows of chastity, poverty, silence, and confinement, they are known for their day-and-night contemplation of the Holy Eucharist. In line with other early and central medieval religious orders, the Poor Claires transferred the silence that mystics had previously maintained in the desert to the indoor world of the monastery. The cloister, introduced in the ninth century, had already become the designated area of spiritual inwardness, a kind of counterpart to the mystic's own soul. Contrary to the idea that one might have of the robustness of monastery walls, the soft sounds and quiet utterances—as though "under one's breath" of the mystic's prayer—entered the composition of the surrounding space like a murmur.[7]

"Look at Meeee..." [*Olha P'ra Mim*], heaved the voices in celebration. The relic had now been placed at the center of the altar. I left the building through a long passageway. In it several TV screens showed a close-up of the Holy Eucharist. I rushed to the spot where I had been told the monastery was located. I rang a bell on the front door, so as to announce my entrance, and waited by a second door upon reading the words, "Do not enter." A nun came out and advised me to move toward a dark cubicle by the hallway. Minutes later another young nun entered the cell, introducing herself as Sister Rita. Only then did I realize—to the great indifference of my tape recorder—that our conversation would have to happen with an iron gate separating us. I was inside the monastery of a thirteenth-century order, although the monastery itself was located inside a Charismatic global multimedia network.

> M.J: I must admit that I'm surprised to find you here, a Poor Claire monastery, in such a place as Canção Nova....
>
> S.R: It started with the inspiration of one of our nuns, in the town of Santa Catarina. She was also called Clara, just like St. Clara. Because of her immobility... her family gave the monastery a TV set for the nursery so that she and the nurse could follow the Mass. One day, on a Thursday, the Holiest appeared on the TV screen.... She was looking at the exposed Jesus on the TV

screen when she received a revelation that a monastery must be built within the Canção Nova Community.... The feeling was so strong that she confessed to the abbess of the monastery. She told her what had happened. First, Sister Clara doubted whether in her condition the sisters would take her seriously. ... She thought they would think she had gone mad. But then they prayed together and discerned that they should contact Padre Jonas (the spiritual founder of Canção Nova). They wrote him a letter and told him about the revelation. When Padre Jonas read the letter, he replied at once to the abbess: "Madre, this is nothing short of an answer to my prayers. I am just returning from Assisi in Italy, where I visited Santa Clara, and asked her to help our community, which is undergoing so much resistance and discredit." And so, at that moment it became clear that Santa Clara was playing a role in mediating our presence here....

M.J.: But why Santa Clara?

S.R.: Santa Clara. Don't you know? ... There was this episode in her life.... On a Christmas night she was bedridden and could not join the other sisters and St. Francis for the Mass. The others went and left her behind alone and sick in her cell. But when the sisters came back from the feast and were about to describe the event, sister Clara told them, "There is no need to tell me anything. For I have seen and heard all through the walls of my cell." So, because of this episode, in 1958, around the time television was invented, Pope Pius XII made her into the patron saint of television.

M.J.: Is that the reason why Padre Jonas went to Assisi?

S.R.: That is the reason why Padre Jonas went to Assisi!

Not surprisingly, the progressive voices of the Catholic Church showed discomfort, disgust even, when they heard about the monastery of Canção Nova. How could such a highly prestigious spiritual order exist alongside such a newly stylized form of mediatized Catholicism? Was this not essentially a contradiction in terms, the depth of the former pitted against the flatness of the latter? Being one of the main facades of the Catholic Charismatic Renewal (CCR) in Brazil and a launcher of the movement into local as well as international spheres, the Canção Nova Media Community had been highly contested by the prevalently Liberationist local church.[8] Arriving in Brazil in 1969, the American-born CCR was damned as "a demon from the north" by partisans of Liberation Theology, in tune with other left-wing intellectual and artistic groups who were opposed both to the military regime and to the injection of American products (including the CCR itself) into the country.[9] The spread of television among the Brazilian population in the 1960s had been accompanied by the massive importation of American entertainment programs, encouraging critics not only to condemn the alienating power of television, but also to oppose the alliance between right-wing policies of the Brazilian state and North American cultural imperialism. Technological alternatives such as community radio, audiocassettes, and a rich production of popular videos were promoted as counter-technologies.[10] Pitted against one another, television and video thus became highly politicized technologies in the Brazil of the 1960s and '70s, comparable with what Sreberny-Mohammed, referring to the Iranian revolution, has described as a battle between "big media" and "small media."[11] The ideological dispute over technology embodied by competing media was very much expressed in terms of a topology of surface and depth. Whereas "big media" could only conjure appearances, "small media" were able to dig deeply into reality in order to reveal the truth behind the surface. Because of its close association with television as a tool for evangelization, the American-born CCR came to further enforce this distinction between surface and depth as reflected in the language of Liberation Theology, whose Marxist orientations and militant spirit revealed the strong influence of Frankfurt School cultural theory on Brazilian intellectuals and activists.

Among the comments expressed to me on various occasions by academic sympathizers or actual Liberationists, it was said that Liberation Theology is grounded in reality, whereas the CCR is ethereal, or that Liberation Theology is for the earth, whereas the CCR is for the air, or that Liberation Theology cares for the political, whereas the CCR cares only for the spiritual. No ideology, only aesthetics; no content, only alienation; no substance, only air. Even though the divide between the two movements became less pronounced after 1985 (the year Brazil regained parliamentary democracy), the tropes of surface and depth still lingered, and even today they come into play as soon as one starts to discuss Catholicism in contemporary Brazil. Indeed, one good illustration of this internal tension within Brazilian Catholicism occurred in 1999, when news spread that a monastery of Poor Claires was going to be built inside Canção Nova. It seemed as if, because they were "older" and "pristine," the Poor Claires were owners of a much deeper spirituality than Canção Nova's "flat" spirituality. With their strict conduct of expiation and recollection, the Poor Ladies represented a much "thicker" body than the *prêt-a-porter* Catholicism of Canção Nova. I have analyzed these disputes within the contemporary Brazilian Catholic Church elsewhere.[12] In this chapter I am moved by more epistemological concerns—namely, to inquire what the tropes of surface and depth tell us about historical perceptions of the air and the conceptual ground. For, as Luce Irigaray has proposed, modern thinking has been prevalently a "grounding" enterprise, within which our perceptions of air have evolved.[13] In a similar vein, I ask, how might we produce an anthropology of the air in which religion and technology leave their legible traces?

Airspace

In a recent interview Steven Connor has argued that the expression "thin air," as used by Shakespeare, references a truly modern idea.[14] As he explains, before Shakespeare, the air was thickly populated and animated by a plethora of entities, substances, odors, humors, voices, and specters. It was only with the advent of the modern period that airspace became, as it were, emptied of all of its life, inhabiting forces, and beings. To paraphrase Connor, air stopped being a substance and became instead a dimension. In order for it to become a measurable dimension, air first had to be emptied and transformed into a vacant, raw kind of space, open to construction: an abstract frame within which movement simply happens. Yet despite this reduction of space to a surface on which things are measured and reality is imprinted, one cannot say that the Renaissance was responsible for having flattened airspace. On the contrary, the modern period marks the advent of depth, linear perspective, and dimensionality, each of which was attained by a concomitant withdrawal of the perceiving subject into an exterior, detached position from which space could be measured and controlled. In other words, in order for it to be deepened, space first had to be flattened. Modern hermeneutics could then grow out of a distrust of the flat character of appearances—not despite, but precisely because of the fact that the activities of writing, reading, painting, and later printing all involve the use of flat surfaces.

Medieval art, on the contrary, is often acknowledged for its flat features and its lack of perspective. Art historians often attribute this to the efforts of medieval artists to depict otherworldly affairs and the teachings of Christ, rather than the world around them, inhabited by people and ideas (as would later become typical of art in the Renaissance period).[15] However, as already mentioned, the air in which the medieval artist lived was densely populated by earthly as well as unearthly entities. Contrary to modern air, medieval air was loaded, charged, thick with events and networked out of the mist, as it were.

Historical shifts in the conception of the air were by no means confined to the European experience. As with many other colonized regions of the world, Brazil underwent its own reform of the air, starting in the late nineteenth century.[16] That reform was intimately associated with the establishment of the new republic in 1889 and the subsequent spread among Brazilians of the slogan *A Conquista do Ar* ("The Conquest of the Air"). Brazil's Conquest of the Air translated into a number of initiatives such as parades, poems praising the skies, incentives to develop aviation technologies (that for a time placed Brazil at the forefront of the history of aircraft inventions, thanks to the pioneering work of Alberto Santos-Dummont),[17] and, most remarkably, the construction in 1931 of the gigantic statue of Jesus Redeemer of the Corcovado, overlooking the bay of Rio de Janeiro. This new fixation with the organization of airspace harnessed the church and the state in a joint effort to tune the newly formed Brazilian republic to the positivist adage *Ordem e Progresso* ("Order and Progress"). Influenced by Auguste Comte's motto "love as a principle; order as the basis; progress as the goal," the statue of the Jesus of the Corcovado powerfully synthesized in a figurative idiom the encounter between politics, art, and religion. It spoke directly to a campaign mobilized by the modern Catholic Church to dissipate Brazil's air from the thick webs of mysticism woven out of four centuries of interaction among Indians, Africans, Christians, and neo-Christians. In the new climate of independence, the call to conquer the air of Brazil through a vast evacuation of its ulterior forces and substances reinforced historical associations of the colonization of Brazil with the thickness of its air. Occupied with cleansing their own air from the mystical Middle Ages, the Iberians had seen Brazil—known then as the Land of the Holy Cross—as a kind of backyard into which all sorts of "matters out of order" could be discarded, not least with the exiling of criminals, heretics, or victims of malaria (literally "bad air"). In this context the project of Brazilian independence and formation of a new nation was intimately bound up with reform of the air.

It is striking, then, that a quarter of a century later the CCR (which went on to infiltrate the entire fabric of Brazilian Catholicism) began working to rearticulate airspace in Brazil, questioning the entrenched republican ideals of airspace and world viewing. Might there be something about this most recent shift in the air that transports us back to the medieval world of St. Claire? This is no negligible point when one considers how, despite the efforts of reformers such as those in Brazil, since at least the second half of the nineteenth century airspace was not emptied, but rather newly populated—if not congested—through the development of new aerial technologies, including aviation machinery, the telegraph, the telephone, the gramophone, radio, television, and satellite technologies. In the contemporary moment, aerial technologies are once again proving to be excellent environments for the spectral. Moreover, surfaces no longer lie still, as evidenced by our animated engagement with interactive screens that seem to be endowed with a will of their own. Does all this loading of the air imply that we are losing our perspective? Have the evacuation of substance and the consequent "dimensionalization" of airspace in the modern period occasioned new calls for depth?

Linear perspective presupposed the idea that movement must always be preceded by position. This scheme allowed knowledge to become standardized—to be as optically consistent as possible. It implied that things had an origin, an end, and a vanishing point, as they were gradually distanced from the eye. The eruption of realistic painting at the dawn of the Renaissance revealed the rise and expansion of this new ocularcentrism. Paintings such as *The Arnolfini Portrait*, painted in 1434 by Jan van Eyck (well known for its utterly detailed depictions of an optical atmosphere, expressed by the "three-dimensionality, presence, individuality and psychological depth lacking in earlier works"), show how "the history of art from that time evolved in intimate relation with the history of optics itself."[18] Western formations of the visible accrued from a rich scientific optical tradition with help of lenses and mirrors. But contemporary regimes of visibility have been enabled just as much by the networking potentials of new media technologies that have expanded our network of sensory perception, encompassing not only the eye, but the entire body. In other words, the project of reconceptualizing the image in an age of technological interactivity has unsettled the laws of geometric perspective that once guaranteed that all parallel lines would meet at a vanishing point, not unlike in the image of the two lines of a railway track.

Whereas modernist analyses of culture were staged according to the rules of perspective and linear time, which foregrounded the separation between subject and object, and between origins and ends, that type of analytical perspective may no longer be suitable to account for the contemporary context of technological interactivity, in which receptors are themselves invited to become part of the production process and viewers are directly implicated in the viewing. Rather than having texts disseminated in linear fashion, receptors are increasingly implicated in the acts of production and of dissemination themselves. As exemplified by the solicitation of homemade video footage by major news corporations such as the BBC and CNN, media products are marked by the traits of their own making. What presents itself as "news" is actually no more than the redundant gesture already produced and captured at the receiving end.[19] News emerges out of the feedback loop of reproduction. Ends are rejoined. Potentiality is the message. One of the main outcomes of this recursivity between the old and the new is that the subject both sees and becomes the seen. Analysts no longer exist in a state of detached "hermeneutic suspicion" from the seen, but are themselves part of what is seen. How, then, can one apply linear terms and one-dimensional measures to a visual culture that is increasingly premised on these new modes of interface between cause and effect and between producer and receiver? When origins and ends are being folded into the middle (read: medium) and into the self-referential aesthetics of "the making-of," in some ways might that process expose and comment upon the very plasticity of the idea of "origin?"[20] If it is the case, as indeed it seems to be, that one of these new conditions of the image presents itself in the folding-in of origins and ends through processes of feedback (and feed-forward), perhaps it would be more useful to disabuse ourselves of the notion of "perspective"—and its corollary aspects of causal linearity—and replace it with "*prospective*," a term that references the present's virtual possibility as something never quite present to itself.

Breathing the Aura

Although contemplation is a term that came to be associated with the artist's aesthetic engagement with a piece of art—as that which positions the subject apart from an object and warrants its aura—it was also a central notion in the religious life of St. Claire, and it certainly influenced later depictions of the saint as an "icon of contemplation." The medieval notion of *contemplationem* referred to "the act of looking attentively" and thus presented an altogether different set of premises. Contemplation in the medieval sense had nothing to do with an idea of waiting—a gazing out into the world, as if from an open window, as presupposed by linear perspectivism. Nor was it simply a matter of passive observation in the pursuit of truth. Rather, in medieval times, to contemplate meant to actively engage in the pursuit of knowledge through augury or divination. Contemplation thus referred to an act of looking forward expectantly to an event, or to one's capacity to anticipate, infer, or extract "information" from the world through its signs and omens.[21] Contemplation in the medieval sense was therefore less about *seeing* than about *seeing through*: less about *per*spective than *pro*spective. Similarly, the word "temple"—from which the word "contemplation" is derived—stood for a demarcated space for auguring. Quite often medieval religious spaces were constructed not in order to allow people to *see* the transcendent, but rather to invite them to transcend the immediate time and space of their existential condition. Paradoxically, the latter was attained by means of a well-cultivated faculty to immerse oneself in the very space one wanted to transcend. To contemplate was essentially to engage in an extramural activity, and in that sense it was an action that, although premised on an idea of seeing, in fact shared more with sound than with vision itself. This was the case not simply because of sound's permeability and indeterminacy (when compared to the image), but also due to sound's immersive quality, as opposed to the "detachment" of vision.[22] Simply put, the medieval contemplative self was an auditory rather than a visual one. As Gaston Bachelard writes, "all profound contemplation is necessarily and naturally a hymn"[23] (and by the way, the name "Canção Nova" means "New Song").

When Hannah Arendt suggests that the advent of the modern age meant the reversal of *vita contemplativa* into *vita activa*, there is a risk that the reader will mistakenly infer that in the Middle Ages there was no such thing as acting, only observing. This would be misleading not simply because it is rather implausible, but because such a differentiation is itself a product of the modern age. The transition to which Arendt refers is precisely the one that created the foundations and technological conditions for accommodating such a distinction. "The point was not that truth and knowledge were no longer important, but that they could be won only by 'action' and not by contemplation. It was an instrument, the telescope, a work of man's hands, which finally forced nature, or rather the universe, to yield its secrets."[24] What was at stake was the reformulation of the notion of contemplation more than its replacement by that of action. The discovery of the telescope and the rediscovery of the Archimedean vantage point reinstated the importance of positioning oneself external to the observed phenomenon. To be contemplative henceforth would mean to engage in an intellectual exercise that could no longer lend itself to being identified with the thing contemplated. It was this dissociation between seer and seen that allowed Renaissance artists to distance themselves from the medieval mode of contemplation in order to depict scenes in a "naturalistic" fashion.

The notion of contemplation went through further alteration through thinkers such as Martin Heidegger—specifically in his famous lecture, "The Age of the World-Picture"—or through Walter Benjamin's views on the progressive loss of the aura with the coming of the age of mechanical reproducibility. Published one year before Heidegger's lecture, Benjamin's thoughts on the auratic share with Heidegger's notion of the "world as picture" the basic presumption of a world that is accessed from a distance ("however close it may be" in the case of Benjamin;[25] however far it may be, in the case of Heidegger). In other words, both authors ground their arguments in the principle of detachment. In Heidegger this is achieved in his analysis of a picturing of the world that (as Arendt also argues) can be traced back to the invention of the telescope and the rise of the Cartesian doubt. In Benjamin detachment is part and parcel of the display of the auratic. Indeed, the auratic depended on a distance between seer and artwork that new media such as film and photography threatened to eliminate. So, for instance, Benjamin compares the painter with a magician whose efficacy depends on the maintenance of "a natural distance" vis-à-vis the spectator, whereas the filmmaker is compared with a surgeon or the projectile of a gun, both of which "penetrate deeply into the fabric of the given"—that is, presuppose an abstinence of distance.[26] However, the more we read Benjamin (indeed, the more we reproduce our readings of Benjamin's texts), the more we come to realize that the dualities of distance and proximity, outside and inside, or rise and decay that inform the relation between seer and seen are not exactly two separate moments in the life of the aura, but rather exist as its constitutive paradox. This idea been thoughtfully captured by Samuel Weber, who writes:

> But if aura, also designated by Benjamin as the "unique appearance of a distance, however close it may be" is inseparable from a certain separation, this can also explain something that Benjamin himself at times seems to have had difficulties coming to terms with: the fact that the aura, despite all its withering away, dilapidation and decline, never fully disappears. Far from it, since it returns with a vengeance, one might say, in those forms of representation that would, according to Benjamin's account, seem hostile to it: film, for instance, and we can now add television as well. The aura would be able to return in the age of technical reproducibility because, as the appearance or apparition of an irreducible separation, *it was never uniquely itself* but always constituted in a process of detachment: detachment from self as demarcation of a self.[27]

As Weber suggests, the form of demarcation through detachment that is characteristic of the aura is equivalent to the process of reproduction. Paradoxically, the best copy is precisely the one that is furthest from the original. Conversely, the closer a copy is to the original, the further it is from being a copy. From the perspective of the contemplator or viewer on the receiving end, the consequences of realizing this paradox are momentous. For, as Benjamin argues, the desire to overcome the uniqueness of every event through reproduction corresponds with a parallel aspiration to bring things spatially and humanly closer. The contemplator is no longer at the receiving end of production, but becomes progressively implicated in it. As Weber points out, with the coming of technical reproducibility, reception and production share fundamental features, which is why, in fact, both ends of the process are placed in Benjamin's writings under the same German designation of *aufnehmen*.[28] But how do these considerations of the auratic connect to the breathing subject and, more broadly, to the aforementioned notion of contemplation? If, following Benjamin, aura in the age of technical reproducibility is the result of a process through which the viewer becomes increasingly implicated in that which he or she contemplates, then aura is less something "to be seen" than something "to be breathed." As Benjamin states, "On a summer afternoon, resting, to follow a chain of mountains on the horizon or a branch casting its shadow on the person resting—that is what it means to breathe in the aura of those mountains, of this branch."[29]

Whereas seeing the aura would imply that the subject exists outside the picture, breathing implies a subject immersed in its substance. The contemplative subject, as Weber suggests, is not detached from the picture it contemplates, but rather is embedded in the scene that it both observes and breathes. As Weber writes, "The only difference between the world of this picture and Heidegger's world picture is that Benjamin's subject is depicted as being 'in the picture' and that being in it, it cannot quite get the picture in its entirety." Precisely this inability to see the picture in its entirety, to secure it with definition, or to fully capture with one's eyes those mountains (for the subject is ensconced in it) helps to explain what it means to contemplate in the age of mechanical reproducibility. In ways that recall medieval monastic practices of devotional contemplation, the visuality inherent in mechanical reproduction is more of a prospectival than a perspectival concern: more like a network of sensory apprehension than a unidirectional vision. Vision, for Benjamin, "shifts from eye to lips, thus taking a detour via the whole body"[30]

What is more, such a detour blasts apart the temporal continuity between past and present as time becomes bound to repetition and convolution. If we accept the idea that—as Catholic Charismatics maintain—St. Claire did not simply see images on the walls of her cell but rather, by means of "the breath of the spirit," was able to *see through* the walls into another place and another time, or if, seven hundred years later, we can say that Sister Clara did not simply see the Holy Body on Canção Nova's TV screen, but rather *through it* saw that a monastery of Poor Claires would be built inside Canção Nova, then perhaps we can say that the two Claires did not see. *Rather, seeing occurred through them.* Indeed, clairvoyantly! Walls and screens conflated in the same pneumatic force. Each moment, each to and fro, prefigured the other, as in a cosmic game of intercalated mirrors. Not as a linear time, as in a cause-effect sequence, but as a kind of convoluted loop: a maelstrom that places time always already in the middle.

Breathing, Indwelling

To be sure, everything about Canção Nova seemed contrary to the logic of the cloister. Canção Nova is a place where loudness was encouraged as a means of reconnection to Biblical myths, such as the sound of Joshua's seven ram-horns in the battle of Jericho or the sounds of the Pentecost in the form of "a rushing wind." The passage of the Pentecost as described in Acts 2:4 is often regarded as the foundational prooftext in the life of a Charismatic. The wind of Pentecost, it is often said, blew up not only the walls of the space in which the apostles were hidden, but also the walls of their own bodies, as they were petrified in fear. This was the moment of the downpouring of charismata, or gifts, through the breath of the Spirit, also known as the baptism in the Holy Spirit. Catholic Charismatics value this Biblical passage for its highly performative aspects. Words are valued not primarily in terms of their referential meaning, but in terms of their materiality. What matters is the vocal strain: the word-bearing air manifested in voicing such that reading, reciting, and praying can all be understood as forms of instilling an aerial animus in things. Once articulated, the "exhaled word" spreads out and enraptures those who are under its spell. Spell and spelling are thus related. Moreover, through its vocal power, the inflamed wind of Pentecost changes the conventional understandings of objects, of their relations in space, and even of space itself. Accordingly, it is no longer about a fixed, positioned body or space merely containing movement. Rather, it is movement—in this case, the movement of sound—that world-builds, creating space.

This symbiotic relation between the breathing body and the making of space through breathing or voicing (as structured breath) is best captured by the concept of bodybuilding. Indeed, it explains why aerobics evolved to become an important liturgical reference in the religious practices of Catholic Charismatics in Brazil. The hugely popular "aerobics of Jesus" invented by the media-savvy Brazilian priest Padre Marcelo Rossi is among the most conspicuous illustrations of this tendency, but there are many other performative instances that show the centrality of *pneuma* within local religious practices of the CCR.[31] Consider, for example, a ritual enacted by Catholic Charismatics in general every year in December. For seven consecutive days, organized prayer groups march in vigil around the main churches of São Paulo, praying, singing, and clapping in allusion to the biblical myth of the breaking of the walls of Jericho (Joshua 6:20). Such public expressions of the Charismatic movement—especially in places like São Paulo, where Liberation Theology was once particularly strong—are still contested. In the past, Charismatics were obliged to meet secretively in private condominiums within the city or to gather only in places outside the city. Starting in the 1980s, however, the Charismatic movement gained new visibility, not only through organized mega-events in football stadiums, parks, and gymnasiums, but also through electronic media. In the face of a recalcitrant church, the ritual of Jericho—expressed in the collective act of singing and clapping around cathedrals for seven days—worked as a diatribe against those local church authorities who refused to accord the CCR a place within its parishes and associated constituencies.[32] What the ritual of Jericho expresses—the possibility of breaking down walls through the power of breath—is a battle between movement and position, symbolized respectively by the CCR and by the local ecclesiastic establishment. This antagonistic relation corresponds to the classic dispute between institution and charisma, which, as Charismatics often say, is personified in St. Peter and St. Paul.

The ritual of Jericho thus enacts a particular conception of space that challenges the idea of a fixed position from which one controls, orders, and calculates movement. Such a conception of space lies outside the Cartesian three-dimensional space that has greatly influenced the standards of modern Western architecture. Whereas Western theories of architecture traditionally relied on modern ideas of "world-viewing," Catholic Charismatics present a particular idea of inhabitancy or "indwelling" that prioritizes movement over fixation. The ideal architectonic model for a Catholic Charismatic draws upon St. Paul's dictum, "your body is the temple of the Holy Spirit."[33] There is perhaps no better architectural form for expressing this Pauline saying about the mediation of body and building than a tent (indeed, St. Paul himself was a tentmaker). Tents are "bodybuildings" in the sense that they are materially like bodies, but with the shape of a building. Tents are made of a resilient, pliant, as well as breathable fabric—much like a body's skin—yet their function and shape resemble those of a house, albeit one that permeates movement and temperature. Tents, like lungs, are pneumatic structures. Thus, to go back to the ritual of Jericho, while some Brazilian Charismatics would go on marathons of marching and singing around the cathedrals of São Paulo, others would remain inside tents that were set up on the patio of the cathedral. Even though these tents were used for practical purposes—namely, to logistically support the seven days of the ritual—they also instantiated a particular ideal of indwelling modeled on the act of breathing. As portable chapels, the tents provided the CCR with a tangible expression of its identity as a religious (pneumatic) movement, in contrast with the "fixity" of cathedrals.

That Thursday . . .

That Thursday, after my visit to the monastery, I again entered the main temple to follow Canção Nova's second part of the liturgical program "Contemplation Day." The ceremony was being transmitted live on radio and TV, reaching all of Brazil as well as Portugal, Italy, Israel, Morocco, and—through Canção Nova's Internet WEB TV—the entire globe.[34] The priest and his acolytes marched to the welcoming sounds of singing and clapping. The priest placed the monstrance at the center of the altar table and joined the singing that was being orchestrated by an animator standing on the right side of the stage. As usual, they performed a few other songs before beginning the liturgy. The idea was to warm up the gathering: *criar um clima* ("to build up an environment"), as Catholic Charismatics like to say, in order to welcome the Holy Spirit into their midst.

With a capacity of four thousand people, the walls of the temple at Canção Nova were for the most part made of brick and cement. However, along one of the lateral wings of the building, the wall had been replaced by a large steel structure, very much like a scaffold. At first glance it seemed as if the scaffold was there to repair the building. Yet on further observation this was obviously not the case. Far from repairing the wall, the gridiron structure was meant to be part of it, as a kind of counter-wall. Rather than barring the passage of air—and everything else carried by it, such as sound, temperature, smell, and light—the mesh-like pattern of the scaffold invited passage between the interior and the exterior of the building.

Simultaneously, and in analogy with architectural space, the devout were invited to allow their bodies to stretch and open up, like a scaffold, in order to host the "Eucharistic waves." Although nowadays the expression "Eucharistic waves" applies more generally to the act of engaging in contemplation and consumption of the Eucharist, it first appeared in connection with St. Claire, who, above all, was recognized as the Lady of Perpetual Contemplation. Legendarily known as the patron saint of television and TV writers,[35] St. Claire is often depicted holding a monstrance in her hand. At Canção Nova the electrification of the monstrance through its lengthy exposure on the screen on Thursday, Adoration Day, further helped to mystify television around the sign of Eucharistic waves. In this context to be "receptive to the Eucharist waves" was very much an expression of convergence of the religious and the technological, and also of convergence of body and space. The process of opening oneself or tuning to the "spiritual waves" is conventionally referred as an act of anointment, the practice of which results in a kind of cosmetic lubrication of the body. One opens up one's pores so that the entire body can breathe and "build up" in breath aerobically.

Catholic Charismatic musical productions are often composed to fit with a particular breathing economy materialized in the strain and timbre of the voice, in the oxygen indebt, or in a specific rhythm of the heart, all of which contribute to generate an ideal atmosphere. On that particular day, the hymn "Look at Me" worked as a romantic ballad dedicated to the Eucharist. Its slow, melodic rhythm, built on four ascending verses, culminated in a high-pitched refrain. With its alternating movements of expansion and contraction, inhaling and exhaling, that music helped to pace the crowd, which for its part gradually converged into a single orchestration of sound and movement. After ceaseless repetitions of the main refrain, the assembled congregation morphed into a kind of gigantic lung, which through its tremulous dance of contraction and expansion pumped air into the Eucharistic Body, which was exposed on the altar and also refracted onto the TV screens that filled the hall. The miracle of Real Presence resembled an act of cardiopulmonary resuscitation. Transubstantiation out of air!

The miracle of Real Presence—the belief among Catholics that Christ is really, and not merely symbolically, present in what was previously just bread and wine—is altered here. Although a priest is the one who performs the ritual, great emphasis is nonetheless placed on the power of breath—air-conditioning the entire space and consummating in the miracle of Real Presence in ways that are not reducible to hierarchical mediation or preexisting sacramental meaning. Because everybody partakes in the rhythm of resuscitation, everybody can become Eucharistic. As a result, not only is the deepest mystery of the church, the miracle of transubstantiation, reconceived in terms of breath, air itself is substantiated. Air is rendered as a substance rather than a dimension.

Breath has the power to summon the presence of the real because it is closer to the heart and implies an existential immediacy, invoking all sorts of feelings of authenticity and spontaneity. But at the same time, this sense of real presence is extended to encompass a virtual presence. The more people partook in the making of the real, by inhaling and exhaling, the more they seemed capable of becoming *virtually* anyone. The singularity of each individual receded into a collectively distributed experience. The concreteness of each body, and of space itself, seemed at once to intensify and to diffuse. As with the medieval space of contemplation, the more immersed the practitioners, the greater their abstraction. Less *per*spective, more *pro*spective. This idea of a distributed identity becomes particularly apparent, and most strikingly so, when one considers the role of notions of autonomy and responsibility during the act of confession. Whereas the traditional technology of confession presupposed a conscious and autonomous subject who engaged in a primarily private and verbal ritual (moreover, one dependent on a mediator), Catholic Charismatics would organize spectacles such as the "Day of Contemplation," where confessions were not only public, but also—primarily—somatic. It was the body that confessed. Lumps, burns, numbness on the skin, knots on the throat, fever, tingling in limbs or sensations of electrical shock were among the possible somatic registers of sin. Yet sins did not surface only in individual bodies. They were also revealed by proxy, as sins committed by others in the past, or by someone far away, or even by somebody standing right next to a person at the show (as if she was not there at all). Each body became metonymically associated with the Eucharistic Body: vacillating between the presence of breath as a "here and now" and as a potential extension to others.[36]

Conclusion

My concern in this chapter has been not so much about the visualization of movement as about the movement by which such vision is possible. My argument is that the desire of St. Claire (or her contemporary counterpart, or, for that matter, the followers of Canção Nova) to contemplate has nothing to do with a look in detachment, but rather is a desire to *actively participate in the movement of what is being contemplated.* Saint Claire did not prefigure television; she became television: TV St. Claire.[37] This desire to partake in movement—to embody the qualities of the medium rather than fixate it according to rules of Euclidean space – changed the basis upon which the modern postulate of depth came into being. Because movement is what literally matters, reality became virtual, fraught with the potential for change, alteration, and even transubstantiation.

The paramount question in this chapter is this: what happens to the quest for depth in the contemporary moment when, instead of operating as one open Albertian window that converges on a single vanishing point, our media surfaces are characterized by multiple, heterogeneous, juxtaposed, and cross-linked "open windows," dazzlingly animated with life and movement? Instead of a one-dimensional relationship between producer and receiver, cause and symptom, old and new, messages today are less referents pointing to an elsewhere than traces of their own itineraries and trajectories, their movements and processes coming into being, only to depart again through bodily detours. Perhaps Benjamin's aura was never meant to be seen, but rather only to be breathed: the movement that *is* through a virtual separation from itself. For what is breath if not the expression of that irreducible process of "taking-leave" that, as Samuel Weber writes, characterizes the aura?[38]

NOTES

INTRODUCTION: RELIGION, TECHNOLOGY, AND THE THINGS IN BETWEEN
Jeremy Stolow

1. See Donald J. Mastronarde, "Actors on High: The Skene Roof, the Crane, and the Gods in Attic Drama," *Classical Antiquity* 9, no. 2 (October 1990): 247–94; Rush Rehm, *Tragic Greek Theatre* (New York and London: Routledge, 1994), 69–71.
2. See, for instance, Aristotle, *Poetics* 1454a–b.
3. Whereas in ancient Greek the term *mēchanê* still reverberated with the connotations of its root word, *mekhos* (literally a "means" or an "expedient," etymologically connected to the proto-Indo-European word *magh-*, "to be able," whence also comes the term "magic"), by Roman times the word *machina* already had expanded its semantic terrain to include "device," "frame," "contrivance," and "trick."
4. David Hume, *Dialogues and Natural History of Religion*, ed. J. C. A. Gaskin (1757–1779; Oxford: Oxford University Press, 1993); Ludwig Feuerbach, *Lectures on the Essence of Religion*, trans. Ralph Manheim (1851; New York: Harper and Row, 1967); Emile Durkheim, *The Elementary Forms of Religious Life*, trans. Karen E. Fields (1912; New York: Free Press, 1995).
5. Bruno Latour, *On the Modern Cult of the Factish Gods* (Durham, N.C.: Duke University Press, 2010), 43; see also Latour, "What Is Iconoclash? Or Is There a World Beyond the Image Wars?" in *Iconoclash: Beyond the Image Wars in Science, Religion, and Art*, ed. Latour and Peter Weibel (Cambridge, Mass.: MIT Press, 2002), 14–37; Latour, *Pandora's Hope: Essays on the Reality of Science Studies* (Cambridge, Mass.: Harvard University Press, 1999), 266–92.
6. Matthew Engelke, "Religion and the Media Turn: A Review Essay," *American Ethnologist* 37, no. 2 (2010): 371–79.
7. A landmark text in the generation of this "media turn" in the study of religion is Hent de Vries and Samuel Weber, eds., *Religion and Media* (Stanford: Stanford University Press, 2001). For overviews of religion and media as a field of research, see David Morgan, ed., *Key Words in Religion, Media and Culture* (New York: Routledge, 2008); and Jeremy Stolow,

"Religion and/as Media," *Theory, Culture & Society* 22, no. 2 (2005): 119–45; see also the many contributions to the journal *Material Religion: The Journal of Objects, Art, and Belief*, which began publishing in 2005.

8. As Hent de Vries argues in his agenda-setting introduction to the volume *Religion and Media*, "We should no longer reflect exclusively on the meaning, historically and in the present, of religion—of faith and belief and their supposed opposites such as knowledge and technology—but concentrate on the significance of the processes of mediation and mediatization without and outside of which no religion would be able to manifest or reveal itself in the first place"; de Vries, "In Media Res: Global Religion, Public Spheres, and the Task of Contemporary Comparative Religious Studies," in *Religion and Media*, ed. de Vries and Weber, 28.

9. On the (mediated) production of immediacy, see Rosalind Morris, "Modernity's Media and the End of Mediumship? On the Aesthetic Economy of Transparency in Thailand," *Public Culture* 12, no. 2 (2000): 457–75; Birgit Meyer, "Mediation and Immediacy: Sensational Forms, Semiotic Ideologies and the Question of the Medium," *Social Anthropology* 19, no. 1 (2010): 23–39; and Mattijs van de Port, "(Not) Made by the Human Hand: Media Consciousness and Immediacy in the Cultural Production of the Real," *Social Anthropology* 19, no. 1 (2010): 74–89.

10. The "conflict thesis" is usually traced back to John William Draper, *History of the Conflict between Religion and Science* (New York: Appleton, 1878). For recent critiques, see John Hedley Brooke, *Science and Religion: Some Historical Perspectives* (Cambridge: Cambridge University Press, 1991); Thomas Dixon, Geoffrey Cantor, and Stephen Pumfrey, eds., *Science and Religion: New Historical Perspectives* (Cambridge: Cambridge University Press, 2010); and Ronald L. Numbers, ed., *Galileo Goes to Jail, and Other Myths about Science and Religion* (Cambridge, Mass.: Harvard University Press, 2009). On "scientific wonders" and the culture of public scientific spectacle, see Bernadette Bensaude-Vincent and Christine Blondel, eds., *Science and Spectacle in the European Enlightenment* (Aldershot, UK: Ashgate, 2008); Lorraine Daston and Katharine Park, *Wonders and the Order of Nature, 1150–1750* (New York: Zone Books, 1998); James Delbourgo, *A Most Amazing Scene of Wonders: Electricity and Enlightenment in Early America* (Cambridge, Mass.: Harvard University Press, 2006); Fred Nadis, *Wonder Shows: Performing Science, Magic, and Religion in America* (New Brunswick, N.J.: Rutgers University Press, 2005); and Simon Schaffer, "Natural Philosophy and Public Spectacle in the Eighteenth Century," *History of Science* 21 (March 1983): 1–43.

11. Jacques Derrida, "Faith and Knowledge: The Two Sources of 'Religion' at the Limits of Reason Alone," in *Religion*, edited by Jacques

Derrida and Gianni Vattimo, 56–57 passim (Stanford: Stanford University Press, 1998).

12. On "cybergnosticism," see Stef Aupers, Dick Houtman, and Peter Pels, "Cybergnosticism: Technology, Religion, and the Secular," in *Religion: Beyond a Concept*, ed. Hent de Vries (New York: Fordham University Press, 2008), 687–703. On the "disembodiment" of information and the dismantling of the humanist subject in cybernetic discourse, see N. Katherine Hayles, *How We Became Posthuman: Virtual Bodies in Cybernetics, Literature, and Informatics* (Chicago: University of Chicago Press, 1999). On the creation of "hybrids," see Ann Balsamo, *Technologies of the Gendered Body: Reading Cyborg Women* (Durham, N.C.: Duke University Press, 1999); Elaine Graham, *Representations of the Post/Human: Monsters, Aliens and Others in Popular Culture* (Manchester, UK: Manchester University Press, 2002); and Donna Haraway, *Simians, Cyborgs and Women: The Reinvention of Nature* (New York: Routledge, 1991).

13. On visual phantasmagoria, especially in the history of photography and early cinema, see Clément Chéroux, ed., *The Perfect Medium: Photography and the Occult* (New Haven: Yale University Press, 2004); Tom Gunning, "Phantom Images and Modern Manifestations: Spirit Photography, Magic Theater, Trick Films, and Photography's Uncanny," in *Fugitive Images: From Photography to Video*, ed. Patrice Petro (Bloomington: Indiana University Press, 1995). 42–71; Gunning, "To Scan a Ghost: The Ontology of Mediated Vision," *Grey Room* 26 (Winter 2007): 94–127; Corey Keller, ed., *Brought to Light: Photography and the Invisible, 1840–1900* (New Haven: Yale University Press, 2007); Marina Warner, *Phantasmagoria: Spirit Visions, Metaphors, and Media into the Twenty-first Century* (Oxford: Oxford University Press, 2006). On the religiosity of "special effects," see de Vries, "Of Miracles and Special Effects," *International Journal for the Philosophy of Religion* 50, no. 1 (December 2001): 41–56. On Pokémon, see Anne Allison, *Millennial Monsters: Japanese Toys and the Global Imagination* (Berkeley: University of California Press, 2006). On "the digital sublime," see Vincent Mosco, *The Digital Sublime: Myth, Power and Cyberspace* (Cambridge, Mass.: MIT Press, 2004). More generally, on the theme of "magic in modernity," ranging from studies of "voodoo economics" to "ghosts in the machine" of modern politics to the hazy borderlands that divide "secular" from "real" magic, see Jean Comaroff, "Occult Economies and the Violence of Abstraction: Notes from the South African Postcolony," *American Ethnologist* 26 (1999): 279–301; Jean Comaroff and John L. Comaroff, "Millennial Capitalism: First Thoughts on a Second Coming," in *Millennial Capitalism and the Culture of Neoliberalism*, ed. Comaroff and Comaroff (Durham, N.C.: Duke University Press, 2001), 1–56; Erik Davis, *Techgnosis: Myth, Magic, and Mysticism in the Age of Information* (New York: Harmony Books, 1998); Derrida, *Specters of*

Marx: The State of the Debt, the Work of Mourning, and the New International, trans. Peggy Kaumpf (New York: Routledge, 1994); Simon During, *Modern Enchantments: The Cultural and Secular Power of Magic* (Cambridge, Mass: Harvard University Press, 2002); Avery Gordon, *Ghostly Matters: Haunting and the Sociological Imagination* (Minneapolis: University of Minnesota Press, 1997); Birgit Meyer and Peter Pels, eds., *Magic and Modernity: Interfaces of Revelation and Concealment* (Stanford: Stanford University Press, 2003); Pels, "Magical Things: on Fetishes, Commodities, and Computers," in *The Oxford Handbook of Material Culture Studies*, ed. D. Hicks and M. C. Beaudry (Oxford: Oxford University Press, 2010), 613–33; Jeffrey Sconce, *Haunted Media: Electronic Presence from Telegraphy to Television* (Durham, N.C.: Duke University Press, 2000); Randall Styers, *Making Magic: Religion, Magic, and Science in the Modern World* (Oxford and New York: Oxford University Press, 2004); Michael Taussig, *The Magic of the State* (New York: Routledge, 1997); Pamela Thurschwell, *Literature, Technology and Magical Thinking, 1880–1920* (Cambridge: Cambridge University Press, 2001).

14. One of the few volumes purporting to offer a comprehensive account of the topic is Jay Newman, *Religion and Technology: A Study in the Philosophy of Culture* (Westport, Conn.: Praeger, 1997), although that book differs from the present work by having silently assumed a Christian vocabulary for defining and distinguishing religion and technology (an issue to which I shall return presently).

15. See, for instance, Lynn White Jr., *Medieval Religion and Technology: Collected Essays* (Berkeley: University of California Press, 1978). An important early foray into this topic is Lewis Mumford, *Technics and Civilization* (New York: Harcourt Brace, 1934); see also the references cited in the chapters by Peters and Ernst in this volume.

16. David F. Noble, *The Religion of Technology: The Divinity of Man and the Spirit of Invention* (New York: Albert A. Knopf, 1997).

17. See, for instance, Robert Merton, "Studies in the Sociology of Science," in idem, *Social Theory and Social Structure*, rev. and enlarged ed. (New York: Free Press, 1957), 531–627; David B. Ruderman, *Kabbalah, Magic and Science: The Cultural Universe of a Sixteenth-Century Jewish Physician* (Cambridge, Mass: Harvard University Press, 1988); Frances A. Yates, *The Rosicrucian Enlightenment* (London: Routledge and Kegan Paul, 1972).

18. On al-Biruni and other Muslim scientists of the medieval period, see George Saliba, *Islamic Science and the Making of the European Renaissance* (Cambridge, Mass.: MIT Press, 2007). On Boyle, see Merton, "Studies." On Newton's relationship with alchemy, see William R. Newman and Anthony Grafton, eds., *Secrets of Nature: Astrology and Alchemy in Early Modern Europe* (Cambridge, Mass.: MIT Press, 2001); Charles Webster, *From Paracelsus*

to Newton: Magic and the Making of Modern Science (Cambridge: Cambridge University Press, 1982); on John Wesley, see Paola Bertucci, "Revealing Sparks: John Wesley and the Religious Utility of Electrical Healing," *British Journal for the History of Science* 33, no. 3 (2006): 341–62. On the role of magic in the construction of European modernity, in addition to the sources cited in note 13, see Carlo Ginzburg, *The Cheese and the Worms: The Cosmos of a Sixteenth-Century Miller* (Baltimore: The Johns Hopkins University Press, 1980); Zakiya Hanafi, *The Monster in the Machine: Magic, Medicine, and the Marvelous in the Time of the Scientific Revolution* (Durham, N.C.: Duke University Press, 2000).

19. See, for instance, Thomas Hankins and Robert Silverman, *Instruments and the Imagination* (Princeton: Princeton University Press, 1995).

20. Norbert Wiener, *God and Golem, Inc.: A Comment on Certain Points where Cybernetics Impinges on Religion* (Cambridge, Mass.: MIT Press, 1964); Dean Hamer, *The God Gene: How Faith Is Hardwired into Our Genes* (New York: Anchor Books, 2005). For a nuanced critique of efforts to reduce religious affects, modes of behavior, and structures of belief to the "hard wiring" of human cognition, see Barbara Herrnstein-Smith, *Natural Reflections: Human Cognition at the Nexus of Science and Religion* (New Haven: Yale University Press, 2009).

21. See, for instance, Lesley Howsam, *Cheap Bibles: Nineteenth-Century Publishing and the British and Foreign Bible Society* (Cambridge: Cambridge University Press, 1991); David Paul Nord, *Faith in Reading: Religious Publishing and the Birth of Mass Media in America* (Oxford: Oxford University Press, 2004). For a more ambitious study of nineteenth-century missionary work, one that seeks to circumvent what I am here calling the "instrumentalist trap," see John Lardas Modern, "Evangelical Secularism and the Measure of Leviathan," *Church History* 77, no. 4 (December 2008): 801–76.

22. For more nuanced accounts of the relationship between diabolization and technological modernity, in particular as they were worked out in the context of colonial encounter, see Meyer, *Translating the Devil: Religion and Modernity Among the Ewe in Ghana* (Edinburgh: Edinburgh University Press, 1999); and Taussig, *The Devil and Commodity Fetishism in South America* (Chapel Hill: University of North Carolina Press, 1980).

23. Latour, *We Have Never Been Modern*, trans. Catherine Porter (Cambridge, Mass.: Harvard University Press, 1993).

24. This argument is elaborated in extensive detail in Styers, *Making Magic*.

25. See especially Meyer and Pels, eds., *Magic and Modernity*. For other treatments of magic that do not so simply perpetuate the divide that locates

"magic" on the far side of rational modernity, see Alfred Gell, "Technology and Magic," *Anthropology Today* 4, no. 2 (1988): 6–9; Stanley Jeyaraja Tambiah, *Magic, Science, Religion, and the Scope of Rationality* (Cambridge: Cambridge University Press, 1990); see also the sources cited in note 13.

26. See Martin Heidegger, "The Question Concerning Technology," in idem, *The Question Concerning Technology and Other Essays* (New York: Harper, 1977), 3–35; Jacques Ellul, *The Technological Society* (New York: Vintage Books, 1964); Ellul, *Jacques Ellul on Religion, Technology and Politics: Conversations with Patrick Troude-Chastenet*, trans. Joan Mendès France (Atlanta, Ga.: Scholars Press, 1998); Paul Tillich, *The Spiritual Situation in Our Technical Society*, ed. J. Mark Thomas (1955–1963; Macon, Ga.: Mercer University Press, 1988). Many so-called "pessimistic" or "antimodern" critiques of modern technology assume a Christian perspective, either explicitly or implicitly; see, for instance, Albert Borgmann, *Power Failure: Christianity in the Culture of Technology* (Grand Rapids, Mich.: Brazos Press, 2003); Michael Breen, Eamonn Conway, and Barry McMillan, eds., *Technology and Transcendence* (Dublin: The Columba Press, 2003); David J. Hawkin, *The Twenty-first Century Confronts Its Gods: Globalization, Technology and War* (Albany, N.Y.: State University of New York Press, 2004); Murray Jardine, *The Making and Unmaking of Technological Society: How Christianity Can Save Modernity From Itself* (Grand Rapids, Mich.: Brazos Press, 2004); Quentin J. Schultze, *Habits of the High-Tech Heart: Living Virtuously in the Information Age* (Grand Rapids, Mich.: Baker Academic, 2002); and William A. Stahl, *God and the Chip: Religion and the Culture of Technology* (Waterloo, Ontario: Wilfred Laurier University Press, 1999).

27. Interview with Heidegger by the German magazine *Der Spiegel*, conducted on 23 September 1966 and published posthumously on 31 May 1976; English translation in *The Heidegger Controversy: A Critical Reader*, edited by Richard Wolin, 91ff (Cambridge, Mass.: MIT Press, 1992).

28. On the other hand, for a brilliant reading of the resonance between Heidegger's critique of technological modernity and mystical and apophatic theological traditions (as represented, *inter alia*, by the writings of Gregory of Nyssa and Nicholas of Cusa), which challenges dominant definitions of humanity, creativity, and world-making, see Thomas A. Carlson, *The Indiscrete Image: Infinitude and the Creation of the Human* (Chicago: University of Chicago Press, 2008).

29. Max Weber, "Science as a Vocation," in *From Max Weber: Essays in Sociology*, ed. H. H. Gerth and C. Wright Mills (1919; New York: Oxford University Press, 1946), 139.

30. Among the many examples of critique of religious fundamentalism inspired (at least implicitly) by Weber's analysis of disenchantment, see

Haym Soloveitchik, "Rupture and Reconstruction: The Transformation of Contemporary Orthodoxy," *Tradition* 28 (1994): 64–130. For an extensive rejoinder to Weber's treatment of the relationship between magic and modernity, both inside and outside the theaters of Western capitalism, industry, politics, and science, see Meyer and Pels, eds., *Magic and Modernity*.

31. Heidegger, "Question," 13f; see also Bernard Stiegler, *Technics and Time, I: The Fault of Epimetheus*, trans. Richard Beardsworth and George Collins (Stanford: Stanford University Press, 1998), 1ff.

32. For a particularly serviceable overview of the history of the word "technology," see Carl Mitcham, *Thinking Through Technology: The Path Between Engineering and Philosophy* (Chicago: University of Chicago Press, 1994).

33. See Amos Funkenstein, *Theology and the Scientific Imagination from the Middle Ages to the Seventeenth Century* (Princeton: Princeton University Press, 1989); Bronislaw Szerszynski, *Nature, Technology and the Sacred* (Oxford: Blackwell, 2005).

34. See André Leroi-Gourhan, *Milieu et techniques* (Paris: Éditions Albin Michel, 1945); Leroi-Gourhan, *Le geste et la parole, Tome 1: Technique et langage* (Paris: Éditions Albin Michel, 1965).

35. Stiegler, *Technics and Time*, 140ff; see also Stiegler, "Derrida and Technology: Fidelity at the Limits of Deconstruction and the Prosthesis of Faith," in *Jacques Derrida and the Humanities: A Critical Reader*, edited by Tom Cohen, 238–70 (Cambridge: Cambridge University Press, 2001).

36. See, e.g., Latour, "Technology Is Society Made Durable," in *A Sociology of Monsters: Essays on Power, Technology and Domination*, ed. John Law (London and New York: Routledge, 1991), 103–31; Latour, "Where Are the Missing Masses? The Sociology of a Few Mundane Artefacts," in *Shaping Technology—Building Society: Studies in Sociotechnical Change*, ed. Wiebe E. Bijker and John Law (Cambridge, Mass.: MIT Press, 1992), 225–58; Latour, "When Things Strike Back," *British Journal of Sociology* 51, no. 1 (2000): 107–23.

37. Alongside Friedrich Kittler and Siegfried Zielinski, Wolfgang Ernst has become a significant contributor to the development of media archaeological methods. In addition to his chapter in this volume, see Ernst, *Digital Memory and the Archive* (Minneapolis: University of Minnesota Press, 2012). For a useful recent overview of media archaeology, see Erkki Huhtamo and Jussi Parikka, eds., *Media Archaeology: Approaches and Implications* (Berkeley: University of California Press, 2011).

38. See Talal Asad, *Genealogies of Religion: Disciplines and Reasons of Power in Christianity and Islam* (Baltimore: The Johns Hopkins University Press, 1993); David Chidester, *Savage Systems: Colonialism and Comparative Religion*

in Southern Africa (Charlottesville, Va.: University Press of Virginia, 1996); Tomoko Masuzawa, *The Invention of World Religions, Or, How European Universalism Was Preserved in the Language of Pluralism* (Chicago: University of Chicago Press, 2005); Guy Strousma, *A New Science: The Discovery of Religion in the Age of Reason* (Cambridge, Mass.: Harvard University Press, 2010).

39. Derrida, "Faith and Knowledge," 29ff.

40. For an extended definition of catachresis, see the French grammarian Pierre Fontanier's magisterial synthesis of classical rhetoric: Fontanier, *Les Figures du discours* (Paris: Flammarion, 1977 [orig. 1821]), 213–19. Interest in the trope of "catechresis" has been revived in recent years, notably by Gayatri Spivak, who uses the term to map the exchange of concepts between the Western metropolis and its former territories, grafting concepts such as "nation," "constitution," and "democracy" into situations where they find no native referents, because these terms are of uniquely Western European provenance; see Gayatri Chakravorty Spivak, *Outside in the Teaching Machine* (New York: Routledge, 1993), 20–38. There is an intended resonance between Spivak's use of the term and its appearance in this text.

41. Mumford, *Technics and Civilization*, 212–67.

CALENDAR, CLOCK, TOWER
John Durham Peters

1. Anthony F. Aveni, *Empires of Time: Calendars, Clocks, and Cultures* (New York: Kodansha America, 1994), chap. 1.

2. Ibid., chap. 2.

3. E. G. Richards, *Mapping Time: The Calendar and its History* (Oxford: Oxford University Press, 1999); and Duncan Steel, *Marking Time: The Epic Quest to Invent the Perfect Calendar* (New York: Wiley, 2000).

4. The calendar riots that are said to have resulted from this shift are more legend than history; see Robert Poole, "'Give Us Our Eleven Days!': Calendar Reform in Eighteenth-Century England," *Past and Present*, no. 149 (1995): 95–139.

5. Eviatar Zerubavel, "Easter and Passover: On Calendars and Group Identity," *American Sociological Review* 47 (1982): 284–89.

6. James W. Carey, "Technology and Ideology: The Case of the Telegraph," in *Communication as Culture* (Boston: Unwin Hyman, 1989), 201–30, at 227.

7. Eviatar Zerubavel, *The Seven Day Circle: The History and Meaning of the Week* (New York: Free Press, 1985).

8. George Dyson, *Darwin among the Machines* (Reading, Mass.: Addison-Wesley, 1997), chap. 10.

9. Stewart Brand, *The Clock of the Long Now* (New York: Basic Books, 1999).

10. Tony Jones, *Splitting the Second: The Story of Atomic Time* (Bristol, UK: Institute of Physics, 2000).

11. Lewis Mumford, *Technics and Civilization* (New York: Harcourt, Brace and Jovanovich, 1934), 12–17.

12. David Landes, *Revolution in Time: Clocks and the Making of the Modern World* (Cambridge, Mass: Harvard University Press, 1983, 2000).

13. E. P. Thompson, "Time, Work-Discipline, and Industrial Capitalism," *Past and Present*, no. 38 (1967): 56–97.

14. Robert Frost, "Acquainted with the Night," in *The Poetry of Robert Frost* (New York: Holt, Rinehart, and Winston, 1969), 255 (lines 11–14).

15. Frances Cornford, "The Watch," in *Literature: An Introduction to Fiction, Poetry, and Drama*, ed. X. J. Kennedy (Boston: Little Brown, 1976), 584 (lines 7–10).

16. Dava Sobel, *Longitude* (New York: Walker, 1995).

17. Derek Howse, *Greenwich Time* (London: Oxford University Press, 1980).

18. Peter Galison, *Einstein's Clocks, Poincaré's Maps* (New York: Norton, 2003).

19. Sybille Krämer, "The Cultural Techniques of Time Axis Manipulation: On Friedrich Kittler's Conception of Media," *Theory, Culture and Society* 23 (2006): 93–109.

20. Roland Barthes, "La Tour Eiffel" (1964), in idem, *Oeuvres Complètes*, ed. Éric Marty (Paris: Seuil, 1993), 1385.

21. Friedrich Kittler, *Optische Medien: Berliner Vorlesung* (Berlin: Merve, 2002).

22. Orhan Pamuk, *My Name Is Red*, trans. Erdağ M. Göknar (New York: Vintage, 2001), 70.

23. Barthes, "La Tour Eiffel," 1384.

24. Volker Aschoff, *Geschichte der Nachrichtentechnik*, vol. 1 (Berlin: Springer, 1989), chap. 3.

25. Alain Corbin, *Village Bells*, trans. Martin Thom (New York: Columbia University Press, 1998).

26. Amos Oz, *A Tale of Love and Darkness*, trans. Nicholas de Lange (New York: Harcourt, 2004), 191.

27. Quoted in Brian Winston, *Media, Technology, and Society: A History from the Telegraph to the Internet* (London: Routledge, 1998), 263.

28. Theodor Reik, "The Shofar," in idem, *Ritual: Psycho-Analytic Studies*, trans. Douglas Bryan (New York: Farrar, Straus, 1946), 221–361.

29. Charles Braibant, *Histoire de la Tour Eiffel* (Paris: Plon, 1964).
30. *Hamlet*, 1.iv.75–78.
31. Marshall McLuhan, *Understanding Media* (New York: McGraw-Hill, 1964), chap. 1.
32. Carl Couch, "Markets, Temples, and Palaces," *Studies in Symbolic Interaction* 7 (1986): 137–59.
33. This essay adapts entries previously published as "Calendar" and "Clock" in *Encyclopedia of Religion, Communication, and Media*, ed. Daniel A. Stout (New York: Routledge, 2006), 57–59, 77–79. I am grateful to the publisher for kind permission to rework this earlier material.

TICKING CLOCK, VIBRATING STRING: HOW TIME SENSE OSCILLATES BETWEEN RELIGION AND MACHINE
Wolfgang Ernst

Significant portions of an earlier version of this text were translated by Michael Darroch (University of Windsor, Canada). The author and editor both thank him for his efforts.

1. For academic definitions of religion, see Hubert Cancik, Burkhard Gladigow, and Matthias Laubscher, eds., *Handbuch religionswissenschaftlicher Grundbegriffe*, vol. 1 (Stuttgart: Kohlhammer, 1988).
2. Rolf F. Nohr, "Rhythmusarbeit," in *Das Spiel mit dem Medium*, ed. Britta Neitzel and Rolf F. Nohr (Marburg: Schüren, 2006), 225; this and all translations hereafter by Michael Darroch unless otherwise noted.
3. Ernst Cassirer, *Zur Logik der Kulturwissenschaft* (Göteborg: Wissenschaftliche Buchgesellschaft, 1942), 25.
4. Kay Kirchmann, *Verdichtung, Weltverlust und Zeitdruck: Grundzüge einer Theorie der Interdependenzen von Medien, Zeit und Geschwindigkeit im neuzeitlichen Zivilisationsprozeß* (Opladen: Leske and Budrich, 1998), 138f.
5. Werner Sulzgruber, *Zeiterfahrung und Zeitordnung vom frühen Mittelalter bis ins 16. Jahrhundert* (Hamburg: Kovac, 1995), 46.
6. Klaus Beck, *Medien und die soziale Konstruktion von Zeit: Über die Vermittlung von gesellschaftlicher Zeitordnung und sozialem Zeitbewußtsein* (Opladen: Westdeutscher Verlag, 1994), 128ff.
7. Letter from Leibniz, 18 May 1696, quoted in *Die Hauptschriften zur Dyadik von G. W. Leibniz: Ein Beitrag zur Geschichte des binären Zahlensystems*, by Hans J. Zacher (Frankfurt am Main: Klostermann, 1973), 209.
8. Michel Foucault, *Discipline and Punish: The Birth of the Prison* (New York: Vintage Books, 1979), 149.
9. Louis de Boussanelle, *Le Bon militaire* (Paris: La Combe, 1770), 2.

10. Peter Gendolla, "Die Einrichtung der Zeit," in *Augenblick und Zeitpunkt*, ed. Christian W. Thomsen and Hans Holländer (Darmstadt: Wissenschaftliche Buchgesellschaft, 1984), 49.

11. Marshall McLuhan, *Understanding Media: The Extensions of Man* (New York: McGraw Hill, 1964), 142.

12. Ibid., 112

13. Ibid., 112.

14. See Arno Borst, *Computus: Zeit und Zahl in der Geschichte Europas* (Berlin: Klaus Wagenbach, 1990), 18–23.

15. Michael. T. Clanchy, *From Memory to Written Record* (London: Arnold, 1979), 78.

16. Friedrich Kittler, *Optische Medien: Berliner Vorlesung* (Berlin: Merve, 2002), 47.

17. Werner Faulstich, *Das Medium als Kult: Von den Anfängen bis zur Spätantike* (Göttingen: Vandenhoeck and Ruprecht, 1997), 297.

18. Vivian Hunter Galbraith, *Historical Research in the Middle Ages* (London: Althone, 1951), 2.

19. Clanchy, *Memory*, 78.

20. Martin Heidegger, "The Age of the World Picture," in idem., *Off the Beaten Track*, ed. and trans. Julian Young and Kenneth Haynes (Cambridge: Cambridge University Press, 2002), 67.

21. On this, see Tatjana Böhme, "Die Zeit macht uns, durch den Gegensatz, die Ewigkeit verständlich: Die Zeit sollte der Freund aller Musiker sein," in *Zeit und Raum in Musik und Bildender Kunst*, ed. Tatjana Böhme and Klaus Mehner (Cologne Weimar and Vienna: Böhlau, 2000), 116.

22. Heidegger, "Age of the World Picture," 58.

23. On this see Barry Powell, *Homer and the Origin of Writing* (Cambridge: Cambridge University Press, 1990).

24. McLuhan, *Understanding Media*, 272.

25. Norbert Wiener, *Cybernetics: or Control and Communication in the Animal and the Machine* (Cambridge, Mass.: MIT Press, 1948).

26. Gerald J. Whitrow, *Die Erfindung der Zeit* (Hamburg: Junius, 1991), 158.

27. See Kurt von Fritz, "The Discovery of Incommensurability by Hippasus of Metapontum," *Annals of Mathematics* 46, no.2 (1945): 242–64.

28. Evanghélos Moutsopoulos, *La musique dans l'oeuvre de Platon*, 2nd ed. (1959; Paris: Presses Universitaires de France, 1989), 374.

29. Wolfgang Scherer, "Musik und Echtzeit: Zu John Cages 4'33"," in *Zeit-Zeichen: Aufschübe und Interferenzen zwischen Endzeit und Echtzeit*, ed. G. Christoph Tholen and Michael O. Scholl (Weinheim: VCH Acta Humaniora, 1990), 351–362, 356.

30. On this topic, see Grete Wehmeyer, *Prestississimo: Die Wiederentdeckung der Langsamkeit in der Musik* (Hamburg: Kellner, 1989), 15.

31. Hermann von Helmholtz, *On the Sensations of Tone as a Physiological Basis for the Theory of Music* (1863; Whitefish, Mont.: Kessinger, 2005), 398; see also Scherer, "Musik und Echtzeit," 362.

32. Nicole Oresme, *Le livre du ciel et du monde*, ed. Albert D. Menot (Madison: University of Wisconsin Press, 1968).

33. Wiener, "Time, Communication, and the Nervous System," *Annals of the New York Academy of Sciences* 50 (1948–50): 207.

34. Ibid.

35. Gerhard Dohrn-van Rossum, *History of the Hour: Clocks and Modern Temporal Orders* (Chicago: University of Chicago Press, 1996), 53.

36. Ibid., 46.

37. Ibid.

38. Ernst Pöppel, "Die Rekonstruktion der Zeit," in *Das Phänomen Zeit in Kunst und Wissenschaft*, ed. Hannelore Paflik (Weinheim: VCH, 1987), 29f.

39. See, e. g., Franz Reuleaux, *Theoretische Kinematik: Grundzüge einer Theorie des Maschinenwesens* (Braunschweig: Vieweg, 1875).

40. Dohrn-van Rossum, *History of the Hour*, 48.

41. Walter Benjamin, *Das Kunstwerk im Zeitalter seiner technischen Reproduzierbarkeit* (Frankfurt: Suhrkamp, 1963), 17; see also Jonathan D. Kramer, *The Time of Music* (New York and London: Schirmer, 1988), 68.

42. Wolfgang Coy, "Der diskrete Takt der Maschine," in *Zeitreise: Bilder, Maschinen, Strategien, Rätsel*, ed. Georg Christoph Tholen, Michael Scholl, and Martin Heller (Frankfurt: Stroemfeld and Roter Stern, 1993), 367–78.

43. Hartmut Böhme, "Vom Cultus zur Kultur(wissenschaft): Zur historischen Semantik des Kulturbegriffs," in *Literaturwissenschaft—Kulturwissenschaft: Positionen, Themen, Perspektiven*, ed. Renate Glaser and Matthias Luserke (Opladen: Westdeutscher Verlag, 1996), 55.

44. Ernst Jünger, "Über den Schmerz," in idem, *Blätter und Steine*, 2nd. ed. (1934; Hamburg: Hanseat. Verlagsanstalt, 1941), 208.

45. Hugo Münsterberg, *Grundzüge der Psychotechnik* (Leipzig: Barth, 1914), 559.

46. John von Neumann, "General and Logical Theory of Automata," in idem, *Collected Works*, vol. 5, *Design of Computers, Theory of Automata and Numerical Analysis*, ed. A. H. Taub (Oxford: Pergamon, 1951), 292.

47. J. D. North, "Monasticism and the First Mechanical Clocks," in *The Study of Time II: Proceedings of the Second Conference of the International Society for the Study of Time*, ed. J. T. Fraser and N. Lawrence (Lake Yamanaka, Japan, Berlin, Heidelberg, and New York: Springer, 1975), 381.

48. For the contrast of media archaeology to media anthropology, see Wolfgang Ernst, "Medienmonastik: Taktung im Widerstreit zwischen Liturgie und Maschine," in *Klosterforschung: Befunde, Projekte, Perspektiven*, ed. Jens Schneider (Munich: Fink, 2006), 163-182.

49. Ibid., 393.

50. Dohrn-van Rossum, *History of the Hour*, 46.

51. Sigfried Giedion, *Mechanization Takes Command* (Oxford: Oxford University Press, 1948).

52. Dohrn-van Rossum, *History of the Hour*, 105.

53. Ibid., 87.

54. Joseph Needham, *The Shorter Science and Civilisation in China*, ed. Colin A. Ronan (Cambridge: Cambridge University Press, 1978), 1:58.

55. Manfred Schukowski, *Die astronomische Uhr der St.-Marien-Kirche zu Rostock*; brochure (Rostock: n.p., 2004), 4.

56. St. Augustine, *The Confessions of St. Augustine, Bishop of Hippo*, book XI, chap. 20, trans. and annot. J. G. Pilkington (Edinburgh: T. and T. Clark 1876), 306.

57. Friedrich Kittler, *Eine Kulturgeschichte der Kulturwissenschaft* (Munich: Fink, 2000), 235f.

58. Henri Lefebvre, *Rhythmanalysis: Space, Time, and Everyday Life* (London and New York: Continuum, 2004), 73.

59. Ibid.

60. Martin Heidegger, "Time and Being," in idem., *On Time and Being*, trans. Joan Stambaugh (Chicago: University of Chicago Press, 2002), 16.

61. Claude Cadoz, *Les réalités virtuelles* (Paris: Flammarion, 1994), 85.

62. Bernhard Siegert, *Passage des Digitalen: Zeichenpraktiken der neuzeitlichen Wissenschaften 1500–1900* (Berlin: Brinkmann and Bose, 2003), 9; see also Claude Elwood Shannon, "A Symbolic Analysis of Relay and Switching Circuits," *Transactions American Institute of Electrical Engineers* 57 (1938): 713-23.

63. William Aspray and Arthur Burks, "Computer Architecture and Logical Design," in *Papers of John von Neumann on Computing and Computer Theory*, ed. William Aspray and Arthur Burks (Cambridge, Mass.: MIT Press, 1987), 5f.

THE ELECTRIC TOUCH MACHINE MIRACLE SCAM: BODY, TECHNOLOGY, AND THE (DIS)AUTHENTICATION OF THE PENTECOSTAL SUPERNATURAL
Marleen de Witte

1. Yigal Mesika, "Real Magic," accessed 22 June 2009, http://www.yigalmesika.com/.

2. Yigal Mesika, personal email correspondence, 4 December 2009.

3. See, for example, "Uganda pastor denies miracle scam," BBC News, 7 July 2007, accessed 22 June 2009, http://news.bbc.co.uk/2/hi/africa/6294666.stm.

4. Hent de Vries, "In Media Res: Global Religion, Public Spheres, and the Task of Contemporary Comparative Religious Studies," in *Religion and Media*, ed. de Vries and Samuel Weber (Stanford: Stanford University Press, 2001), 3–42; see also Dennis Tedlock, "The Shaman as Magician," *Journal of Shamanic Practice* 1 (2008): 16–20.

5. De Vries, "In Media Res," 29.

6. Ibid., 27–28, emphasis in original.

7. Chris Shilling and Philip A. Mellor, "Cultures of Embodied Experience: Technology, Religion, and Body Pedagogics," *The Sociological Review* 55, no. 3 (2007): 531–49.

8. Several authors have identified the dialectics between mediation and immediacy as central to the intersection of media technologies and religious traditions; see, for example, Patrick Eisenlohr, "Technologies of the Spirit: Devotional Islam, Sound Reproduction and the Dialectics of Mediation and Immediacy in Mauritius," *Anthropological Theory* 9, no. 3 (2009): 273–96; Matthew Engelke, *A Problem of Presence: Beyond Scripture in an African Church* (Berkeley: University of California Press, 2007); Birgit Meyer, "Introduction: From Imagined Communities to Aesthetic Formations; Religious Mediations, Sensational Forms and Styles of Binding," in *Aesthetic Formations: Media, Religion and the Senses in the Making of Communities*, ed. Meyer (New York: Palgrave MacMillan, 2009), 1–28, and several contributions to that volume; Mattijs van de Port, "Visualizing the Sacred and the Secret: Televisual Realities and the Religious Imagination in Bahian Candomblé," *American Ethnologist* 33, no. 3 (2006): 444–61.

9. De Vries, "In Media Res"; Eisenlohr, "Technologies"; Meyer, "Introduction: From Imagined Communities"; Jeremy Stolow, "Religion and/as Media," *Theory, Culture and Society* 22, no. 4 (2005): 119–45.

10. Friedrich Kittler, *Gramophone, Film, Typewriter* (Stanford: Stanford University Press, 1999), 13.

11. Marcel Mauss, "Techniques of the Body," *Economy and Society* 2, no. 1, trans. Ben Brewster (1973): 70–88; Maria José A. de Abreu, "Breathing into the Heart of the Matter: Why Padre Marcello Needs No Wings," *Postscripts* 1, nos. 2–3 (2005): 325–49; de Abreu, "Goose Bumps All Over: Breath, Media, and Tremor," *Social Text* 3, no. 96 (2008): 59–78; Charles Hirschkind, *The Ethical Soundscape: Cassette Sermons and Islamic Counterpublics* (New York: Columbia University Press, 2006).

12. Marshall McLuhan, *Understanding Media: The Extensions of Man*, 2nd ed. (London: Routledge and Kegan Paul, 1966). On the tactile qualities of modern technologies of mass reproduction, see also Walter Benjamin, "The Work of Art in the Age of Mechanical Reproduction," in *Illuminations*, trans. Harry Zohn (New York: Schocken, 1968), 238.

13. McLuhan, *Understanding Media*, 336.

14. Ibid., 333.

15. In the field of cinema studies, Laura Marks and Vivian Sobchack have focused on the bodily sensuality of film experience and the relation between audiovisuality and tactility; see Laura Marks, *Touch: Sensuous Theory and Multisensory Media* (Minneapolis: University of Minnesota Press, 2002); Vivian Sobchack, *Carnal Thoughts: Embodiment and Moving Image Culture* (Berkeley: University of California Press, 2004); see also Jojada Verrips, "'Haptic Screens' and Our 'Corporeal Eye,'" *Etnofoor* 15, nos. 1–2 (2002): 21–46.

16. Meyer, "Introduction: From Imagined Communities."

17. With 24.1 percent of the total population and 45.8 percent of all Christians in Accra regarding themselves as charismatic-Pentecostal, charismatic-Pentecostalism has become the main religious orientation; *Population and Housing Census* 2000 (Accra: Ghana Statistical Service, 2000).

18. Kwabena Asamoah-Gyadu, *African Charismatics: Current Developments within Independent Indigenous Pentecostalism in Ghana* (Leiden: Brill, 2005); Marleen de Witte, "Spirit Media: Charismatics, Traditionalists, and Mediation Practices in Ghana" (Ph.D. diss., University of Amsterdam, 2008); Paul Gifford, *Ghana's New Christianity: Pentecostalism in a Globalising African Economy* (London: Hurst, 2004); Meyer, "Christianity in Africa: From African Independent to Pentecostal-Charismatic Churches," *Annual Review of Anthropology* 33 (2004): 447–74.

19. De Witte, "The Spectacular and the Spirits: Charismatics and Neo-Traditionalists on Ghanaian Television," *Material Religion* 1, no. 3 (2005): 314–35; Asamoah-Gyadu, "Of Faith and Visual Alertness: The Message of 'Mediatized' Religion in an African Pentecostal Context," *Material Religion* 1, no. 3 (2005): 336–57; Meyer, "'Praise the Lord:' Popular Cinema and Pentecostalite Style in Ghana's New Public Sphere," *American Ethnologist* 31, no. 1 (2004): 92–110.

20. See Emmanuel Larbi, *Pentecostalism: The Eddies of Ghanaian Christianity* (Accra: Centre for Pentecostal and Charismatic Studies, 2001).

21. Interview, "Clifford" (full name not disclosed), member of media staff, International Central Gospel Church, 2 April 2002.

22. Richard Gyamfi Boakye, *Invisibility to Visibility: How You Can Release Things from the Spiritual Realm* (Kumasi, Ghana: Willas Press, 2001), 1:4.

23. Ibid., 4–5.

24. Emmanuel Abrahams Abrahams, *Spiritual Electronics: The Principles of Giving to Release the Blessings of God* (New Achimota, Ghana: Power of God Mission, 2000), preface.

25. For a description of discursive images of antennas or satellite dishes deployed by Catholic Charismatics in Brazil, see de Abreu, "Breathing," 345.

26. For a description of how computer technology increased the plausibility of witchcraft among young Sowetans in South Africa, see also Adam Ashforth, *Witchcraft, Violence, and Democracy in South Africa* (Chicago: University of Chicago Press, 2005). On Afa divination as computer technology, see Chigbo Josep Ekwealo, "African Divinatory System (Afa) and Computer Technology: The Meta-physics of the New Past and an Old Future," paper presented to the Karl Popper Centenary Congress (University of Vienna, 3–7 July 2002).

27. Interview, Kofi Hande, 29 April 2002.

28. See de Witte, "Altar Media's Living Word: Televised Charismatic Christianity in Ghana," *Journal of Religion in Africa* 33, no. 2 (2003): 172–202; de Witte, "Spirit Media: Charismatics, Traditionalists, and Mediation Practices in Ghana" (Ph.D. diss., University of Amsterdam, 2008).

29. Interview, Pastor Dan, May 8, 2002.

30. Benny Hinn, *Good Morning, Holy Spirit* (Nashville: Thomas Nelson, 1990), 22.

31. De Abreu, "Goose Bumps."

32. Gifford, *Ghana's New Christianity*.

33. "Miracle Days Are Here" (Accra: Lighthouse Chapel International, n.d.), videotape.

34. Asamoah-Gyadu, "Anointing through the Screen: Neo-Pentecostalism and Televised Christianity in Ghana," *Studies in World Christianity* 11, no. 1 (2005): 20.

35. Ibid., 23.

36. Ibid., 23.

37. De Witte, "Accra's Sounds and Sacred Spaces," *International Journal of Urban and Regional Research* 32, no. 2 (2008): 690–709; Meyer, "'There is a Spirit in that Image': Mass-Produced Jesus Pictures and Protestant-Pentecostal Animation in Ghana," *Comparative Studies in Society and History* 52, no. 1 (2010): 100–30.

38. Dag Heward-Mills, "Catch the Anointing" (Accra: Dag's Tapes and Publications, 2000), front cover.

39. Ibid., 12.

40. Ibid., 34.

41. See de Witte, "Altar Media's Living Word."

42. Interview, "Kofi" (full name not disclosed), editor of *Living Word*, 4 June 2002.

43. See, for instance, Vivian Sobchack's description of "mimetic sympathy" as a bodily process of posture, tension, and intention, in *Carnal Thoughts*, 76.

44. Of course there is a difference between the effect intended by the editors and the actual audience experience. Although letters of testimony sent to the church in response to the media ministry indicate that some people indeed experience the Holy Spirit through a media broadcast, this is certainly not always the case, and much depends on factors beyond the editors' control, such as a person's background, context of reception, intention, and desire.

45. Jesse Weaver Shipley, "Comedians, Pastors, and the Miraculous Agency of Charisma in Ghana," *Cultural Anthropology* 24, no. 3 (2009): 523–52.

46. Mr. Adu, director of Channel R, in an interview with *Radio and TV Review* 28 (2001): 50.

47. Enoch Darfah Frimpong, "Welcome to Kumasi, the Garden City of Africa," last accessed 25 January 2010, http://enochdarfahfrimpong.blogspot.com/2008/06/otsunoko-speaks-i-will-expose-fake.html.

48. "Crackdown on Nigeria TV Miracles," *BBC News*, April 30, 2004, last accessed 25 January 2010, http://news.bbc.co.uk/2/hi/africa/3672805.stm.

49. Interview, Yaw Boadu-Ayeboafo, executive secretary of the National Media Commission, 13 November 2002.

50. De Witte, "Fans and Followers: Marketing Charisma, Making Religious Celebrity in Ghana," *Australian Religion Studies Review* 24, no. 3 (2011).

51. Interview Osofo Boakye, Afrikania Mission priest, 25 October 2002.

52. David Chidester, "The American Touch: Tactile Imagery in American Religion and Politics," in *The Book of Touch*, ed. Constance Classen (Oxford: Berg, 2005), 59.

53. De Witte, "'Insight,' Secrecy, Beasts, and Beauty: Struggles over the Making of a Ghanaian Documentary on 'African Traditional Religion,'" *Postscripts* 1, no. 2–3, (2005): 277–300.

54. Jeffrey Sconce, *Haunted Media: Electronic Presence from Telegraphy to Television* (Durham, N.C.: Duke University Press, 2000).

55. Ibid.; see also Jeremy Stolow, "Salvation by Electricity," in *Religion: Beyond a Concept*, ed. de Vries (New York: Fordham University Press, 2008), 668–86; see also Stolow in this volume.

56. See John Durham Peters, *Speaking into the Air: A History of the Idea of Communication* (Chicago: University of Chicago Press, 1999).

57. Leo Marx, *The Machine in the Garden: Technology and the Pastoral Ideal in America* (London, Oxford, and New York: Oxford University Press, 1964); David E. Nye, *American Technological Sublime* (Cambridge, Mass.: MIT Press, 1994).

58. See also de Abreu, "Breathing."

THE SPIRITUAL NERVOUS SYSTEM: REFLECTIONS ON A MAGNETIC CORD
DESIGNED FOR SPIRIT COMMUNICATION
Jeremy Stolow

Research for this paper was conducted with the support of the Social Sciences and Humanities Research Council of Canada. I wish to thank Maria José de Abreu, Courtney Bender, Cornelius Borck, Ann Taves, Ghislain Thibault, and Angela Zito for their incisive comments on earlier versions of this text. I also greatly benefited from questions and comments from audience members at the following presentations: at *Authorizing Inscriptions* (University of California—Davis, April 2008); at the Instituto do Filosofia e Ciências Humanas (State University of Rio de Janeiro, August 2008); at the Concordia University Mobile Media Lab (September 2008); at *Invidious Distinctions and Ambiguous Attachments* (Social Science Research Council, New York, October 2008); at the Center for Religion and Media (New York University, November 2008); and at the American Academy of Religion (Chicago, November 2008). A special word of thanks goes to Carly Machado, who has been collaborating with me on research into nineteenth-century Spiritualism for the past few years; the idea for this paper was first conceived during conversations with her.

1. Andrew Jackson Davis, *The Philosophy of Spiritual Intercourse, Being an Explanation of Modern Mysteries*, 2nd rev. ed. (1853; Boston: Colby and Rich, 1890), 164. Davis's magnetic cord is discussed briefly in Catherine L. Albanese, *A Republic of Mind and Spirit: A Cultural History of American Metaphysical Religion* (New Haven: Yale University Press, 2007), 225–26. I am indebted to Albanese for drawing attention to Davis's cord, although, as I hope becomes clear in the following pages, my own discussion elaborates a different set of concerns.

2. Davis, *Philosophy of Spiritual Intercourse*, 164–65, italics in original.

3. Ibid., 165. Davis revised these instructions some thirty years later in *The Present Age and Inner Life: Ancient and Modern Spirit Mysteries Classified and Explained* (Boston: Colby and Rich, 1886), 101–03.

4. Davis, *Philosophy of Spiritual Intercourse*, 166.

5. Ibid.

6. Ibid., 168.

7. This is not to detract from the strong commitment among Spiritualists to a form of scientific positivism, which held that the veracity of paranormal and supernatural experiences during séance rituals could be established through controlled observation. In this respect, it is important to recall the highly publicized efforts of a number of prominent scientists—both those sympathetic with and those skeptical of Spiritualism's basic tenets—to conduct experiments during séances, treating the séance chamber as a sort of laboratory for controlled observation and evidentiary analysis. Among the many scientists who entered the séance chamber and documented their findings were Robert Hare, Michael Faraday, Alfred Russell Wallace, Edmund Carpenter, Cromwell Varley, and Oliver Lodge; see Peter Lamont, "Spiritualism and a Mid-Victorian Crisis of Evidence," *The Historical Journal* 47, no. 4 (2004): 897–920; Richard J. Noakes, "Telegraphy Is an Occult Art: Cromwell Fleetwood Varley and the Diffusion of Electricity to the Other World," *British Journal for the History of Science* 32, no. 4 (1999): 421–59; Jon Palfreman, "Between Skepticism and Credulity: A Study of Victorian Scientific Attitudes to Modern Spiritualism," in *On the Margins of Science: The Social Construction of Rejected Knowledge*, ed. Roy Wallis (Keele, UK: University of Keele, 1979), 210–23; Peter Pels, "Spirits and Modernity: Alfred Wallace, Edward Tylor, and the Visual Politics of Facts," in *Magic and Modernity: Interfaces of Revelation and Concealment*, ed. Birgit Meyer and Peter Pels (Stanford: Stanford University Press, 2003), 241–71; Elisabeth Wadge, "The Scientific Spirit and the Spiritualist Scientist: Moving in the Right Circles," *The Victorian Review* 26, no. 1 (2000): 24–42.

8. See, for instance, Ernst Benz, *The Theology of Electricity: On the Encounter and Explanation of Theology and Science in the Seventeenth and Eighteenth Centuries* (Allison Park, Penn.: Pickwick, 1989); Paola Bertucci, "Revealing Sparks: John Wesley and the Religious Utility of Electrical Healing," *British Journal for the History of Science* 33, no. 3 (2006): 341–62.

9. See Bret E. Carroll, *Spiritualism in Antebellum America* (Bloomington: Indiana University Press, 1997), 61–65, 129–40.

10. Davis, *Philosophy of Spiritual Intercourse*, 168f.

11. Some of the most trenchant critiques of the "conflict thesis" between science and religion have been voiced by historians of Victorian science, who have pointed out how many of the narrative elements that made up the so-called "war" waged by inquiring scientific minds on religious superstition were rooted in the aspirations of secular iconoclasts, eager to enlist "modern science" in their struggle for dominance over the newly created domain of state education in the late nineteenth century; see Frank M. Turner, "The Victorian Conflict Between Science and Religion: A Professional Dimension," *Isis* 69 (1978): 356–76; John Hedley Brooke, *Science and Religion:*

Some Historical Perspectives (Cambridge: Cambridge University Press, 1991); Thomas Dixon, Geoffrey Cantor, and Stephen Pumfrey, eds., *Science and Religion: New Historical Perspectives* (Cambridge: Cambridge University Press, 2010).

12. Exemplary studies of popular science in the nineteenth century include Roger Cooter, *The Cultural Meaning of Popular Science: Phrenology and the Organization of Consent in Nineteenth-Century Britain* (Cambridge: Cambridge University Press, 1984); Robert Darnton, *Mesmerism and the End of Enlightenment in France* (Cambridge, Mass.: Harvard University Press, 1968); Aileen Fyfe, *Science and Salvation: Evangelical Publishing in Victorian Britain* (Chicago: University of Chicago Press, 2004); Craig James Hazen, *The Village Enlightenment in America: Popular Religion and Science in the Nineteenth Century* (Urbana: University of Illinois Press, 2000). On the history of the relationship between professional electrical engineers and late-nineteenth-century American popular culture, see Carolyn Marvin, *When Old Technologies Were New: Thinking About Electrical Communication in the Late Nineteenth Century* (New York and Oxford: Oxford University Press, 1988), especially chap. 1. For an extended treatment of the neglect of popular science as a serious topic of investigation, see Roger Cooter and Stephen Pumfrey, "Separate Spheres and Public Places: Reflections on the History of Science Popularization and Science in Popular Culture," *History of Science* 32, no. 3 (1994): 237–67.

13. Key histories of nineteenth-century Spiritualism in the English-speaking world include Ann Braude, *Radical Spirits: Spiritualism and Women's Rights in Nineteenth-Century America* (Boston: Beacon Press, 1989); Robert S. Cox, *Body and Soul: A Sympathetic History of American Spiritualism* (Charlottesville: University of Virginia Press, 2003); Molly McGarry, *Ghosts of Futures Past: Spiritualism and the Cultural Politics of Nineteenth-Century America* (Berkeley: University of California Press, 2008); Laurence Moore, *In Search of White Crows: Spiritualism, Parapsychology, and American Culture* (New York: Oxford University Press, 1977); Janet Oppenheim, *The Other World: Spiritualism and Psychical Research in England, 1850–1914* (Cambridge: Cambridge University Press, 1985); Alex Owen, *The Darkened Room: Women, Power, and Spiritualism in Late Victorian England* (Chicago: University of Chicago Press, 1989). On the French variant of Spiritualism, known as Spiritism, see John Warne Monroe, *Laboratories of Faith: Mesmerism, Spiritism, and Occultism in Modern France* (Ithaca, N.Y.: Cornell University Press, 2008); Lynn L. Sharp, *Secular Spirituality: Reincarnation and Spiritism in Nineteenth-Century France* (Lanham, Md.: Lexington Books, 2006).

14. Albanese, *Republic of Mind and Spirit*.

15. The term "kinetic revolution" is borrowed from Catherine Albanese's discussion of the mid-century American Transcendentalist movement, which included figures such as Ralph Waldo Emerson; see Albanese, "The Kinetic Revolution: Transformation in the Language of the Transcendentalists," *New England Quarterly* 48, no. 3 (1975): 319–40. For the applicability of the notion of a "kinetic revolution" to American Spiritualism, see Carroll, *Spiritualism*, 62–64.

16. See Jeremy Stolow, "Salvation by Electricity," in *Religion: Beyond a Concept*, ed. Hent de Vries (New York: Fordham University Press, 2008), 668–86. I am hardly the first to point out the intimate relationship between Spiritualism and telegraphy; see also Albanese, *Republic of Mind and Spirit*, 225–27; Braude, *Radical Spirits*, 4–5, 23–24; Jeffrey Sconce, *Haunted Media: Electronic Presence from Telegraphy to Television* (Durham, N.C.: Duke University Press, 2000), 21–37; Werner Sollors, "Dr. Benjamin Franklin's Celestial Telegraph, or Indian Blessings to Gas-lit American Drawing Rooms," *Social Science Information* 22, no. 6 (1983): 992.

17. On Spiritualist appropriations of the technologies of their day, see Stolow, "Salvation," 668–86; Steven Connor, "The Machine in the Ghost: Spiritualism, Technology, and the 'Direct Voice,'" in *Ghosts: Deconstruction, Psychoanalysis, History*, ed. Peter Buse and Andrew Stott (London: Macmillan, 1999), 203–25; Sheri Weinstein, "Technologies of Vision: Spiritualism and Science in Nineteenth-Century America," in *Spectral America: Phantoms and the National Imagination*, ed. Jeffrey Andrew Weinstock (Madison: University of Wisconsin Press, 2004), 124–40.

18. My use of the term "purification" draws upon Bruno Latour's famous account of the place of scientific knowledge within what he calls the "Modern Constitution," a historical effort to achieve the (impossible and therefore always paradoxical) goal of distinguishing nature and culture as two ontologically distinct zones, and thereby to secure for modern science its status as objective and value-neutral; see Latour, *We Have Never Been Modern* (Cambridge, Mass.: Harvard University Press, 1993), 10–48 *et passim*.

19. See George H. Daniels, "The Process of Professionalization in American Science: The Emergent Period, 1820–1860," in *Science in America Since 1820*, ed. Nathan Reingold (New York: Science History Publications, 1976), 63–78. On the death of natural philosophy and the invention of modern science, see Simon Schaffer, "Scientific Discoveries and the End of Natural Philosophy," *Social Studies of Science* 16 (1986), 387–420. On the growing demand, over the course of the nineteenth century, to reorganize medical knowledge and practice through professional specialization (not least in the domain of neurology, which took shape as an institutionally

distinct branch of medical practice only in the final third of the century), see George Weisz, "The Emergence of Medical Specialization in the Nineteenth Century," *Bulletin of the History of Medicine* 77, no. 3 (2003): 536–74.

20. See, for instance, Donald Zochert, "Science and the Common Man in Ante-Bellum America," *Science in America Since 1820*, ed. Reingold (New York: Science History Publications, 1976), 7–32. For an exemplary study of popular science publishing in nineteenth-century Britain, see Fyfe, *Science and Salvation*.

21. On the history of electrical display in eighteenth- and nineteenth-century America, see especially James Delbourgo, *A Most Amazing Scene of Wonders: Electricity and Enlightenment in Early America* (Cambridge, Mass.: Harvard University Press, 2006), 87–128 *et passim*; Fred Nadis, *Wonder Shows: Performing Science, Magic, and Religion in America* (New Brunswick, N.J.: Rutgers University Press, 2005), 3–82. More broadly, on public displays of electricity in the late eighteenth and early nineteenth centuries, see Iwan Rhys Morus, *Frankenstein's Children: Electricity, Exhibition, and Experiment in Early Nineteenth-Century London* (Princeton: Princeton University Press, 1998); Rhys Morus, "Radicals, Romantics and Electrical Showmen: Placing Galvanism at the End of the English Enlightenment," *Notes and Records of the Royal Society* 63, no. 3 (2009): 263–75; Schaffer, "Natural Philosophy and Public Spectacle in the Eighteenth Century," *History of Science* 21 (March 1983): 1–43; Schaffer, "The Consuming Flame: Electrical Showmen and Tory Mystics in the World of Goods," in *Consumption and the World of Goods*, ed. John Brewer and Roy Porter (New York: Routledge, 1993), 489–526; and Bernadette Bensaude-Vincent and Christine Blondel, eds., *Science and Spectacle in the European Enlightenment* (Aldershot, UK: Ashgate, 2008).

22. Donald M. Scott, "The Popular Lecture and the Creation of a Public in Mid-Nineteenth Century America," *Journal of American History* 66, no. 4 (1980): 791–809.

23. The popular Spiritualist organizer and contemporary historian of American Spiritualism, Emma Hardinge, hailed Davis as a John the Baptist–type figure, who had prepared the way for the blossoming of the movement (cited in Albanese, *Republic of Mind and Spirit*, 206).

24. On Davis's biography, career, and literary output, see Albanese, "On the Matter of Spirit: Andrew Jackson Davis and the Marriage of God and Nature," *Journal of the American Academy of Religion* 60, no. 1 (1992): 1–17; Robert W. Delp, "Andrew Jackson Davis: Prophet of American Spiritualism," *The Journal of American History* 54, no. 1 (1967): 43–56.

25. On popular science publishing in the nineteenth century, see Geoffrey Cantor, Gowan Dawson, Richard Noakes, Sally Shuttleworth,

and Jonathan R. Topham, eds., *Science in the Nineteenth-Century Periodical: Reading the Magazine of Nature* (Cambridge: Cambridge University Press, 2004); Louise Henson, Geoffrey Cantor, Gowan Dawson, Richard Noakes, Sally Shuttleworth, and Jonathan R. Topham, eds., *Culture and Science in the Nineteenth-Century Media* (Aldershot, UK: Ashgate, 2004); Susan Sheets-Pyenson, "Popular Science Periodicals in Paris and London: The Emergence of a Low Scientific Culture, 1820–1875," *Annals of Science* 42 (1985): 549–72.

26. On Hare, see Craig James Hazen, *The Village Enlightenment in America: Popular Religion and Science in the Nineteenth Century* (Urbana: University of Illinois Press, 2000), 65–112. On Spear, see John Benedict Buescher, *The Remarkable Life of John Murray Spear: Agitator for the Spirit Land* (Notre Dame, Ind.: University of Notre Dame Press, 2006). William Denton's classic work on psychometry appeared in his book *The Soul of Things: Psychometric Experiments for Re-Living History* (Boston: 1863).

27. Davis, "The Soul's Telegraphic Faculty," *The Herald of Progress* 1, no. 23 (28 July 1860): 1.

28. Davis, *Great Harmonia*, vol. 4, *The Reformer, Concerning Physiological Vices and Virtues, and the Seven Phases of Marriage*, 8th ed. (Boston: Colby and Rich, 1884), 286; emphasis in the original.

29. Davis, "The Soul's Telegraphic Faculty," 1.

30. Ibid.

31. Ibid.

32. Davis, *Present Age and Inner Life*, 281–82.

33. *The Spiritual Telegraph* was founded by S. B. Brittan and Charles Partridge and published in New York from 1852 to 1860, until it merged into Davis's own paper, *The Herald of Progress*.

34. Cox, *Body and Soul*, 20.

35. Alex Owen recounts how British Spiritualists typically conceived the relationship of mediumistic healer and patient in terms of a transfer of energy, often described as a magnetic or electro-biological force that the healer could exchange for the patient's "depleted vitality" during the acts of intimate coupling, which could consist of diagnosis during trance states or the laying of hands; see Owen, *Darkened Room*, 109–10.

36. Quoted in Cox, *Body and Soul*, 88.

37. Quoted in Cox, *Body and Soul*, 89.

38. As reported in Cox, *Body and Soul*, 101.

39. Although a voluminous literature on the role of telegraphy in the nineteenth century has developed in its wake, the "classic" statement on the revolution inaugurated by telegraph is James Carey, "Technology and Ideology: The Case of the Telegraph," in idem, *Communication as Culture:*

Essays on Media and Society, rev. ed. (1989; New York and London: Routledge, 2009), 155–76.

It is always risky business to try to periodize processes of rapid technological change (not least because the effects of new media technologies are experienced according to the uneven geography in which they spread), but roughly speaking, the year 1890 serves as a useful threshold dividing us from our nineteenth-century forebears, whose thoughts and actions were encased in the representational architecture of the nervous system. I invoke 1890 as the inaugural moment of yet another technocultural shift, based on emerging principles of wireless connectivity, spark gaps, harmonic resonances, and other modes of representing interstitial spaces between bodies (dramatized through laboratory experiments and through the introduction of new media technologies such as the radio transmitter, the electroencephalograph, and the spectroscope). To the extent that those developments heralded new alignments of legitimate and marginal sciences, technoinstitutional arrangements, and cultural practices (including a new cosmological vocabulary), they mark a distinct departure from the preoccupations of the present discussion. On the affinity between fin-de-siècle Spiritualism and the emerging technoculture of "wireless," see especially Anthony Enns, "Psychic Radio: Sound Technologies, Ether Bodies, and Spiritual Vibrations," *Senses and Society* 3, no. 2 (2008): 137–52.

40. Davis, *Philosophy of Spiritual Intercourse*, 173–74.

41. Davis, *Mental Disorders; Or, Diseases of the Brain and Nerves, Developing the Origin and Philosophy of Mania, Insanity, and Crime, With Full Directions for their Treatment and Cure* (New York: American News Company, 1871), 128–29.

42. Davis, *Mental Disorders*, 103–04.

43. Ibid., 114.

44. On the history of conceptions of the nervous system from antiquity to modernity, and especially the key shifts instigated by the development of neurology, neuro-anatomy, and physiology in the early nineteenth century, see Pietro Corsi, ed., *The Enchanted Loom: Chapters in the History of Neuroscience* (New York and Oxford: Oxford University Press, 1991); Laura Otis, *Networking: Communicating with Bodies and Machines in the Nineteenth Century* (Ann Arbor: University of Michigan Press, 2001); George S. Rousseau, *Nervous Acts: Essays on Literature, Culture and Sensibility* (Houndsmills, UK: Palgrave-Macmillan, 2004); Laura Salisbury and Andrew Shail, "Introduction," in *Neurology and Modernity: A Cultural History of Nervous Systems, 1800–1950*, ed. Laura Salisbury and Andrew Shail (London: Palgrave-Macmillan, 2010), 1–40; Gordon M. Shepherd, *Foundations of*

the *Neuron Doctrine* (Oxford: Oxford University Press, 1991). As James Delbourgo documents, there were eighteenth-century predecessors to the "reinvention" of nerves as an electrical mediation system, although the tendency was still to describe the nerves as conduits of an electrical *fluid*; see Delbourgo, *Most Amazing Scene*, 223–24, 235.

45. Salisbury and Shail, "Introduction," in *Neurology and Modernity*, 13.

46. As Müller proposed, the sensation of "seeing light," for instance, could be produced by the emanations from the external world, but just as readily could be produced by internal processes, such as when chemical agents (such as narcotics) are introduced into the bloodstream; see Johannes Müller, *Elements of Physiology*, trans. William Baly, 2nd ed. (Philadelphia: Lean and Blanchard, 1843), 714f. Müller's text first appeared in 1833, and went through multiple editions. For discussion of this text and its influence, with particular reference to evolving theories of sense perception, see Jonathan Crary, *Techniques of the Observer: On Vision and Modernity in the Nineteenth Century* (Cambridge, Mass.: MIT Press, 1992), 88–93; Jonathan Sterne, *The Audible Past: Cultural Origins of Sound Reproduction* (Durham, N.C.: Duke University Press, 2003), 60–62.

47. On this point, see Sterne, *Audible Past*, 61–62.

48. Hermann von Helmholtz, *On the Sensations of Tone as a Physiological Basis for the Theory of Music*, trans. Alexander J. Ellis, 2nd English ed., based on the 4th German ed. [1877] (London: Longmans, Green, 1885), 149. Helmholtz's text was first published in 1862. This passage is also discussed by Jonathan Crary in relation to Müller's doctrine of the "separation of the senses"; see Crary, *Techniques*, 93; cf. Sterne, *The Audible Past*, 62f.

49. See Otis, *Networking*, 10–14 *et passim*.

50. Despite their enthusiasm for comparing nerves with telegraph messaging systems, mid-century physiologists were hardly unaware of the significant differences between biological and mechanical media. As reported by Otis, in 1850 Helmholtz measured the velocity of nervous impulses at a rate of 26.4 meters per second, in marked contrast with the conduction of electricity through metal wiring, as Charles Wheatstone, the inventor of the British needle telegraph system, had demonstrated in 1834, when he calculated that electricity could reach a velocity of over 250,000 miles per second. "Clearly," Otis concludes, "the living and the telegraphic communications systems were not functioning in the same way"; Otis, *Networking*, 27.

51. See Otis, *Networking*, 120–36; Rhys Morus, "'The Nervous System of Britain': Space, Time, and the Electric Telegraph in the Victorian Age," *British Journal for the History of Science* 33, no. 4 (2000): 455–75.

52. Quoted in Salisbury and Shail, "Introduction," in *Neurology and Modernity*, 16.

53. As argued by the botanist and comparative anatomist William Lauder Lindsay (1829–1880), "the old doctrine or assumption of the phrenologists ... that, namely, which regards the brain as the sole organ of the mind— must unquestionably be given up. We must henceforth regard the true site, seat, or organ of mind as the whole body; and this is the only sound basis on which the comparative psychologist can begin his studies"; Lindsay, *Mind in the Lower Animals*, vol. 2, *Mind in Disease* (London: Kegan Paul, 1879), 4. Lindsay's argument rested on what by the final third of the nineteenth century was regarded as incontrovertible evidence derived from comparative anatomy and experiments with the body parts of lower animals, such as the legs of decapitated frogs, the muscles of which were long known to be made to react to excitation of the nerves. This unseating of the brain even led some comparative anatomists to suggest that the brain of higher animals was merely the "upward extension" of the more fundamental and more universal system of nerves located around the spinal cord. Long before Lindsay's writing, the most famous scientist to experiment with frogs' legs was of course Luigi Galvani, whose theory of "animal electricity" was subsequently discredited by Alessandro Volta; see Marcello Pera, *The Ambiguous Frog: The Galvani-Volta Controversy on Animal Electricity* (Princeton: Princeton University Press, 1992).

54. See, for instance, Edwin Lee, *A Treatise on Some Nervous Disorders: Being Chiefly Intended to Illustrate those Varieties which Stimulate Structural Disease* (London: Burgess and Hill, 1833); cf. John O'Reilly, *The Anatomy and Physiology of the Placenta: The Connection of the Nervous Centres of Animal and Organic Life* (New York: Hall, Clayton, 1860), especially 11–15, which provides a typical account of the "battery-like" functioning of the brain.

55. On the efforts of nineteenth-century neurologists to investigate and diagnose such phenomena as somnambulism and trance states, see Edward M. Brown, "Neurology and Spiritualism in the 1870s," *Bulletin of the History of Medicine* 57, no. 4 (1983): 563–77. More generally, on the history of medical responses to Spiritualism (which generally took the form of alarmism and hostility toward spirit mediums on the part of the medical establishment), see Braude, *Radical Spirits*, 142–61; Owen, *Darkened Room*, 139–67.

56. Cox, *Body and Soul*, 27–35 et passim.

57. Adam Smith, *The Theory of Moral Sentiments*, ed. Knud Haakonssen (1759; Cambridge: Cambridge University Press, 2002).

58. Cox, *Body and Soul*, 31–33; see also Christopher Lawrence, "The Nervous System and Society in the Scottish Enlightenment," in *Natural Order: Historical Studies of Scientific Culture*, ed. Barry Barnes and Steven

Shapin (London: Sage, 1979), 19–40; Margaret Schabas, "Adam Smith's Debts to Nature," *History of Political Economy* 35, no. 2 (2003): 262–81.

59. Cox, *Body and Soul*, 30.

60. Cox, *Body and Soul*, 70.

61. Davis, *Great Harmonia*, vol. 1, *The Physician, Being a Philosophical Revelation of the Natural, Spiritual, and Celestial Universe*, 4th ed. (Boston: Benjamin B. Mussey, 1850), 282–83.

62. David Hume, *An Enquiry Concerning the Principles of Morals* (London: A. Millar, 1751), 99. For an insightful comparison of Hume and Smith on spatial dimensions of sympathy, see Fonna Forman-Bazilai, "Sympathy in Spaces: Adam Smith on Proximity," *Political Theory* 33, no. 2 (2005): 189–217.

63. On Franklin's conception of electricity as a balance of positive and negative charges, see Delbourgo, *Most Amazing Scene*, 31–41 *et passim*.

64. For a clear discussion of how Faraday conceptualized gravity, radiation, and electricity, and their possible relationships with the transmission medium, transmission propagation, and the receiving entity, see Michael Faraday, "On the Physical Character of the Lines of Magnetic Force," in idem, *Experimental Researches in Electricity* (London: Bernard Quaritch, 1855), 3:407–37; originally published in *Philosophical Magazine* (June 1852).

65. By the 1880s, even further steps were taken that contributed to a dismantling of the linear model of electrical energy transfer and its replacement with more "radiant" models. In 1884, for instance, John Henry Poynting (1852–1914) demonstrated that electrical currents do not flow *inside* conducting wires, but rather in the empty space surrounding them. On Poynting and his contemporary students of Maxwell, see Bruce J. Hunt, "Lines of Force, Swirls of Ether," in *From Energy to Information: Representation in Science and Technology, Art and Culture*, ed. Bruce Clarke and Linda Dalrymple Henderson (Stanford: Stanford University Press, 2002), 99–103; cf. Enns, "Psychic Radio," 142.

66. Several historians of nineteenth-century Spiritualism have noted the equation of femininity with negative magnetic polarity, which in turn served as a rhetorical legitimation for associating mediumship with irrationality (among both advocates and detractors of the movement, for opposing reasons); see, for instance, Braude, *Radical Spirits*, 24; McGarry, *Ghosts of Futures Past*, 46, 51, 158–59; and Owen, *Darkened Room*, 14–15.

67. Davis, "Pathological Offices of the Sympathetic Ganglia," *The Herald of Progress* 1, no. 22 (21 July 1860): 4–5.

68. Davis, *Views of Our Heavenly Home: A Sequel to a Stellar Key to the Summer Land* (Boston: Colby and Rich, 1878), 81–82.

69. Ibid., 93–94.

70. Davis, *Death and the After-Life: Eight Evening Lectures on the Summer-Land* (New York: A. J. Davis, 1865), 36–37.

71. See, for instance, Delbourgo, *Most Amazing Scene*, 87–128; Nadis, *Wondr Shows*, 21–47.

72. Steven Connor, for instance, has commented on "the peculiarly persistent anachronism of the technologies borrowed by the séance," identifying such devices as levitating trumpets and cat's whisker diodes as "imaginary technologies [that] are always slightly out of date, slightly awkward and klunky"; Connor, "Machine in the Ghost," 223 *et passim*.

73. Latour, *We Have Never Been Modern*, 29–48 *et passim*.

74. As Carolyn Marvin has noted, electrical engineers were among the very last engineering professionals to consolidate their legitimacy in the form of a professional association: the American Institute for Electrical Engineers, which was created in 1884; see Marvin, *When Old Technologies Were New*, 10–15.

75. For discussion of popular science writing in the nineteenth century, see the references listed in note 25.

76. Robert Whytt, *Observations on the Nature, Causes, and Cure of those Disorders which have been Commonly Called Nervous, Hypochondriac, or Hysteric: To which are Prefixed Some Remarks on the Sympathy of the Nerves*, 2nd ed. (Edinburgh: J. Balfour, 1765), 2; quoted in Salisbury and Shail, "Introduction," in *Neurology and Modernity*, 12.

77. Thomas Trotter, *A View of the Nervous Temperament*, 3rd ed. (Newcastle: Edward Walker, 1812), 213; quoted in Salisbury and Shail, "Introduction," in *Neurology and Modernity*, 7.

78. Helmholtz, *Sensations of Tone*, 149, emphasis added.

79. Nor was it the case that "professional" scientists enjoyed exclusive access to such instruments, as is evident from the long history of domestic consumption of apparatuses for the sake of "parlor science." Consider, in this regard, the role of microscopes in American popular culture, beginning in the 1850s; see John Harley Warner, "'Exploring the Inner Labyrinths of Creation': Popular Microscopy in Nineteenth-Century America," *Journal of the History of Medicine and Allied Sciences* 37, no. 1 (1982): 7–33. At the other extreme of the visible spectrum, for an eclectic and thought-provoking set of discussions of the role of telescopes and popular astronomy in the nineteenth-century Atlantic world, see David Aubin, Charlotte Bigg, and H. Otto Sibum, eds., *The Heavens on Earth: Observatories and Astronomy in Nineteenth-Century Science and Culture* (Durham, N.C.: Duke University Press, 2010).

80. Davis, *Death and the After-Life*, 36.

81. Davis, *Death and the After-Life*, 35.

82. Davis, "Pathological Offices of the Sympathetic Ganglia," *The Herald of Progress* 1, no. 22 (21 July 1860): 4.

AN EMPOWERED WORLD: BUDDHIST MEDICINE
AND THE POTENCY OF PRAYER IN JAPAN
Jason Ānanda Josephson

I'd like to thank the participants of Buddhism's Occult Technologies Conference for their helpful comments and particularly the insights provided by my respondent Mark Rowe. I'd also like to thank Healan Gaston and Andrew Jewett for reading drafts of the paper.

1. For a history of Kotohira Shrine, see Sarah Thal, *Rearranging the Landscape of the Gods: The Politics of a Pilgrimage Site in Japan, 1573–1912* (Chicago: University of Chicago Press, 2005), 324f and 55–56.

2. Ian Reader and George Tanabe, *Practically Religious: Worldly Benefits and the Common Religion of Japan* (Honolulu: University of Hawai'i Press, 1998), 175.

3. See, e.g., *Medicine Buddha Sutra*, Taishō 14:450.

4. For example, "Prince [Shōtoku] ordered his attendant, Ichii of Tomi, to pray to the Four Deva Kings and had him shoot an arrow, which hit Moriya in the chest"; *The Konjaku Tales*, trans. Yoshiko Kurata Dykstra, 6 vols. (Osaka: Kansai Gaidai University, 1998–2003), 5. For the drowning of the wicked official, see ibid., 116.

5. Miyata Noboru and Tsukamoto Manabu, eds., *Minkan shinkō to minshkū shkūkykō* (Tokyo: Yoshikawa Kōbunkan, 1994), 108–19.

6. *Qikākānsh òu qikākāny àn gukānshìykīn púsà zhìbìng héyào jkīng*, Taishō 1059. Although some small adjustments were made in consultation with the Chinese source, the translation above is based on Paul Unschuld, *Medicine in China: A History of Ideas* (Berkeley: University of California Press, 1985), 317.

7. A. Bhattacharya N. Pakrashi, "Abortifacient Principle of *Achyranthes aspera* Linn.," *Indian Journal of Experimental Biology* 15, no. 10 (1977): 856–85; Sumeet Dwivedi, Dubey Raghvendra, and Kushagra Mehta, "*Achyranthes aspera* Linn. (Chirchira): A Magic Herb in Folk Medicine," *Ethnobotanical Leaflets* 12 (2008): 670–76.

8. Unschuld, *Medicine in China*, 320.

9. Demiéville, "Byō," 257f; Duncan Ryūken Williams, *The Other Side of Zen: A Social History of Soto Zen Buddhism in Tokugawa Japan* (Princeton: Princeton University Press, 2005), 88.

10. Williams, *Other Side of Zen*, 88.

11. For some examples of the range of Buddhist medical practices in early modern Japan, see Hattori Toshirō, *Edo jidai igakushi no kenkykū* (Tokyo: Yoshikawa Kōbunkan, 1978); Yamada Keiji and Kuriyama Shigehisa, eds., *Rekishi no naka no yamai to igaku* (Kyoto: Kokusai Nihon Bunka Kenkyū Senta, 1997); Williams, *The Other Side of Zen*.

12. See particularly the translation of the *Laṅkkāvatkā ra Sutra* attributed to Siksānanda Taisho 16:672 and the *Mahā prajñāparamitā sūtra*, translated by Xuanzang Taisho, 5–7:220.

13. Skt. *Mahāvairocanbhisaṃbodhi-vikurvitā dhiṣṭhā na-vaipulyasūtra*, *Taishō*, 18:848.

14. Kūkai, *Kōbō daishi Zenshū*, 15 vols. (Tokyo: Yoshikawa Kōbunkan, 1911), 1:516; Yoshito Hakeda, *Kūkai: Major Works* (New York: Columbia University Press, 1972), 232; Rolf W. Giebel and Dale A. Todaro, *Shingon Texts*, BDK English Tripitaka (Berkeley, Calif.: Numata Center for Buddhist Translation and Research, 2004), 79; Robert Sharf, *Coming to Terms with Chinese Buddhism: A Reading of the Treasure Store Treatise* (Honolulu: University of Hawai'i Press, 2002), 125.

15. As discussed by Sharf, *Chinese Buddhism*, 125.

16. *Sammitsu kaji sureba sokushitsu ni arawaru*; Kūkai, *Kōbō daishi Zenshū*, 1:507; Yoshito Hakeda, *Kūkai: Major Works* (New York: Columbia University Press, 1972), 227; Giebel and Todaro, *Shingon Texts*, 67. Later Shingon priests, such as Kakuban (1095–1143), continued to refine Kūkai's terminology using both kaji in the sense Kūkai intended, as a bridge between Buddha and practitioner, and also as reference to the body of the Buddha that interacts with sentient beings (skt. *nirmā ṇakā ya*, jpn. *kajishin*), literally "the empowerment body" of the Buddha. In this terminology, the bridge metaphor behind kaji is interpreted as a bidirectional phenomenon, in which the Buddha is also empowered by kaji to preach in the human world; see Hendrik Van der Veere, *A Study into the Thought of Kġyō Daishi Kakuban* (Leiden: Hotei, 2000), 205–7 and 90–92.

17. Murasaki Shikibu, *Genji Monogatari*, in *Shinpen Nihon koten bungaku zenshu*, ed. Abe Akio, 86 vols. (Tokyo: Shōgakkan, 1994–1998), 20:199–200. For another example of Heian period usage of kaji in childbirth, see Murasaki Shikibu, *Izumi Shikibu nikki; Murasaki Shikibu nikki; Sarashina nikki; Sanuki no Suke no nikki*, ed. Fujioka Tadaharu, vol. 26, *Shinpen Nihon koten bungaku zenshū* (Tokyo Shōgakkan, 1994), 226.

18. For an example, see Gerald Groemer, "The Arts of the Gannin," *Asian Folklore Studies* 58, no. 2 (1999): 278.

19. For another example of a kaji practice, see Ashihara Jakushō, *Sahūshū* (Osaka: Taiyūji, n.d.), 4.

20. For more details on the process of creating empowered fragrant water see Tomita Gakujun, ed., *Himitsu jirin* (Tokyo: Kaji Sekai Shisha, 1911), 135.

21. Ashihara, *Sahōshū*, 6.

22. See, e.g., Kusaka Shodō, *Shingon himitsu kaji kitō no okuden* (Tokyo: Rekishi Toshosha, 1930); Ono Kiyohide, *Kaji kitō himitsu taizen* (Osaka: Daibunkan, 1954). Evil spirits were nonetheless perceived as one of the main causes of illness, so these two categories of effects are clearly connected by the belief that kaji enabled one to participate in the invisible world and defend against negative influences.

23. Fabio Rambelli, "Secret Buddhas: The Limits of Buddhist Representation," *Monumenta Nipponica* 57, no. 3 (2002): 285.

24. Naimushō Keishikyoku, *Keishi Ruijū Kisoku* (Tokyo: Keishikyoku, 1879), 1:385f. For further discussion, see also Jason Ānanda Josephson, *The Invention of Religion in Japan* (Chicago: University of Chicago Press, 2012).

25. *The Record of Rites* is a Chinese text based on a compilation of Zhou Dynasty materials (1050 BCE–256 BCE), which traditionally was believed to have been edited by Confucius. However, the edition that made it into the Confucian classics was the product of significantly later editing. The extent of this editing and the exact dates under which it occurred are contested. However, it probably reached something like its current form in the Han Dynasty (202 BCE–220 CE); from *The Record of Rites*, *Quli*, section 2.

26. Sugawara Michizane, *Hakuran Kogen* (1785; Tokyo: Hakubunkan, 1894), 4:5.

27. Similar arguments persisted in China and were used by both Taoist and Confucian critics of popular movements; see Terry Kleeman, "Licentious Cults and Bloody Victuals: Sacrifice, Reciprocity and Violence in Traditional China," *Asia Major* 7, no. 1 (1994): 185f.

28. Chihara Tei, "Bōsō Manroku," *Nihon zuihitsu taisei* (Tokyo: Yoshikawa Kōbunkan, 1976), 303; see also Josephson, "Evil Cults, Monstrous Gods, and the Labyrinth of Delusion: Rhetorical Enemies and Symbolic Boundaries in the Construction of 'Religion' in Japan," *Bochumer Jahrbuch zur Ostasienforschung* 33 (2009): 39–59.

29. Martin Heidegger, "The Question Concerning Technology," in idem, *The Question Concerning Technology and Other Essays* (New York: Harper, 1977), 3–35.

30. See Josephson, "Fissures in the World-Mountain: Science and Cosmological Conflict in Early Modern Japan," unpublished manuscript (n.p., n.d.).

31. See Josephson, *Invention*, 108–9.

32. Translated in Thomas C. Smith, "The Introduction of Western Industry to Japan During the Last Years of the Tokugawa Period," *Harvard Journal of Asiatic Studies* 11, nos. 1–2 (1948): 136.

33. Josephson, *Invention*, 108.

34. The phrase was first popularized in the Muromachi Era (1392–1573) text, the *Kanke Ikai*, a collection of thirty-three lines used in writing practice and falsely attributed to Sugawara no Michizane.

35. For a discussion of this Shinto-scientific hybridity as the "Shinto secular," see Josephson, *Invention*, 132–63.

36. For example, Japanese kanpō medicine viewed tuberculosis as a contagious bacterium (or animalcule) long before it was recognized as such in Western medicine, and thus the embrace of the new medical system may have actually contributed to the tuberculosis epidemic; William Johnston, *The Modern Epidemic: A History of Tuberculosis in Japan* (Cambridge, Mass.: Harvard University Press, 1995), 42–43.

37. "While Western medical technology has been previously opposed, its beneficial aspects shall be employed henceforth"; Dajōkan 3.3.3, *Hōrei Zensho*, 139 vols. (Tokyo: Naikakukan Pōkyoku, 1887–1912).

38. See Josephson *Invention*, 145–47.

39. Johnston, *Modern Epidemic*, 178–79.

40. Ibid., 179. For a discussion of the parallels in the creation of a hygienic state in Britain, see Dorothy Porter, *Health, Civilization, and the State: A History of Public Health from Ancient to Modern Times* (New York: Routledge, 1999), 128f; and for the United States and the changing status of medicine, see Paul Starr, *The Social Transformation of American Medicine* (New York: Basic Books, 1982).

41. Michel Foucault, *The History of Sexuality: An Introduction*, trans. Robert Hurley (New York: Vintage, 1990), 139f.

42. Translated in Johnston, *Modern Epidemic*, 179. For a further discussion of Nagayo's impact on China's version of hygienic modernity, see Ruth Rogaski, *Hygienic Modernity* (Berkeley: University of California Press, 2004), 136f.

43. William Steslicke, "Doctors, Patients, and Government in Modern Japan," *Asian Survey* 12, no. 11 (1972): 915.

44. Naibushō 9.1.12, *Hōrei Zensho*.

45. See Gotō Shinpei, *Kokka eisei genri* (Tokyo: Gotō Shinpei, 1889).

46. Kyōbushō 22, 7.6.7, *Hōrei Zensho*.

47. Shihōshō, *Keihō* (Tokyo: Dajōkan Insatsu Kyoku, 1880).

48. Kenneth Mark Anderson, "The Foreign Relations of the Family State: The Empire of Ethics, Aesthetics, and Evolution in Meiji Japan" (PhD diss., Cornell University, 1999), 248.

49. Takeda Dōshō, "The Fall of Renmonkyō and Its Place in the History of Meiji-Period Religions," in *New Religions: Contemporary Papers on Japanese Religion 2*, ed. Inoue Nobutaka (Tokyo: Institute for Japanese Culture and Classics, Kokugakuin University, 1991), 25–57; see also Josephson, *Invention*, 238–39.

50. Ibid.; Watanabe Masako and Igeta Midori, "Healing in the New Religions: Charisma and 'Holy Water,'" in *New Religions*.

51. Takeda, "Fall of Renmonkyō."

52. Ibid.; Jōdokyōhō [Pure Land News], 32:179.

53. It should be noted that the truth of these claims was never verified.

54. Discussed in detail in Josephson, *Invention*.

55. Kaigo Tokiomi, ed., *Shūshin* (Tokyo: Kōdansha, 1962), 168f.

56. Kokutei Shōgaku Kyōkasho Kyōzai Kenkyūkai, ed., *Kokutei Shōgaku Kyōkasho Kakushina Kyōzai Jiten* (Tokyo: Jūbunkan, 1904); Monbushō, ed., *Jinjō Shōgaku Shūshinsho*, 2 vols. (Kando: Kumagai Kyūeidō, 1904); Futsū Kyōiku Kenkyūkai, ed., *Jinjō Shōgaku Kokugo Kyōju Saian: Maiji Haitō* (Tokyo: Mastumara Sanshōdō, 1910); Kyōiku Gakujutsu Kenkyūkai, ed., *Shūshinka Kyōju Yōrō: Kaitei Kokutei Kyōkasho 1–4 Gakunen*, 4 vols. (Tokyo: Dōbunkan, 1910); Tōkyō Kyōikukai, ed., Jinjō Shōgaku Zenka Shōkai Dai 4–6 Gakunen, 3 vols. (Tokyo: Shinonomedō, 1912).

57. Monbushō, *Jinjō Shōgaku Shūshinsho*, 53. The official dictionary of educational materials, *Kokutei Shōgaku Kyōkasho Kakushina Kyōzai Jiten*, issued in 1904, reproduced this list in a slightly altered form, adding ghosts, monsters, the Dog-God, and human-foxes. Kokutei Shōgaku Kyō kasho Kyōzai Kenkyūkai, *Kokutei Shōgaku Kyōkasho Kakushina Kyōzai Jiten*, 543.

58. Futsūkyōiku, *Jinjō Shōgaku Kokugo Kyōju Saian: Maiji Haitō*, 4:58–59 (emphasis added).

59. Hōritsu Kenkyūkai, *Kaisei Teikoku Roppōzensho* (Tokyo: Kokubunkan, 1911); see also Kawamura Kunimitsu, *Genshisuru Kindaikūkan* (Tokyo: Seikyūsha, 1997), 39.

60. Takeda, "Fall of Renmonkyō,"

61. Inoue Enryō, "Meishinkai," in *Yōkaigaku Zenshū* (1904; Tokyo: Kashiwa Shoten, 2000), 639.

62. Ibid.

63. Ibid.

64. Ibid., 640.

65. Ibid. The term Inoue uses here for "intermingling," in the period he was writing, had a negative connotation similar to that of miscegenation.

66. Ibid.

67. Inoue Enryō, "Meishin to Shōkyō," in *Yōkaigaku Zenshū* (1916; Tokyo: Kashiwa Shoten, 2000), 267. The term *seishin* also could be translated as "psychological."

68. Kōon, "Meishin to Shōshin ni Tsukite," *Kaji Sekai* 1, no.1 (1900): 15.

69. Ibid.

70. A key Buddhist conceptual hermeneutic is the distinction between absolute and conventional truth. Although a complex concept with a range of possible nuances, in general "absolute truth" is the view of reality as understood by the enlightened mind, but which is inexpressible linguistically, while "conventional truth" is the ordinary or commonsense view of the truth as grasped by those still trapped in the world of sense phenomena.

71. Kōon, "Meishin to Shōshin ni Tsukite," 15.

72. Ibid.

73. Kobayashi, "Kaji Sekai no Igi,"1.

74. Kobayashi, "Kaji Sekai no Igi," 5.

75. For example, see *Manganji (kajikitō goma)* http://www.geocities.jp/fudoumanganji/kajikitou.html, accessed 17 August 2009.

76. In 1957 the issue of the relationship between Buddhist healing and medicine again came to the surface when a mentally ill woman died while a Buddhist priestess performed empowered prayer intended to exorcise a possessing evil spirit. In a case that went all the way to the Japanese Supreme Court, the priestess was charged with negligent homicide, a verdict that the Supreme Court ultimately upheld in 1963; see Koizumi Yoichi, "Shinkyō no Jiyū to Kaji Kitō," in *Kenpo' hanrei hyakusen*, ed. Kazuyuki Takahashi, Hasabe Yasuo, and Ishikawa Kenji (Takahashi. Tokyo: Yūhikaku, 2007)

77. Oda, *Kaji*, 92.

78. See Ikeguchi Ekan, *Shingon Mikkyō no Shinpi: Gyō to kaji ryoku* (Osaka: Toki Shobo, 1990).

79. *Daikokuji Shingon Buddhist Temple Homepage*, accessed 17 August 2009; no longer available.

DOES SUBMISSION TO GOD'S WILL PRECLUDE BIOTECHNOLOGICAL INTERVENTION?
LESSONS FROM MUSLIM DIALYSIS PATIENTS IN CONTEMPORARY EGYPT
Sherine F. Hamdy

Thanks to Jeremy Stolow for encouraging me to submit to this volume, and to *Anthropology Quarterly* for allowing me to reprint pieces from the article "Islam, Fatalism, and Medical Intervention: Lessons from Egypt on the Cultivation of Forbearance (Sabr) and Reliance on God (Tawakkul)," 82, no. 1 (2009): 97–120. I benefited from the discussion of Michael Fischer at the panel on "Islam and Science" at the American Anthropological Association's 105th annual meeting in San José, California, in December 2006, and from feedback on previous drafts of this piece from Ian Straughn, Jessaca Leinaweaver, and Zareena Grewal.

1. Tanta is the capital of the Nile Delta province Gharbiyya, located less than 100 km north of Cairo. I conducted fieldwork in five different private and public dialysis centers there. I omit the full names of patients and physicians to protect their privacy. All interviews were conducted in colloquial Egyptian Arabic.

2. Although the poor receive government compensation for dialysis, this does not mean that all poor patients in need of dialysis receive it. Major obstacles include high rates of underdiagnosis of kidney failure, the lack of access to dialysis clinics, and the lack of know-how to obtain the necessary paperwork for government compensation.

3. This illustrates the ways in which physicians in Egypt act as social gatekeepers. In this instance, the physicians did not confine their role to intervening in the health of Muhammad, their patient, but also intervened in the larger social consequences of his family, including of a potential wife.

4. As I lay out in my larger study on organ transplantation in Egypt, the lack of agreement over the legality of extracting organs from brain-dead patients means that transplantation (of the kidney and liver lobe) depends entirely on living donors; see Sherine F. Hamdy, *Our Bodies Belong to God: Islam and Bioethics in Egypt* (Berkeley: University of California, 2012).

5. See, for example, Renée C. Fox and Judith P. Swazey, *"The Courage to Fail": "A Social View of Organ Transplants and Dialysis"* (Piscataway, N.J.: Transaction, 2002).

6. See, for example, Thomas Scully and Celia Scully, *Playing God: The New World of Medical Choices* (New York: Simon and Schuster, 1987); and Ronald Munson, *Raising the Dead: Organ Transplants, Ethics, and Society* (Oxford: Oxford University Press, 2002).

7. Shaykh al-Sha'arawi was a popular Egyptian television figure who died in 1998, and who hosted several Qur'anic commentary programs on state-run television (after President Sadat gave him his own television slot). More than a decade after his death, his programs continue to be watched, and he is deeply respected throughout Egyptian society. His greatest contribution was to translate the classical archaic Arabic of the Qur'an into the colloquial Egyptian dialect used in everyday life.

8. Minufiyya is a rural province in the Nile Delta, from which Ali commutes to Tanta thrice weekly for his dialysis treatment.

9. Armando Salvatore discusses what he calls the hyperobjectification of Islam among both Western observers and contemporary Muslims who draw on Islamic rhetoric for political ends. In his politicized form of Muslim identity, Ali stands out from the other patients (many from rural backgrounds) when he makes statements such as "Religion is the only thing stopping me." Most of his fellow patients do not articulate "religion" as an autonomous agent

in this way. I argue in this chapter that Ali does not generally view "religion" as an object external to himself, but in the quote above, he is participating in an increasingly dominant discourse that represents the role of religion in one's life in this objectified way; see Salvatore, *Islam and the Political Discourse of Modernity* (Reading, UK: Garnet, 1997).

10. On Mexican post-transplant patients' sense of liminality between illness and recovery, and how they never quite achieve the promise of returning to "normal," see Megan Crowley-Matoka, "Desperately Seeking 'Normal': The Promise and Perils of Living with Kidney Transplantation," *Social Science and Medicine* 61 (2005): 821–31.

11. Crowley-Matoka (ibid.) notes that much unlike the situation in the United States, in Mexico (and in Egypt, as well) it is the medical professionals who create the desire and demand for kidney transplantation among patients.

12. The more powerful generation of immunosuppressant drugs that is now available in Egypt (at higher cost) makes complete tissue match less necessary, and many in Ali's position might have proceeded with their transplants anyway. In Ali's case, his refusal to proceed was a combination of reluctance on his part and on the part of his physicians. Because the number of patients needing transplants far exceeds the facilities available, physicians in Egypt (in state hospitals) are disinclined to proceed with transplants without a full tissue match to increase chances of graft survival. On the relationship between donating kin and immunosuppressant drugs, see Lawrence Cohen, "The Other Kidney: Biopolitics Beyond Recognition," *Body and Society* 7, nos. 2–3 (2001): 9–29.

13. The particular patterns of kidney-giving along kin relations are detailed in Hamdy, *Our Bodies Belong to God*.

14. The process is much more mystified in the contemporary United States, where kidneys are procured through a complex medical industry and the minutia of procurement are rendered less visible to the waiting patients. This is especially the case with organs procured from brain-dead patients. Yet living kidney donation is currently on the rise in the United States, exceeding cadaver donation for the first time in 2001; see Sharon Kaufman, Ann. J. Russ, and Janet Shim, "Aged Bodies and Kinship Matters: The Ethical Field of Kidney Transplant," *American Ethnologist* 33, no. 1 (2006): 82.

15. In her work on kidney transplantation in Mexico, Crowley-Matoka argues that with each step (finding a kidney, testing, paperwork) desire for the transplant is created and substantiated in the patient. Ali's case also shows that with each step, a patient's hopes can be quickly dashed. North American kidney-failure patients also face these dilemmas of finding their own kidneys when they feel that the waiting lists are too long and that they

cannot sustain life on dialysis while waiting; see Kaufman, Russ, and Shim, "Aged Bodies," 82.

16. While the buying and selling of organs is officially illegal in Egypt, hospital administrators and doctors generally turn a blind eye to the practice, which has proliferated in Cairo, and hospital laboratories often facilitate tissue-compatible donors willing to sell their kidneys to potential recipients.

17. I argue elsewhere that wives' bodies are generally seen as more "expendable" than those of men, and that wives generally donate kidneys to their husbands at much higher rates than the other way around; see Hamdy, *Our Bodies Belong to God*.

18. This verse comes from *The Qur'an*, chap. 57 (*Al-Hadid*), verse 4. For English translations, see Muhammad Asad's *The Message of the Holy Qur'an* (Gibraltar: Dar Al-Andalus, 1980) and M. A. S. Abdel Haleem, *The Qur'an: A New Translation* (Oxford: Oxford University Press, 2004).

19. *The Qur'an*, chap. 2 (*Al-Baqara*), verse 115.

20. This hadith is well-known and oft-cited among Egyptians. It is cited in the modern Islamic scholar Sayyid Sabiq's compendia of hadith traditions, *Fiqh al-Sunna*; see al-Sayyid Sabiq, *Fiqh al-Sunna*, 3 vols. (Cairo: Maktabat al-Qahira, 1994).

21. In line with this critique, see Talal Asad, *Genealogies of Religion: Discipline and Reasons of Power in Christianity and Islam* (Baltimore: Johns Hopkins University Press, 1993); Talal Asad, *Formations of the Secular: Christianity, Islam, Modernity* (Stanford: Stanford University Press, 2003); Saba Mahmood, *Politics of Piety: the Islamic Revival and the Feminist Subject* (Princeton: Princeton University Press, 2005); Charles Hirschkind, *The Ethical Soundscape: Cassette Sermons and Islamic Counterpublics* (New York: Columbia University Press, 2006).

22. Hania Sholkamy, "Conclusion: The Medical Cultures of Egypt," in *Health and Identity in Egypt*, ed. Hania Sholkamy and Farha Ghannam (Cairo: American University in Cairo Press, 2004), 111–28.

23. Hence my slight difference from Hania Sholkamy's important discussion of forbearance in Egyptian medical experiences, where she writes, "God, as the ultimate source, is a formula that helps ex post facto acceptance but is not one which precipitates an a priori fatalism. It is a tenet that leaves plenty of room for people to take initiative in defining, managing, and protecting their health and well-being"; Sholkamy, "Conclusion," in *Health and Identity*, 122. For Ali, what was important was a continual alignment of himself and his own desires with what he understood to be God's will.

24. Paul Farmer, *Aids and Accusation: Haiti and the Geography of Blame* (Berkeley: University of California Press, 1992); Farmer, "On Suffering and

Structural Violence: A View from Below," in *Social Suffering*, ed. Veena Das, Arthur Kleinman, and Margaret Lock (Berkeley: University of California Press, 1997), 261–284; Farmer, *Infections and Inequalities: The Modern Plagues* (Berkeley: University of California Press, 1999).

25. For example, artificial insemination with donor sperm is rejected as a treatment for male infertility, but not because it is seen as inefficacious or inaccessible. Infertile couples in Egypt appeal to God in cultivating steadfastness in their difficult situations rather than resorting to practices that rely on third-party semen, ova, or wombs, for they consider those practices to be unethical for introducing foreign reproductive elements into a marriage and "confusing" the blood lineage of the offspring. These practices, notably, do not achieve the desired goal, which is defined as producing biological offspring of both husband and wife; see Hamdy, "God's Gift to Women: Ideologies of Motherhood, Womanhood, and Fertility in Egypt," (unpublished master's thesis, Stanford University, 1998); Marcia Inhorn, *Infertility and Patriarchy: The Cultural Politics of Gender and Family Life in Egypt* (Philadelphia: University of Pennsylvania Press, 1996); Inhorn, *Local Babies, Global Science: Gender, Religion, and In Vitro Fertilization in Egypt* (New York and London: Routledge, 2003).

THE CANARY IN THE GEMEINSCHAFT? DISABILITY, FILM, AND THE JEWISH QUESTION
Faye Ginsburg

I want to thank Jeremy Stolow for inviting me to be part of the "Deus in Machina" conference and patiently waiting for this piece, and for his excellent editorial skills. I am, as always, indebted to my longstanding colleague Rayna Rapp; many of the ideas of this paper emerged from our intertwined work on disability and its changing social framework. Thanks as well to the insights, creativity, and commitments of extraordinary activist/filmmakers Judith Helfand and Ilana Trachtman, as well as conversations with friends and scholars Barbara Kirshenblatt-Gimblett and Jeffrey Shandler, and to Patsy Spyer for her thoughtful comments on the penultimate version. The ideas for this paper first started to develop in a workshop with the title "The Canary in the Gemeinschaft" that I organized jointly for the Working Group on Jews/Religion/Media and the Working Group on Bioethics and Religion that I ran with Rayna Rapp in 2005–2006 as part of the activities of the Center for Religion and Media at NYU. Finally, I owe my interest in this area and perhaps my most important understandings to my daughter Samantha, who has opened up worlds for me that I never knew existed, and whose joyous exuberance, despite her complex life with familial dysautonomia, is a daily parable of possibility. The section in this paper on Samantha's excursions into media activism is drawn from a 2001 work written with Rayna Rapp: "Enabling Disability: Rewriting Kinship, Reimagining Citizenship," *Public Culture* 13, no. 3 (2001): 533–55.

1. According to Tönnies, who first introduced the categories of Gemeinschaft/Gesellschaft into sociological discourse in 1887, people living in Gemeinschaft are linked by shared belief and kinship and a "unity of will"; see Ferdinand Tönnies, *Community and Civil Society*, ed. José Harris (Cambridge: Cambridge University Press, 2001), 22.

2. Caryn Aviv and David Shneer, *New Jews: The End of the Jewish Diaspora* (New York: New York University Press, 2005).

3. If one were to date the inauguration of this work, it would be 1979, when Ira Wohl's direct cinema documentary *Best Boy*—focusing on the fate of his cousin, the developmentally disabled "Philly" Wohl, who spent his first fifty years at home with Max and Pearl, his aging working-class Jewish parents in Queens—won the Academy Award for Best Documentary. The documentary, which follows Philly as he eventually moves to a group home where he thrives, brought unexpected visibility to the hidden question of disability in the Jewish community. Twenty years later Ira Wohl made a follow-up film, *Best Man*, focused on the story of Philly's Bar Mitzvah at age seventy. In the quarter century since then, a number of landmark documentaries have been made that continue to explore the sometimes perplexing questions raised by disability in the Jewish American post-war culture, a gemeinschaft that valorizes intelligence and middle-class achievement in its children.

4. Holocaust scholar Lucy Dawidowicz argues that the term the "Jewish Question" was not only associated with Nazi genocidal policy; it was a neutral expression for the negative attitude toward the apparent and persistent singularity of the Jews as a people on the background of the rising political nationalisms and new nation-states; see Dawidowicz, *The War Against the Jews, 1933–1945* (Bantam: New York, 1975), 10.

5. "Bio-power," a term introduced by Michel Foucault, refers to the ways that modern states regulate their subjects through practices such as the control of heredity, public health, and of populations; see Foucault, *The History of Sexuality*, vol. 1, *The Will to Knowledge* (London: Penguin, 1988), 12.

6. Foucault, "Technologies of the Self," in *Technologies of the Self*, ed. L. H. Martin, H. Gutman, and P. H. Hutton (Amherst: University of Massachusetts Press, 1988), 12.

7. Toby Miller, *The Well-Tempered Self: Citizenship, Culture, and the Postmodern Subject* (Baltimore: The Johns Hopkins University Press, 1993).

8. Rayna Rapp, *Testing Women, Testing the Fetus* (New York: Routledge, 1999). The question of "who is in?" addresses biopolitics, while the second

question ("who is out?") raises questions about narrative invention, although one might argue that the same concerns are evident in both arenas. On biopolitics, see Deborah Heath and Paul Rabinow, "Biopolitics: The Anthropology of the New Genetics Immunology," *Journal of Culture, Medicine, and Psychiatry* 17 (1993): 1–2. On narrative invention, see Alisa Lebow, *First Person Jewish* (Minneapolis: University of Minnesota Press, 2008); Laura Levitt, *American Jewish Loss After the Holocaust* (New York: New York University Press, 2007); and Mary Jo Maynes, Jennifer Pierce, and Barbara Laslett, *The Use of Personal Narratives in the Social Sciences and History* (Ithaca: Cornell University Press, 2008).

9. See Rapp, *Testing Women*, 5.

10. Sander Gilman, "The New Genetics and the Old Eugenics: The Ghost in the Machine," *Patterns of Prejudice* 36, no. 1 (2002). The phrase "the ghost in the machine" was first introduced by Gilbert Ryles to critique the Cartesian concept of mind in his book *The Concept of Mind* (Chicago: University of Chicago Press, 1949), and then taken up by Arthur Koestler in his book *The Ghost in the Machine* (London: Penguin Group, 1967) where he discusses the human tendency to self-destruction.

11. Gilman, "The New Genetics," 2.

12. Eric Parens and Adrienne Asch, eds., *Prenatal Testing and Disability Rights* (Washington, D.C.: Georgetown University Press, 2000).

13. Rayna Rapp and Faye Ginsburg, "Enabling Disability: Rewriting Kinship, Reimagining Citizenship," *Public Culture* 13, no. 3 (2001): 533–56.

14. Of course, there are those who may not be aware that their ancestry is Ashkenazi, but who carry the genes associated with that community nonetheless, making the question of boundaries and categories particularly complex. For example, the British filmmaker Stephen Frears had no idea about his own lineage until his son, born in 1972, was diagnosed with familial dysautonomia. As Frears commented in a 2001 interview, "I may not have known I was Jewish, but I carried the gene"; see Naomi Pfefferman, "Hidden Heritage Inspires Director," *Jewish Journal.com*, 27 September 2001, accessed 16 June 2012, http://www.jewishjournal.com/arts/article/hidden_heritage_inspires_director_20010928/.

15. See Gina Kolata, "Nightmare or the Dream of a New Era in Genetics?" *New York Times*, 7 December 1993, accessed 20 July 2009, http://www.nytimes.com/1993/12/07/health/nightmare-or-the-dream-of-a-new-era-in-genetics.html. In the Ashkenazi Jewish population (those of Eastern European descent), estimates suggest that one in four individuals is a carrier of one of eight genetic conditions for which genetic testing is now available. These diseases include Tay-Sachs disease, Canavan, Niemann-Pick, Gaucher, familial dysautonomia,

Bloom syndrome, Fanconi anemia, cystic fibrosis, and mucolipidosis IV. Some of these diseases may be severe, and may result in the early death of a child. For those in the very orthodox or Hasidic communities, for whom abortion is not an option, and for whom knowledge that a genetic disease runs in their family creates a profound reduction in their "kinship capital," creative alternatives to secular forms of genetic testing were developed. Rabbi Josef Ekstein, who had four of his own children die of Tay-Sachs disease, realized his community needed to take advantage of the testing available and founded Dor Yeshorim in the early 1980s. Hebrew for "generation of the righteous," Dor Yeshorim is a premarital genetic testing program for Ashkenazi Jews in Israel and the United States. This service is usually used by orthodox Jewish couples whose marriages have been arranged by their families and the community's rabbi. The prospective partners are tested for carrier status. Individuals are tested anonymously, using a code. The rabbi compares the results by code, and if both people are carriers for the same disorder, the families are informed that the marriage may not take place. If only one person is a carrier, then the marriage can go forward, since the couple cannot have a child with the disease. Which person is a carrier is not divulged, to avoid stigmatization; see Mary Kugler, R.N., "Jewish Genetic Testing for Rare Disorders," *About.com/Rare Diseases*, accessed 14 January 2007, http://www.rarediseases.about.com/od/geneticdisorders/a/doryeshorim.htm.

16. Benedict Anderson, *Imagined Communities* (New York: Verso, 1991).

17. Gilman, "Private Knowledge," *Patterns of Prejudice* 36, no. 1 (2002): 6.

18. Gilman, "The New Genetics," 16.

19. In "The Question Concerning Technology," Heidegger draws on the etymology of *techne*: its roots are in the Greek *techne*, which is "the name not only for the activities and skills of the craftsman but also for the arts of the mind and the fine arts." For the Greeks *techne* was intimately linked to *poiesis*, the poetic, and thus linked to the "bringing forth" so essential in the pursuit of *aletheia/veritas*/truth; see Martin Heidegger, "The Question Concerning Technology," in idem, *The Question Concerning Technology and Other Essays* (New York: Harper, 1977), 13 *et passim*.

20. On Mengele and his practices, photographic and otherwise, see Robert Jay Lifton, *The Nazi Doctors: Medical Killing and the Psychology of Genocide* (New York: Basic Books, 2000). On the resignification and recirculation of photographs, see Susan Crane, "Choosing Not to Look: Representation, Repatriation, And Holocaust Atrocity Photography," *History and Theory* 47, no. 3 (2008): 309–30.

21. See Ginsburg, "Screen Memories: Resignifying the Traditional in Indigenous Media," in *Media Worlds: Anthropology on New Terrain*, ed. F.

Ginsburg, B. Larkin, and L. Abu Lughod (Berkeley: University of California Press, 2002), 39–56.

22. See, for instance, Alisa Lebow, *First Person Jewish* (Minneapolis: University of Minnesota Press, 2008); Michael Renov, *The Subject of Documentary* (Minneapolis: University of Minnesota Press, 2004); and Catherine Russell, *Experimental Ethnography: The Work of Film in the Age of Video* (Durham, N.C.: Duke University Press, 1999).

23. See Liem Deanne Borshay, *First Person Plural* (San Francisco: Center for Asian American Media, 2000), DVD, 56 min.; Lebow, *First Person Jewish*.

24. For a full discussion of this idea, and of "media worlds" more generally, see the introduction to *Media Worlds*, ed. Ginsburg, Larkin, and Lughod, 5.

25. Joe Berlinger, *Gray Matter* (New York: New Video, 2004), DVD, 56 min.

26. For details, see Virginia Heffernan, "'Gray Matter': A Driven Filmmaker and His Grim Subject," *New York Times*, 23 April 2005, accessed 20 July 2009, http://www.nytimes.com/2005/04/12/arts/television/12heff.html?pagewanted=print.

27. Steve Erlanger, "Vienna Buries Child Victims of the Nazis," *New York Times*, 29 April 2002, http://www.nytimes.com/2002/04/29/world/vienna-buries-child-victims-of-the-nazis.html.

28. Shahar Rozen, *Liebe Perla* (Tel Aviv: Eden Productions, 1999), DVD, 53 min.

29. In her excellent article on the film, Barbara Duncan writes that Hannelore Witkofski, in an interview for the film magazine, *Documenter* [http://www.documenter.com/issue04/041acgb.htm] clarified her conditions for being filmed, drawing the line at the privacy of her home: "I didn't want any type of 'home story,' because of my experiences with how disabled persons are presented in the media, how they are shown. So imagine, this cute . . . picture of a short-statured woman cooking on a very short oven with a small soup. It would be a kind of children's movie, like a fairytale. So it was for me, very important to save my privacy. . . . And on the other side, [I wanted] to bring my work to the center, because working people with disability, this is absolutely uncommon in the public view. Disabled people are poor, they suffer, but they don't work"; Duncan, "Liebe Perla: A Complex Friendship and Lost Disability History Captured on Film," *Disability World: A Bi-Monthly Webzine of International Disability News and Views* 9 (July–August 2001), accessed 20 July 2009, http://www.disabilityworld.org/07-08_01/arts/perla.shtml.

30. Quoted in Yehuda Koren and Eilat Negev, *In Our Hearts We Were Giants: The Remarkable Story of the Lilliput Troupe* (New York: Da Capo, 2005), 274.

31. In a thoughtful and provocative essay that includes discussion of *Liebe Perla*, Susan Crane, writing from an ethical and historical-critical perspective, asks: "Have Holocaust atrocity photographs reached the limits of their usefulness as testimony?" She argues for their repatriation rather than for unconditional public access, given that "few of the victims of the Shoah pictured in either the best known or the least circulated images were willing subjects"; Crane, "Choosing Not to Look: Representation, Repatriation, and Holocaust Atrocity Photography," *History and Theory* 47, no. 3 (2008): 309.

32. Sara Eigen, "Liebe Perla, Memento Mori: On Filming Disability and Holocaust History," *Women In German Yearbook: Feminist Studies in German Literature and Culture* 22 (2006). Eigen ends her article with this eloquent articulation of closure around the question of the missing film: "Perla Ovici died in 2001, the last of her immediate family, the only known remaining witness to the film that she hoped to locate and destroy"; Eigen, "Liebe Perla," 18.

33. Ibid. For an excellent overview of the role that the Kaiser Wilhelm/Max Planck Institutes played in Nazi science before, during, and after the war, see William Seidman, "Science and Inhumanity: The Kaiser-Wilhelm/Max Planck Society," *If Not Now* 2 (Winter 2000), http://www.baycrest.org/journal/ifnoto1w.html; revised 18 February 2001, accessed 21 July 2009, http://www.doew.at/thema/planck/planck1.html. The apology on behalf of the institute's role in such projects occurred at a conference sponsored by the Max Planck Presidential Commission, which was established to investigate the Institute's activities from 1933–1944. On 7 June 2001, Max Planck president Hubert Markl offered survivors of concentration-camp experiments "the deepest regret, compassion, and shame at the fact that crimes of this sort were committed, promoted, and not prevented within the ranks of German scientists. . . . The Max Planck Society, as the Kaiser Wilhelm Society's 'heir,' must face up to these historical facts and its moral responsibility." Markl's admission was followed by emotional speeches by two victims of Nazi physician Josef Mengele's infamous "twins" experiments at the Auschwitz-Birkenau death camp; see Robert Koenig, "Max Planck Offers Historic Apology," *Science*, 12 June 2001, accessed 21 July 2009, http://sciencenow.sciencemag.org/cgi/content/full/2001/612/3.

34. Quoted from Jona Laks' speech in his role as the Chairman of the "Organization of the Mengele Twins" on the occasion of the opening of the symposium entitled "Biomedical Sciences and Human Experimentation at Kaiser Wilhelm Institutes—The Auschwitz Connection," Berlin, 7 June 2001, accessed 10 October 2009, http://www.mpg.de/english/illustrationsDocumentation/documentation/pressReleases/2001/bs_laks_e.htm.

35. Susie Korda, *One of Us* (Producer, Susie Korda, 1999), DVD, 56 min.

36. Rapp and Ginsburg, "Enabling Disability," 544.

37. This particular myth played out in a *New York Magazine* article by Jennifer Stout entitled "Are Jews Smarter?" about a controversial 2005 study. As Stout wrote, "[did] Jewish intelligence evolve in tandem with Jewish diseases as a result of discrimination in the ghettos of medieval Europe? That's the premise of a controversial new study that has some preening and others plotzing"; Stout, "Are Jews Smarter?" *New York Magazine*, 16 October 2009, accessed 20 July 2009, http://nymag.com/nymetro/news/culture/features/1478/.

38. Of course, the questions raised here are guilty of many sins—notably, of overgeneralizing Jewish practices, which span the spectrum from Hasidic to orthodox all the way to the secular and cultural, and of overdetermining as cultural or religious the practice of hiding the presence of disability in a family when it was widespread sociologically.

39. The defective gene causes the body to produce unusually thick, sticky mucus that clogs the lungs and leads to life-threatening lung infections, obstructs the pancreas, and stops natural enzymes from helping the body break down and absorb food. In the 1950s few children with cystic fibrosis lived to attend elementary school. Today, many people with the disease can now expect to live into their thirties, forties, and beyond.

40. Andrea Eisenman, comments at Limmud screening of her film trailer, 15 January 2005; author's transcript.

41. Dianne Cohler-Esses, "In God's Image?" *The Jewish Week*, December 2006, 17.

42. Ibid.

43. Barbara Kirshenblatt-Gimblett, "A Parable in Context: A Social Interactional Analysis of Storytelling Performance," in *Folklore: Performance and Communication*, ed. Dan Ben-Amos and Kenneth S. Goldstein (The Hague: Mouton 1975), 107; see also 123. The term "parable of possibility" has been used in quite different contexts, for instance, by the economist Russell Roberts in his novella about the virtues of the free market and the creativity of the American economy: Roberts, *The Price of Everything: A Parable of Possibility and Prosperity* (Princeton: Princeton University Press, 2008). It also appears in the literary scholar Terence Martin's study of the American literary fixation with "beginnings"; see Martin, *Parables of Possibility: The American Need for Beginnings* (New York: Columbia University Press, 1995).

44. Ilana Tractman, "Director's Statement," *Praying with Lior*, accessed 20 July 2009, http://www.prayingwithlior.com/directorsstatement.html.

45. Trachtman, *Praying with Lior* (2007), DVD, 56 min., http://www.prayingwithlior.com.
46. Quote from author's notes taken at post-screening discussion, 1 February 2008.
47. Ibid.
48. Ibid.
49. See Aviv and Shneer, *New Jews*.
50. "The independent living movement has been an important part of this broader movement for disability rights. It is based on the premise that people with even the most severe disabilities should have the choice of living in the community. This can be accomplished through the creation of personal assistance services allowing an individual to manage his or her personal care, to keep a home, to have a job, go to school, worship, and otherwise participate in the life of the community. The independent living movement also advocates for the removal of architectural and transportation barriers that prevent people with disabilities from sharing fully in all aspects of our society. . . . Although there were earlier experiments with this concept, it wasn't until 1972 that the first Center for Independent Living was founded by disability activists in Berkeley, California"; Regents of the University of California, "Introduction," *History of Disability Rights and Independent Living Movement*, accessed 10 October 2009, http://bancroft.berkeley.edu/collections/drilm/introduction.html.
51. Randi Sherman, "Setting The Wheelchairs In Motion," *The Jewish Week*, 12 March 2008, accessed 13 July, 2009, http://www.thejewishweek.com/viewArticle/c36_a4850/News/New_York.html#.
52. Quoted in Carolyn Slutsky, "Getting Reel on Disabilities," *The Jewish Week*, 23 January 2008, accessed 13 July 2009, http://www.thejewishweek.com/viewArticle/c36_a3543/News/New_York.html#.
53. See Kolata, "Parents Take Charge, Putting Gene Hunt Onto the Fast Track," *New York Times*, 16 July 1996, accessed 20 July 2009, http://www.nytimes.com/1996/07/16/science/parents-take-charge-putting-gene-hunt-onto-the-fast-track.html; Susan Lindee, *Moments of Truth in Genetic Medicine* (Baltimore: The Johns Hopkins University Press, 2008). For the most up-to-date information on FD, see Family Dysautonomia Foundation, "History and Statistics," accessed 20 July 2009, http://www.familialdysautonomia.org/history.htm#history.
54. For more information on the Make-A-Wish Foundation, see http://www.wish.org/ (accessed 14 February 2007).
55. For more on Samantha's Make-A-Wish experience, see "Samantha Meyers: All About My Life," http://samanthamyers.typepad.com/. For

more on her Bat Mitzvah and fundraising efforts, see Family Dysautonomia Foundation, "Samantha Myers Dedicates Bat Mitzvah to Foundation," *Family Matters* (Winter 2003), accessed 14 February 2007, http://www.familialdysautonomia.org/Fammat/winter03_samantha_myers.htm.

56. See, for instance, Robert Bogdan, *Freak Show: Presenting Human Oddities for Amusement and Profit* (Chicago: University of Chicago Press, 1990); Rosemarie Garland Thomson, *Extraordinary Bodies* (New York: Columbia University Press, 1997).

57. Along with parent-activists who worked in the mainstream media, such as Emily Kingsley, a writer for Sesame Street, whose son Jason was the first child with Down syndrome to appear on television, there were people such as Mary Johnson and Cass Irvin, who in 1980 founded the alternative journal *The Disability Rag*; see Barnett Shaw, ed., *The Ragged Edge: The Disability Experience from the Pages of the Disability Rag* (Louisville, Ky.: Advocado Press, 1994).

58. See, for example, the public exhibition by Nancy Burson, "Seeing and Believing: The Art of Nancy Burson," *Grey Art Gallery* (New York: New York University, 12 February–20 April 2002). One of the longest-running disability film festivals in the United States is SuperFest Film Festival, started in 1998, in Berkeley, California, http://www.culturedisabilitytalent.org/superfest/sf2009.html. For a helpful listing of disability film festivals worldwide, see the National Arts and Disability Center website at http://nadc.ucla.edu/filmfest.cfm.

59. Rapp and Ginsburg, "Enabling Disability."

60. For a discussion of these forms of mediation, see Faye Ginsburg, "Found in Translation," *In Media Res: A Media Commons Project*, 28 March 2007, http://mediacommons.futureofthebook.org/imr/2007/03/28/found-in-translation.

61. The January 2007 meeting attracted over five hundred Jews from all walks of life, multiple generations, and a range of Jewish backgrounds who came to take part in lectures, workshops, text-study sessions, discussions, exhibits, performances and much more—all planned by a community of volunteers.

62. "Learning Without Limits," program, Limmud, N.Y., 2005, accessed 10 October 2009, http://apps.zebra.limmudny.org/lny_2005/limmud_pub_schedule/schedule_v1.pl?op=p&id=405; see also Editorial Board, "Here and There," 2*LifeMagazine*, October 2007.

63. According to Jewish law, there are specific times when this prayer should be said. However, it is also recited when people experience something unique, new, and good for the first time: *Baruch Atah Hashem,Elokeinu Melach Haolam,shehechiyanu,v'keyamanu v'heigeanu lazman ha zeh* ["I am grateful to

the source of life, that I have been kept alive and brought to this moment so that I may share life with those I love and experience the blessings and goodness that life has to offer"].

64. *Second Life* [SL, or 2Life] is a virtual world developed and launched in 2003, and is accessible via the Internet. A free client program called the *Second Life Viewer* enables its users, called Residents, to interact with each other through avatars. Built into the software is a three-dimensional modeling tool based around simple geometric shapes that allows a resident to build virtual objects. Residents can explore, meet other residents, socialize, participate in individual and group activities, and create and trade virtual property and services with one another, or travel throughout the world, which residents refer to as the grid. New York University's Working Group on Jews, Religion and Media has an active website, *Modiya*, that includes an active section on new media (including *Second Life*); see http://modiya.nyu.edu/handle/1964/412.

65. On Chava Weissler's research, see Michael Lando, "'Second Life's' Virtual Judaism Gains a New Congregation," *Jerusalem Post*, 12 July 2007, accessed 16 June 2012, http://www.jpost.com/JewishWorld/JewishFeatures/Article.aspx?id=84611.

THINKING ABOUT MELVILLE, RELIGION, AND MACHINES THAT THINK
John Lardas Modern

1. Quoted in Roland Marchand, *Advertising the American Dream: Making Way for Modernity*, 1920–1940 (Berkeley: University of California Press, 1985), 3.
2. Floyd W. Parsons, "Everybody's Business," *Advertising and Selling* 5 (1927): 5.
3. Alfred B. Kuttner, "Nerves," in *Civilization in the United States: An Enquiry by Thirty
Americans*, ed. Harold E. Stearns (New York: Funk and Wagnalls, 1922), 439–40.
4. Martin E. Marty, *Modern American Religion*, vol. 2, *The Noise of Conflict*, 1919–1941 (Chicago: University of Chicago Press, 1991), 4.
5. Frederick Winslow Taylor, *The Principles of Scientific Management* (New York: Harper and Brothers, 1911), 7.
6. W. B. Riley, "The Faith of the Fundamentalists," *Current History* 26, no. 2 (1927): 438.
7. Attorney General Palmer, "The Case Against the 'Reds,'" *The Forum: A Magazine of Constructive Nationalism* 63, no. 2 (1920): 173.

8. Walter Benjamin, "One-Way Street," in *Selected Writings: Volume 1, 1913–1926*, ed. Marcus Bullock and Michael W. Jennings (Cambridge, Mass.: Harvard University Press, 1996), 454.

9. David Jaffe, "The Village Enlightenment in New England, 1760–1820," *The William and Mary Quarterly* 47, no. 3 (1990): 328.

10. In avoiding the radical skepticism of a David Hume, Arminians and enlightened villagers alike idealized order (a *central* believer/observer), symmetry (a God/world that *was* centered) and security (*desire for* this symmetry). And both reasonable faith and faith in reason promised adherents something tangible and permanent—in the form of salvation of the soul and/or certain knowledge of the material world. From an epistemological perspective, Congregationalist minister Jonathan Mayhew's claim "that men are naturally endowed with faculties proper for the discerning" of moral differences and judging "for themselves in things of a religious concern" was not antithetical to Bacon's admission of "nothing but on the faith of eyes . . . so that nothing is exaggerated for wonder's sake"; from Mayhew, "Concerning the Difference Between Truth and Falsehood, Right and Wrong," in *Seven Sermons* (Boston: Rogers and Fowle, 1749), 5; and Francis Bacon, *The Works of Francis Bacon*, ed. James Spedding, Robert Leslie Ellis, and Douglas Denon Heath (New York: Hurd and Houghton, 1870), 8:49. For triumphal accounts in the nineteenth century that linked Bacon, disenchantment, and the "true religion" of Protestantism, see Rufus Blakeman, *A Philosophical Essay on Credulity and Superstition* (New York: D. Appleton, 1849); and Samuel M. Hopkins, "Religious Character of Lord Bacon," *The Biblical Repository and Classical Review* 3 (1847): 127–42. On the relationship between the epistemic and political stances of antebellum Protestantism, see John Lardas Modern, "Ghosts of Sing Sing; or, the Metaphysics of Secularism," *Journal of the American Academy of Religion* 75, no. 3 (2007): 615–50; and Modern, "Evangelical Secularism and the Measure of Leviathan," *Church History: Studies in Christianity and Culture* 77, no. 4 (2008): 801–76.

11. Henry F. May, *The Enlightenment in America* (New York: Oxford University Press, 1976), 56–58, 342; Harry S. Stout, "Religion, Communications, and the Ideological Origins of the American Revolution," *The William and Mary Quarterly* 34, no. 4 (1977): 520; and Charles Sellers, *The Market Revolution: Jacksonian America, 1815–1846* (New York: Oxford University Press, 1991), 202–03.

12. Max Weber, "Science as a Vocation," in *From Max Weber: Essays in Sociology*, ed. H. H. Gerth and C. Wright Mills (New York: Oxford University Press, 1958), 139.

Notes to pages 187–190   329

13. W. H. Worrell, "Do Brains or Dollars Operate your Set?" *Radio Broadcast* 2 (1922), 70.

14. On the genealogy of secularism in the modern West, see Talal Asad, *Formations of the Secular: Christianity, Islam, Modernity* (Stanford: Stanford University Press, 2003). Undergirding this chapter is the fact that 1851, the year *Moby-Dick* was published, also marked one of the first prescriptive uses of the term "secularism" (often attributed to George Jacob Holyoake's address to the London Hall of Science and his founding of the "Society of Reasoners") to connote a self and a world that ultimately made sense without the rhetorical need for divine sanction; from Owen Chadwick, *The Secularization of the European Mind in the Nineteenth Century* (Cambridge: Cambridge University Press, 1975), 9.

15. Herman Melville, *The Writings of Herman Melville*, vol. 14, *Correspondence*, ed. Lynne Horth (Evanston and Chicago: Northwestern University Press, 1993), 212.

16. Melville, *Moby-Dick or The White Whale* (New York: Grosset and Dunlap, 1925), 5.

17. Ibid., 422, 149, 402.

18. "Though I wrote the Gospels in this century," Melville was resigned to the fact that he "should die in the gutter" (Melville, *Correspondence*, 192). *Moby-Dick* was, and is, a work of embedded resistance—taking the measure of its own history and culture—not as forces, per se, that impinge upon the individual, that determine her decisions or condition his actions—but as the generative resources of self.

19. Paul Lauter, "Melville Climbs the Canon," *American Literature* 66 (1994): 6–10.

20. "Your World Has Changed," advertisement, *Advertising and Selling*, 29 June 1927.

21. David A. Mindell, *Between Human and Machine: Feedback, Control, and Computing Before Cybernetics* (Baltimore: The John Hopkins University Press, 2002), 6.

22. Norbert Wiener, *The Human Use of Human Beings: Cybernetics and Society*, 2nd ed. (Garden City, N.Y.: Doubleday Anchor, 1954), 32–34.

23. Otto Mayr, *The Origins of Feedback Control* (Cambridge, Mass.: MIT Press, 1970), 11–52.

24. See, for example, the role feedback technologies have played in the development of the information society and "control revolution" in James R. Beniger, *The Control Revolution: Technological and Economic Origins of the Information Society* (Cambridge, Mass.: Harvard University Press, 1986), 344–89; and in the development of twentieth-century social science in

George P. Richardson, *Feedback Thought in Social Science and Systems Theory* (Philadelphia: University of Pennsylvania Press, 1991).

25. On spiritualist "ambivalence about where to locate authoritative agency in the interface between humans and machines," see Jeremy Stolow, "Salvation by Electricity," in *Religion: Beyond a Concept*, ed. Hent de Vries (New York: Fordham University Press, 2008), 685; see also Lisa Gitelman, *Scripts, Grooves, and Writing Machines: Representing Technology in the Edison Era* (Stanford: Stanford University Press, 1999), 211–13.

26. Walter Rauschenbusch, *A Theology for the Social Gospel* (New York: Macmillan, 1917), 110, 143.

27. George Albert Coe, *A Social Theory of Religious Education* (New York: Charles Scribner's Sons, 1917), 168, 131.

28. Such irony pervades evangelical history and may be found in Jonathan Edwards's "Sinners in the Hands of an Angry God" (1741). A rich and contradictory sermon, it instructs parishioners to recognize their always already abject relation to God while simultaneously demanding that they willingly submit to his will.

29. William Jennings Bryan, *In His Image* (New York: Fleming H. Revell, 1922), 97.

30. Marty, *Modern American Religion*, 2:66–79.

31. Warren I. Susman, *Culture as History: The Transformation of American Society in the Twentieth Century* (New York: Pantheon, 1984), 133.

32. Beniger, *The Control Revolution*, 317.

33. Bruce Barton, *The Man Nobody Knows: A Discovery of the Real Jesus* (Chicago: Ivan R. Dee, 2000), 4, 10, 13, 6.

34. Benjamin, "The Work of Art in the Age of Its Technological Reproducibility, Third Version," in *Selected Writings: Volume 4, 1938–40*, ed. Howard Eiland and Michael W. Jennings (Cambridge, Mass.: Harvard University Press, 2003), 252.

35. Josephine A. Jackson and Helen M. Salisbury, *Outwitting Our Nerves: A Primer of Psychotherapy* (New York: Century, 1922), 296, 360.

36. George A. Dorsey, *Why We Behave Like Human Beings* (New York: Blue Ribbon, 1925), 302, 301.

37. Waldo Frank, *Our America* (New York: Boni and Liveright, 1919), 66, 150, 68.

38. H. M. Tomlinson, "Two Americans and a Whale: Some Fruits of a London Luncheon," *Harpers Magazine*, April 1926.

39. Raymond M. Weaver, "The Centennial of Herman Melville," *Nation*, 2 August 1919.

40. Weaver, *Herman Melville: Mariner and Mystic* (New York: George H. Doran, 1921), 19, 331.

41. Leigh Eric Schmidt, "The Making of Modern 'Mysticism,'" *Journal of the American Academy of Religion* 71, no. 2 (2003): 288.

42. Hans G. Kippenberg, *Discovering Religious History in the Modern Age*, trans. Barbara Harshav (Princeton: Princeton University Press, 2002), 175–86.

43. Charles A. Bennett, *A Philosophical Study of Mysticism: An Essay* (New Haven: Yale University Press, 1923), 6; and Rufus M. Jones, "Mysticism in Present-Day Religion," *Harvard Theological Review* 8, no. 2 (1915): 156, 161.

44. H. A. Murray Jr., "Review of Lewis Mumford's *Herman Melville*," *The New England Quarterly* 2 (1929): 526.

45. Weaver, *Herman Melville*, 15, 19, 21, 24–29.

46. Mumford, *Technics and Civilization* (New York: Harcourt, Brace, 1934), 45, 321, 227, 212, 254.

47. Ibid., 239, 241, 322, 324; italics in original.

48. Ibid., 213

49. Mumford, *Herman Melville* (New York: Literary Guild of America, 1929), 5, 64–65.

50. Mumford, *Sticks and Stones: A Study of American Architecture and Civilization* (New York: Horace Liveright, 1924), 67–68, 101, 74–75, 105, 81.

51. Mumford, *Technics and Civilization*, 331.

52. Public relations and advances in advertising were the latest instances of the "control revolution" in which technology of interchangeability, so integral to the American system of manufacturing, had extended its field of operations under the auspices of consumer capitalism. Machines were not simply making parts for other machines, but were integral to the form and content of social reproduction. Public relations was a particular (and less reliable) version of feedback control. Instead of maintaining a fixed variable on the inside by responding to fluctuations on the outside, "counselors" stoked the flames of consumer desire in order to justify an accelerating rate of production and, ideally, consumption.

53. Edward L. Bernays, *Crystallizing Public Opinion* (New York: Liverlight, 1923), 62.

54. Marchand, *Advertising the American Dream*, 94–95.

55. E. L. Grant Watson, "Moby Dick," reprinted in *Moby-Dick as Doubloon: Essays and Extract (1851–1970)*, ed. Hershel Parker Harrison Hayford (1920; New York: Norton, 1970), 136; and J. W. N. Sullivan, "Herman Melville," reprinted in *Moby-Dick as Doubloon* (1923; New York: Norton, 1970), 163.

56. Mumford, *Herman Melville*, 184–86.

57. D. H. Lawrence, *Studies in Classic American Literature* (New York: T. Seltzer, 1923), 216.

58. Guy Debord, *Society of the Specatcle*, trans. Donald Nicholson-Smith (New York: Zone Books, 1995), 13.

59. Walter Lippmann, *Public Opinion* (New York: T. Seltxer, 1922), 108, 15.

60. Debord, *Society of the Spectacle*, 19.

61. Ibid., 92.

62. A similar point is made by Lisa Costanzo Cahir in "Routinizing the Charismatic: Melville and Hollywood's Three *Moby-Dicks*," *Melville Society Extracts* 110 (1997): 11–17. Although I agree with her assessment that *The Sea Beast* is about Ahab's "real pursuit of identity," I take issue with her argument that *The Sea Beast* validates autonomous, *autotelic* forms of masculine identity.

63. Sigmund Freud, *The Interpretation of Dreams*, trans. A. A. Brill (New York: Macmillan, 1913).

64. Quoted in John Kobler, *Damned in Paradise: The Life of John Barrymore* (New York: Atheneum, 1977), 213.

65. Carol Stein Hoffman, *The Barrymores: Hollywood's First Family* (Lexington: University of Kentucky Press, 2001), 73.

66. Ibid., 74.

67. S. R. Buchman, "*Moby-Dick*—the Book and *The Sea Beast*—the Picture: An Appreciation," in *Moby-Dick or The White Whale*, by Herman Melville (New York: Grosset and Dunlap, 1925), x.

68. Judith Butler, *Bodies That Matter: On the Discursive Limits of "Sex"* (New York: Routledge, 1993), xi.

69. Benjamin, "The Work of Art," 260.

70. Donna Haraway, "A Manifesto for Cyborgs: Science, Technology, and Socialist Feminism in the 1980s," in *The Haraway Reader* (New York: Routledge, 2004), 8; emphasis in Haraway.

71. Benjamin, "The Work of Art," 262.

72. Ibid., 254.

73. Ibid., 269.

74. Ibid., 266; see Johann Wolfgang von Goethe, *Goethe's Theory of Colours*, trans. Charles Lock Eastlake (London: John Murray, 1840).

75. Benjamin, "The Work of Art," 254.

76. Mumford, *Technics and Civilization*, 333–34.

77. Martin Heidegger, "The Age of the World-Picture," in *The Question Concerning Technology and Other Essays*, trans. William Lovitt (New York: Harper and Row, 1977), 135.

78. Benjamin, "The Work of Art," 255.

79. Melville, *Correspondences*, 186.

80. Mumford, *The Golden Day: A Study in American Literature and Culture* (New York: Boni and Liveright, 1926), 150–51.

81. Dickran Tashjian, *Skyscraper Primitive: Dada and the American Avant-Garde, 1910–1925* (Middletown: Wesleyan University Press, 1975), 116–34.

82. Melville, *Moby-Dick*, 4.
83. Emmy Veronica Sanders, "American Invades Europe," *Broom* 1, no. 1 (1921): 89–90.
84. David O'Neil, "The New Broom," *Broom* 1, no. 1 (1921): 96.
85. Quoted in Benjamin, "The Work of Art," 269.
86. Blaise Cendrars, "Profound Today," *Broom* 1, no. 1 (1922): 265.
87. Jean Epstein, "The New Conditions of Literary Phenomena," *Broom* 2, no. 1 (1922): 6–7.
88. Haraway, "A Manifesto for Cyborgs," 9.
89. Enrico Prampolini, "The Aesthetic of the Machine and Mechanical Introspection in Art," *Broom* 3, no. 3 (1922): 236.
90. Mayr, *The Origins of Feedback*, 11–26.
91. Jane Heap, "Dada," *Little Review* 7, no. 2 (1922): 46.
92. Abraham A. Davidson, "The European Art Invasion," in *Making Mischief: Dada Invades New York*, ed. Francis M. Naumann, with Beth Vann (New York: Whitney Museum of Art, 1996), 223–24.
93. Irene Gammel, *Baroness Elsa: Gender, Dada, and Everyday Modernity—A Cultural Biography* (Cambridge, Mass.: MIT Press, 2002), 195.
94. Francis M. Naumann, *New York Dada, 1915–23* (New York: Harry N. Abrams, 1994), 171; and Gammel, *Baroness Elsa*, 220.
95. One is reminded here of Melville's letter to Nathaniel Hawthorne in April of 1851: "We incline to think that God cannot explain His own secrets, and that He would like a little more information upon certain points Himself. We mortals astonish Him as much as He us"; from Melville, *Correspondences*, 186.
96. Quoted in Gammel, *Baroness Elsa*, 229.
97. Grant Overton, *The Philosophy of Fiction* (New York: Appleton, 1928), 231.
98. Shortly after the publication of *Moby-Dick* in November of 1851, reports began to reach America about the August sinking of the *Ann Alexander* by a whale in the South Pacific. It was the first "attack of a whale upon a ship" since the destruction of the *Essex* in 1820. The story about the *Ann Alexander* originally appeared in the Panama *Herald* on October 16 and was reprinted the following month in the *New-York Daily Tribune* and *Littell's Living Age*. The sperm whale that destroyed the *Ann Alexander* had first turned upon starboard and larboard boats, seizing both in its jaws and crushing them to pieces. It then rushed toward the Ann Alexander "at the rate of fifteen knots! *In an instant the monster struck the ship with tremendous violence, shaking her from stem to stern*"; from "A Ship Sunk by a Whale," *Littell's Living Age*, 29 November 1851. Upon reading the article Melville remarked to his publisher,

"the Whale had almost completely slipped me for the time (& I was the merrier for it) when Crash! comes Moby Dick himself . . . It is really & truly a surprising coincidence—to say the least. I make no doubt it is Moby Dick himself . . . I wonder if my evil art has raised this monster"; Melville, *Correspondences*, 209.

99. Thomas A. Carlson, *The Indiscrete Image: Infinitude and the Creation of the Human* (Chicago: University of Chicago Press, 2008), 18.

100. William Jennings Bryan, for example, that standard bearer of fundamental faith, equated faith to a particular kind of technology—"there is that in each human life," he wrote, "that corresponds to the mainspring of a watch—that which is absolutely necessary if the life is to be what it should be, a real life and not a mere existence. That necessary thing is *a belief in God*"; Bryan, *In His Image*, 86. Faith, for Bryan, was that which repeated without difference. It was a dependable, rational, and utterly rationalizing process. It was not, however, self-regulating. It affirmed the "realness" of the individual believer precisely because it ignored the conditions imposed from outside the self. But how might faith be viewed in terms of feedback and reproducibility rather than repetition, a process that does not reaffirm a centered individual with every tick but adjusts accordingly to external fluctuations?

101. Sydney E. Ahlstrom, *A Religious History of the American People* (New Haven: Yale University Press, 1972); Mark A. Noll, *America's God: From Jonathan Edwards to Abraham Lincoln* (New York: Oxford University Press, 2002); and Catherine L. Albanese, *A Republic of Mind and Spirit: A Cultural History of American Metaphysical Religion* (New Haven: Yale University Press, 2007).

102. Ahlstrom, *A Religious History*, 1052.

103. Such a possibility is very much at odds with the Geertzian model of "thick description" and its formidable legacy in the humanities and social sciences. Without questioning the degree to which the self can ever become entirely legible to the self, Geertz claimed that every society and individual life, and by extension, every belief and every practice, "contain their own interpretations. One has only to learn how to gain access to them"; from Clifford Geertz, "Deep Play: Notes on the Balinese Cockfight," in *The Interpretation of Cultures* (New York: Basic Books, 1973), 453.

104. The ambiguities of agency during the "machine age" have been the subject of a number of elegant critical studies; see, for example, Anson Rabinbach, *The Human Motor: Energy, Fatigue, and the Origins of Modernity* (New York: Basic Books, 1990); Mark Seltzer, *Bodies and Machines* (New York: Routledge, 1992); Martha Banta, *Taylorized Lives: Narrative Productions in the Age of Taylor, Veblen, and Ford* (Chicago: University of Chicago Press, 1993);

Carolyn Thomas de la Peña, *The Body Electric: How Strange Machines Built the Modern American* (New York: New York University Press, 2003); and Joel Dinerstein, *The Swinging Machine: Modernity, Technology, and African American Culture Between the World Wars* (Amherst: University of Massachusetts Press, 2003). Dinerstein's work is particularly relevant to the issue of religious combinativeness, given his emphasis on how African American artists strove to refigure "machine aesthetics" in and through their artistry. Dinerstein's work suggests that the self is located—i.e., the self happens—somewhere between resistance and assimilation, between choice and coercion—a lesson that many Anglo-Americans were not willing to consider in their triumphal theorizing about the human in relation to the machine. The possibility for consideration, argues Dinerstein, existed in African American jazz, swing, and dance.

105. Hayles defines reflexivity as "the movement whereby that which has been used to generate a system is made, through a changed perspective, to become part of the system it generates"; N. Katherine Hayles, *How We Became Posthuman: Virtual Bodies in Cybernetics, Literature, and Informatics* (Chicago: University of Chicago Press, 1999), 8–9.

106. Larry Hirschhorn, *Beyond Mechanization: Work and Technology in a Postindustrial Age* (Cambridge, Mass.: MIT Press, 1984), 27.

107. Michel Foucault, *The Archaeology of Knowledge and the Discourse on Language*, trans. A. M. Sheridan Smith (New York: Pantheon, 1972).

AMAZING STORIES: HOW SCIENCE FICTION SACRALIZES THE SECULAR
Peter Pels

1. William Gibson, *Neuromancer* (New York: Ace, 1984); Gibson, *Count Zero* (New York: Ace, 1986); Vernor Vinge, *True Names . . . and Other Dangers* (New York: Baen, 1987); Neal Stephenson, *Snow Crash* (New York: Bantam, 1992).

2. Margaret Wertheim, *The Pearly Gates of Cyberspace: A History of Space from Dante to the Internet* (London: Virago, 1999).

3. Erik Davis, *TechGnosis: Myth, Magic and Mysticism in the Age of Information* (London: Serpent's Tail, 1998).

4. N. Katherine Hayles, *How We Became Posthuman: Virtual Bodies in Cybernetics, Literature, and Informatics* (Chicago: University of Chicago Press, 1999).

5. See Mark Pesce, "True Magic," in *"True Names" and the Opening of the Cyberspace Frontier*, ed. James Frenkel (New York: Tom Doherty Associates, 2001), 221–38; Timothy Leary and Eric Gullichsen, "Digital Polytheism,"

American Buddha Online Library, http://www.american-buddha.com/digital.polytheism.htm.

6. Bruno Latour, *We Have Never Been Modern* (Cambridge, Mass.: Harvard University Press, 1993).

7. See, for example, Bryan Wilson, *Contemporary Transformations of Religion* (Oxford: Oxford University Press, 1976), 88.

8. Bruce Sterling, "Introduction," in *Mirrorshades: The Cyberpunk Anthology*, ed. Bruce Sterling (New York: Arbor House, 1986).

9. On posthumanism, see Hayles, *How We Became Posthuman*.

10. Peter Pels, "Spirits of Modernity: Alfred Wallace, Edward Tylor and the Visual Politics of Fact," in *Magic and Modernity: Interfaces of Revelation and Concealment*, ed. Birgit Meyer and Peter Pels (Stanford: Stanford University Press, 2003), 241–71; Jeremy Stolow, "Salvation by Electricity," in *Religion: Beyond a Concept*, ed. Hent de Vries (New York: Fordham University Press, 2008), 668–86; Stolow, in this volume.

11. A focus on American science fiction is appropriate in the sense that the U.S. trajectory of SF can be seen as representative for the dominant version of popular modernism. A comparative cultural analysis, however, would show that the trajectories of twentieth-century British, French, Japanese, Polish and Soviet SF were all usually less optimistic. This will have to await another essay.

12. See Stef Aupers, Dick Houtman, and Peter Pels, "Cybergnosis, Technology, Religion and the Secular," in *Religion: Beyond a Concept*, ed. de Vries (New York: Fordham University Press, 2008), 687–703.

13. Alfred Bester, *The Stars My Destination* (New York: Vintage, 1996), 27–28.

14. Adam Roberts, *Science Fiction* (London: Routledge, 2000), 146.

15. Cf. George Mann, *The Mammoth Encyclopedia of Science Fiction* (London: Robinson, 2001), 5; and James Blish, as quoted in *Screening Space: The American Science Fiction Film*, by Vivian Sobchak, 2nd ed. (New Brunswick, N.J.: Rutgers University Press), 19.

16. See Wilson, *Contemporary Transformations*, 88.

17. Frank Herbert, *Dune* (London: New English Library, 1989).

18. Bester, *The Stars*, 256.

19. Cf. Wouter Hanegraaff, *New Age Religion and Western Culture* (Leiden: Brill, 1996).

20. See Gillian Bennett, *Traditions of Belief: Women and the Supernatural* (Harmondsworth, UK: Penguin, 1987); Ann Braude, *Radical Spirits: Spiritualism and Women's Rights in Nineteenth-Century America* (Boston: Beacon, 1989); Alex Owen, *The Darkened Room: Women, Power and Spiritualism in Late Victorian England* (London: Virago, 1989); Pels, "Spirits of

Modernity." Perhaps the best-known case of female-led Western esotericism is that of Madame Blavatsky and the Theosophical Society; see Peter Washington, *Madame Blavatsky's Baboon: Theosophy and the Emergence of the Western Guru* (London: Secker and Warburg, 1993).

21. R. Lawrence Moore, *Selling God: American Religion in the Marketplace of Culture* (New York: Oxford University Press, 1994); Benedict Anderson, *Imagined Communities: Reflections on the Origin and Spread of Nationalism* (London: Verso, 1983), 40.

22. Aupers, Houtman, and Pels, "Cybergnosis," 691; Talal Asad, *Formations of the Secular: Christianity, Islam, Modernity* (Stanford: Stanford University Press, 2003), 14n15.

23. Both are also inescapably global: nationalism arose partly from the confrontation of New World colonies with European powers, and theosophy from that between European Christianity and Hinduism, Buddhism, and Jewish mysticism; see Jocelyn Godwin, *The Theosophical Enlightenment* (Albany: State University of New York Press, 1994), showing that "modernity," indeed, does not originate in Europe or the West only; see Timothy Mitchell, "The Stage of Modernity," in *Questions of Modernity*, ed. Timothy Mitchell (Minneaopolis: University of Minnesota Press, 2000), 1–34. I hesitate to use "the market" here, since that is not an (empirically identifiable) institution, but a Western cultural model, often one with salvationist overtones; see Mitchell, *Rule of Experts: Egypt, Technoscience, Modernity* (Berkeley: University of California Press, 2002), 244–71.

24. Jules Verne, *Journey to the Centre of the Earth*, trans. W. Butcher (1864; Oxford: Oxford University Press, 2008); Edward Bulwer Lytton, *The Coming Race* (1871; Stroud, UK: Alan Sutton, 1995). On Madame Blavatsky's theosophy, see S. B. Liljegren, *Bulwer-Lytton's Novels and Isis Unveiled* (Upsala: Lundequistska Bokhandeln; Copenhagen: Munksgaard; Cambridge, Mass.: Harvard University Press, 1957; Christopher F Roth, "Ufology as Anthropology: Race, Extraterrestrials, and the Occult," in *E.T. Culture: Anthropology in Outerspaces*, ed. Deborra Battaglia (Durham, N.C.: Duke University Press, 2005), 38–93, esp. 50.

25. Arthur Conan Doyle, *The Lost World* (New York: Pyramid, 1960).

26. Bulwer Lytton's advanced race (see Bulwer Lytton, *The Coming Race*) used the extraordinary mental power of *vril*, a term he took from the anthropology of religion and from Max Müller's descriptions of Hinduism in particular (and which was copied by Blavatsky: Roth, "Ufology"); Haggard moved from colonial rule and ethnography in Zululand (H. Rider Haggard, *King Solomon's Mines* [Oxford: Oxford University Press, 1989]) to the description of Egyptian/African magic (Haggard, *She* [Oxford: Oxford University Press, 1991]) and a kind of Tibetan theosophy (Haggard, *Ayesha:*

The Return of "She" [New York: Dover, 1978]); Mark Twain's *A Connecticut Yankee in Arthur's Court* used telephony as the model of time travel (David Ketterer, "Introduction," in *Tales of Wonder*, by Mark Twain, ed. David Ketterer, xiii–xxxiii [Lincoln: University of Nebraska Press, 2003]); Luis B. Senarens set fantastic machines (such as robots) among aboriginal Australians or native Americans (Frank Robinson, Robert Weinberg, and Randy Broecker, *Art of Imagination: 20th Century Visions of Science Fiction, Horror, and Fantasy* [Portland, Ore.: Collectors Press, 2002], 26); Conan Doyle's *The Lost World* (and its travel back to the dinosaur age) was based on the actual exploits of anthropologist/geographer Everard im Thurn (see Rosamund Dalziell, "Everard im Thurn in British Guiana and the Western Pacific," in *Writing, Travel and Empire In the Margins of Anthropology*, ed. P. Hulme and R. McDougall [London: I. B. Tauris, 2007], 97–116).

27. As suggested by Dorien Zandbergen during one of the discussions within our "cyberspace salvations" research project; see *Cyberspace*, http://www.cyberspacesalvations.nl. This may, however, turn out to be too simple when we consider the gender politics of the masculine styles adopted by female "gurus" of many occultist associations; see Washington, *Madame Blavatsky's Baboon*, or the "feminine aura" sometimes associated with SF; Gary Westfahl, quoted in Roberts, *Science Fiction*, 29.

28. Asad, *Formations of the Secular*.

29. This is what analysts of the "spiritual supermarket" (such as Steve Bruce, echoing Thomas Luckmann and Bryan Wilson) often tend to forget: the diagnosis of an eclectic "do-it-yourself" religion is based on an ideological abstraction. For a related critique, see Stef Aupers and Dick Houtman, "Beyond the Spiritual Supermarket: The Social and Public Significance of New Age Spirituality," *Journal of Contemporary Religion* 21, no. 2 (2006): 201–22.

30. On occultism, see Theodor Adorno, *The Stars Down to Earth and Other Essays in the Irrational in Culture* (London: Routledge, 1994).

31. A view that may be distilled from the work of de Certeau; see Michel de Certeau, *The Practice of Everyday Life* (Berkeley: University of California Press, 1984).

32. Roth, "Ufology"; Tom Wolfe, *The Electric Kool-Aid Acid Test* (New York: Bantam, 1999). This essay is itself a preparation for a more ethnographic study of SF, the research for which still has to be done.

33. Sobchak, *Screening Space*.

34. Ibid., 20.

35. See Fredric Jameson, *Archaeologies of the Future: The Desire Called Utopia and Other Science Fictions* (London: Verso, 2005), 68.

36. Sobchak, *Screening Space*, 63.

37. Bronislaw Malinowski, *Magic, Science and Religion, and Other Essays* (Garden City, N.Y.: Doubleday, 1954).

38. On the "secular" categories of nature, history and the human, see Asad, *Formations of the Secular,* 192. On "modern magic," see Pels, "Introduction: Magic and Modernity," in *Magic and Modernity: Interfaces of Revelation and Concealment,* ed. Meyer and Pels (Stanford: Stanford University Press, 2003), 1–38.

39. Robert R. Marett, *The Threshold of Religion,* 2nd ed. (London: Methuen, 1914), ix, 12, 22.

40. Ibid., xxxi.

41. I discuss the sacralization of space without claiming that this exhausts possible circumscriptions of what SF is about. Robotics and time travel, for example, cannot be dealt with in this essay.

42. Darko Suvin, *Metamorphoses of Science Fiction: On the Poetics and History of a Literary Genre* (New Haven: Yale University Press, 1979).

43. C. S. Lewis, *Out of the Silent Planet* (New York: Avon, 1949).

44. Ibid., 153.

45. Ibid., 159.

46. Ibid., 27. Lewis explicitly refers—in a negative vein—to the terminology of British colonization by having one of the abductors of his protagonist state that, even on Mars, there is a "native question."

47. Verne, *From the Earth to the Moon,* trans. W. Butcher (Oxford: Oxford University Press, 2008); H. G. Wells, *The War of the Worlds* (Mineola, N.Y.: Dover, 1997).

48. Rudy Rucker, *White Light* (New York: Four Walls Eight Windows, 2001); Andy Wachowski and Larry Wachowski, *The Matrix: Film Script* (Burbank: Warner Bros., 1999).

49. Emile Durkheim, *The Elementary Forms of the Religious Life,* trans. Joseph Ward Swain (New York: Free Press, 1965), 52.

50. Suvin, *Metamorphoses.*

51. I think this is globally true, even in societies that have produced SF against a background that includes much less of a battle between science and Christianity than in Europe or the United States, but the different parameters of this global spreading of SF still remain to be explored.

52. Arthur C. Clarke, *Childhood's End* (New York: Ballantine, 1974), 74.

53. Leo Marx, *The Machine in the Garden: Technology and the Pastoral Ideal in* (New York: Oxford University Press, 1964), 190–226.

54. On Thoreau and Melville, see Marx, *Machine in the Garden.*

55. See, for example, L. Ron Hubbard, *Battlefield Earth: A Saga of the Year 3000* (Los Angeles: Bridge, 1982), ix; Mann, *Encyclopedia,* 12; Roberts, *Science Fiction,* 146.

56. Mann, *Encyclopedia*, 271.
57. Roberts, *Science Fiction*, 73; E. E. "Doc" Smith, quoted in Roberts, *Science Fiction*, 74.
58. Smith, *The Skylark of Space* (New York: Pyramid, 1958), 5 (emphases mine).
59. Ibid., 49 (emphases mine).
60. Ibid., 83.
61. Mann, *Encyclopedia*, 510.
62. For example, when watching a rerun of one of the second series of *Star Wars* films in an Amsterdam bar in 2006, I was struck by the hoots of recognition of the audience titillated by its opening, "technologically sublime" shots of battlestars and swift spaceships.
63. Isaac Asimov, *Foundation* (London: Panther, 1960), 10 (emphases mine).
64. This may have been triggered by the original story format, perhaps, as it was published by the pulp magazines, another symptom of the commercial circuits in which these ideas were materialized.
65. Pioneered in many ways by Fritz Leiber's *The Wanderer* (New York: Tom Doherty Associates, 1983); see John Clute and Peter Nicholls, eds., *The Encyclopedia of Science Fiction* (London: Orbit, 1993), 706. Another stylistic solution to the contradiction between the vastness of scale and the need for identifiable human agency was the "helpless hero," a figure particularly cultivated by Robert Heinlein.
66. Mann, *Encyclopedia*, 45.
67. Asimov, *Foundation*; Asimov, *Foundation and Empire* (London: Panther, 1962); Asimov, *Second Foundation* (London: Panther, 1964).
68. Asimov restarted the Foundation stories in 1982 by connecting them up with his Robot stories and made robots into the agents of telepathy. As indicated in the conclusion, I cannot go into the relationship between telepathy and artificial life in detail in this paper.
69. Bester, *Stars*, 11.
70. Paul Heelas, *The New Age Movement* (Oxford: Blackwell, 1996).
71. Hanegraaff, *New Age Religion*.
72. Asimov, *Pebble in the Sky* (London: Corgi, 1958).
73. Bester, *The Demolished Man* (New York: Vintage, 1996); Bester, *Stars*.
74. James Blish, *ESPer* (New York: Avon, 1952); A. E. van Vogt, *SLAN* (New York: Ballantine, 1961); van Vogt, *The World of Null-A* (New York: Tom Doherty Associates, 2002).
75. Korzybski became, of course, once more popular during the rise of New Age in the 1970s, especially as mediated by the work of Gregory Bateson.
76. Hayles, *How We Became Posthuman*.

77. A less superhuman version of this can be found in Robert Heinlein, *Revolt in 2100* (London: New English Library, 1972). Heinlein's version of mental indoctrination by mathematics, however, is closer to the contemporary scare about psychic manipulation by "scientific" advertising (see, especially, Heinlein, *The Moon Is a Harsh Mistress* [London: New English Library, 1969]), and was most hauntingly and humorously worked out by Frederik Pohl and C. M. Kornbluth in *The Space Merchants* (New York: Ballantine, 1953); and by John Brunner in *Stand on Zanzibar* (London: Gollancz, 1999).

78. Blish, *ESPer*, 53.

79. C. M. Kornbluth, "The Cosmic Charge Account," in *The Marching Morons and Other Famous Science Fiction Stories* (New York: Ballantine, 1959), 109–35, esp. 127.

80. Arthur C. Clarke, *A Fall of Moondust* (London: Pan, 1961), 176–77.

81. Hubbard, *Battlefield Earth*, xi.

82. Mann, *Encyclopedia*, 300.

83. Blish, *ESPer*, 53.

84. Roth, "Ufology," 48.

85. Erich von Däniken, *Chariots of the Gods*, trans. M. Heron (New York: Berkley Books, 1999); for Bulwer-Lytton and Blavatsky, see note 26.

86. Roth, "Ufology," 55.

87. On "antinomian agnosticism," see Roth, "Ufology," 68. On antinomian "cybergnosis," see Aupers, Houtman, and Pels, "Cybergnosis." I cannot go into the extent to which "agnosticism" is closer to "gnosis" than we may think, but its religious roots go back at least to Thomas Huxley's invention of the former term; see Pels, "The Modern Fear of Matter: Reflections on the Protestantism of Victorian Science," *Material Religion* 4, no. 3 (2008): 264–83.

88. Heinlein, *Stranger in a Strange Land* (London: New English Library, 1965).

89. The conversation is mostly conducted by Mike's friends, who try to understand his Martian way of thinking—along the culturally relativist lines sketched by anthropologist Ruth Benedict in *Patterns of Culture*, whose work is cited without reference in the book; Heinlein, *Stranger*, 290–91; Benedict, *Patterns of Culture* (New York: Mentor, 1949).

90. Tom Wolfe, *The Electric Kool-Aid Acid Test* (New York: Bantam, 1999).

91. Ibid., 415. The word "grok(king)" occurs seventeen times in Wolfe's 400-page report.

92. See David Samuels, "Alien Tongues," in *E.T. Culture. Anthropology in Outerspaces*, ed. Deborra Battaglia (Durham, N.C., and London: Duke University Press, 2005), 94–129, esp. 104.

93. Wolfe, *Electric Kool-Aid*, 137.

94. See ibid., 194, 195, 232–33, 246, 259, 260, 271.

95. Ibid., 403.

96. Ibid., 410.

97. Sterling, "Preface," in *Burning Chrome*, ed. Gibson (New York: Ace, 1986), ix–xii, x.

98. John Shirley, *Eclipse* (New York: Warner, 1985).

99. If only because they share a technophile countercultural position not much affected by the "back to nature" attitude of the majority of post-"Summer of Love" hippies. One of the first cyberpunk novels, Rudy Rucker's *White Light*, explicitly cited Neal Cassady and the other Merry Pranksters (Rucker, *White Light*, 9). Rucker and Timothy Leary became some of the most prominent, but also most technolatrous "cybergnostics" in the 1990s; Aupers, Houtman, and Pels, "Cybergnosis."

100. Samuel R. Delany, *Dahlgren* (New York: Bantam, 1975); Philip K. Dick, *Do Androids Dream of Electric Sheep?* (London: Orion, 1999); Brunner, *Stand on Zanzibar*.

101. Andrew M. Butler, *Cyberpunk* (Harpenden, UK: Pocket Essentials, 2000), 15.

102. Gibson, *Neuromancer*, 76 (emphasis in original); Stephenson, *Snow Crash*; Pat Cadigan, *Synners*, 10th ed. (New York: Four Walls Eight Windows, 2001); see also Boutros's chapter in this volume.

103. See, for example, Pesce, "Magic Mirror: The Novel as a Software Development Platform" (Cambridge, Mass.: MIT, October 8–10, 1999), available at *MIT Communications Forum*, last accessed 16 June 2012, http://web.mit.edu/comm-forum/papers/pesce.html.

104. Gibson, *Neuromancer*, 5, 258, 268; Gibson, *Mona Lisa Overdrive* (New York: Bantam, 1988), 16; Gibson, *Count Zero*, 38.

105. Vinge, *True Names*, 48; Ursula Le Guin, *A Wizard of Earthsea* (New York: Bantam, 1975).

106. This may ignore aspects of the more mathematically inspired among cyberpunks (e.g. Rucker, Vinge)—partly because their mathematical fantasies are often beyond me.

107. Sterling, *Schismatrix* (New York: Ace Science Fiction, 1985); Vinge, *A Fire upon the Deep* (New York: Tom Doherty Associates, 1992); Vinge, *A Deepness in the Sky* (New York: Tom Doherty Associates, 1999).

108. See Mark Dery, *Escape Velocity: Cyberculture at the End of the Century* (New York: Grove, 1996).

109. Pels, "Spirits of Modernity"; Stolow, "Salvation by Electricity."

110. See, for the role of futurism in theories about globalization, Anna Lowenhaupt Tsing, "The Global Situation," *Cultural Anthropology* 15, no. 3

(2000): 327–60; for its roots in late medieval techno-millenarian thinking, see David Noble, *The Religion of Technology: The Divinity of Man and the Spirit of Invention* (New York and London: Penguin, 1997); for the nineteenth-century triumph of techno-determinism, see Michael Adas, *Machines as the Measure of Man* (Ithaca, N.Y.: Cornell University Press, 1989); on the malleability of the future, see Reinhart Koselleck, *Futures Past: On the Semantics of Historical Time* (New York: Columbia University Press, 2004).

VIRTUAL VODOU, ACTUAL PRACTICE: TRANSFIGURING THE TECHNOLOGICAL
Alexandra Boutros

1. For further discussion of the relationship between Vodou and Catholicism, see Leslie Desmangles, *The Faces of the Gods: Vodou and Roman Catholicism in Haiti* (Chapel Hill and London: University of North Carolina Press, 1992).

2. For instance, the global dissemination of *mizik rasin* (or roots music), a Haitian popular music movement that incorporates the signifiers, rhythms, and languages of Haitian Vodou into popular music, has certainly contributed to the visibility of Vodou in the North American public sphere; see Laënnec Hurbon, "Current Evolution of Relationships Between Religion and Politics in Haiti," in *Nation Dance: Religion, Identity and Cultural Difference in the Caribbean*, ed. Patrick Taylor (Bloomington: Indiana University Press, 2001), 118–25. For further discussion of *rasin* (roots) culture and its relationship to Haitian popular music, see Elizabeth McAlister, *Rara! Vodou, Power, and Performance in Haiti and Its Diaspora* (Berkeley: University of California Press, 2002). For a discussion of the politics of *mizik rasin*, see Gage Averill, *A Day for the Hunter, A Day for the Prey: Power and Politics in Haitian Popular Music* (Chicago and London: University of Chicago Press, 1997). For a discussion of the circulation of *mizik rasin* in North America, see George Lipsitz, *Dangerous Crossroads: Postmodernism and the Poetics of Place* (London and New York: Verso, 1994).

3. Wade Clark Roof, *A Generation of Seekers: The Spiritual Journeys of the Baby Boom Generation* (San Francisco and New York: HarperCollins, 1993).

4. The U.S.–based Catholic League for Religious and Civil Rights, for instance, published a booklet, with the full support of the Catholic Church; see William A. Donohue, *Angels and Demons: More Demonic Than Angelic* (New York: The Catholic League, 2009).

5. For example, PBS, *Closer to Truth*, "Can Religion Withstand Technology? How the Clash Between Religion and Technology Reshapes Our Search for Meaning," last accessed 18 February 2009, http://www.pbs.org/kcet/closertotruth/explore/show_14.html.

6. Jacques Ellul, *The Technological Society*, trans. John Wilkinson (New York: Alfred A. Knopf, 1964); Lewis Mumford, *The Myth of the Machine* (New York: Harcourt, Brace and World, 1970).

7. See for example, Talal Asad, *Formations of the Secular: Christianity, Islam, Modernity* (Stanford: Stanford University Press, 2003). The narrative of technological progress, or what scholars such as Deleuze and Guattari might call "techno-evolutionism," emerges from a historical determinism prevalent in histories of technology that interpret social change as being determined by technology and interpret that change as "progress."

8. Anna Everett, "The Revolution Will Be Digitized: Afrocentricity and the Digital Public Sphere," *Social Text* 20, no. 2 (2002): 127.

9. John Percy Barlow, "A Declaration of the Independence of Cyberspace," *Electronic Frontier Foundation*, 1996, last accessed 1 December 2009, http://homes.eff.org/~barlow/Declaration-Final.html.

10. Alondra Nelson, "Introduction: Future Texts," *Social Text* 20, no. 2 (2002): 1–15.

11. CÉGEP, a term used predominantly in Quebec, Canada, is the acronym derived from *Collège d'enseignement général et professionnel* (College of General and Vocational Education). CÉGEP is a level of post-secondary education undertaken by students after they graduate from grade 11 of secondary school; it offers preparatory programs for university or entry into the job market.

12. Everett, "Revolution," 133.

13. Julian Dibbell, "A Rape in Cyberspace: Or How an Evil Clown, a Haitian Trickster Spirit, Two Wizards, and a Cast of Dozens turned a Database into a Society," *High Noon on the Electronic Frontier: Conceptual Issues in Cyberspace*, ed. Peter Ludlow (Cambridge, Mass.: MIT Press, 1996), 376–95.

14. For further discussion of the manifestation of characteristics and attributes of "Voodoo" in the online community described by Dibbell, see Barbara Browning, *Infectious Rhythms: Metaphors of Contagion and the Spread of African Culture* (London and New York: Routledge, 1998).

15. Erzulie is the name for a group of goddesses, or *lwa*, in the Vodou pantheon. While the purview of gods and goddesses in Vodou is extensive and multifaceted, Erzulies are popularly understood as having domain over romantic relationships.

16. Legba is said to have domain of the "crossroads," or the junction at which the "real" world and the world of the *lwa* intersect. Legba is the first *lwa* "called" or engaged in most Vodou rituals.

17. Emily Apter, *Continental Drift: From National Characters to Virtual Subjects*, (Chicago: University of Chicago Press, 1999), 217.

18. Ibid., 216.

19. Browning, *Infectious Rhythms*, explores how Vodou/Voodoo has been figured as a form of "contagion" structuring the framing of race and gender in a variety of texts, including Gibson's work.

20. William Gibson, *Count Zero* (New York: Penguin Putnam, 1986), 114.

21. Browning, *Infectious Rhythms*, 122.

22. Allucquère Rosanne Stone, "Will the Real Body Please Stand Up? Boundary Stories About Virtual Cultures," *Cyberspace: First Steps*, ed. Michael Benedikt (Cambridge, Mass.: MIT Press, 1991), 108.

23. Scott McQuire, "Space for Rent in the Last Suburb," in *Prefiguring Cyberculture: An Intellectual History*, ed. Darren Tofts, Annemarie Jonson, and Alessio Cavallaro (Cambridge, Mass.: MIT Press and Power Publications, 2003), 167.

24. Ibid., 167.

25. Gibson, *Neuromancer* (New York: Penguin Putnam, 1984), 167.

26. Site no longer available; last accessed on 6 July 2009; http://www.sentence-ov-desire.net/Pazuzu/voodoo.html.

27. "Vodou Lessons," *Roots Without End Society*, last accessed 1 December 2009, http://www.rootswithoutend.org/racine125/index1.html#lessons.

28. "Haitian Vodou," *Wikipedia*, last accessed 1 December 2009, http://en.wikipedia.org/wiki/Haitian_Vodou.

29. The top two results brought up when you type "Vodou" into the Google search engine are the Wikipedia articles for "Haitian Vodou" and "Voodoo"; last accessed 1 December 2009.

30. Gede.org, last accessed 1 December 2009, http://www.gede.org/about.html.

31. Much has been written about identity play in online environments and the connection of participatory media users to their "real life" identities; see, for example, Sherry Turkle, *Life on the Screen: Identity in the Age of the Internet* (New York: Simon and Schuster, 1995).

32. *Mamma kanzo* or *papa kanzo* is a familiar way of referring to the priestess or priest who conducted one's initiation in Vodou.

33. Gede.org, last accessed 18 February 2009, http://www.gede.org/about.html.

34. For a critical discussion of the praxis and ethics of online community, see Darin Barney, "The Vanishing Table, Or Community in a World That Is No World," in *Community in the Digital Age: Philosophy and Practice*, ed. Andrew Feenberg and Darin Barney (New York: Rowman and Littlefield, 2004), 31–52.

35. N. Katherine Hayles, "Foreword," in *Prefiguring Cyberculture: An Intellectual History*, ed. Darren Tofts, Annemarie Jonson, and Alessio Caval (Cambridge, Mass.: MIT Press and Power Publications, 2003), xiii.

36. Much has been written on how cooperative, trust-based e-commerce networks such as eBay work; see, for example, Josh Boyd, "In Community We Trust: Online Security Communication at eBay," *Journal of Computer Mediated Communication* 7, no. 3 (2002), http://jcmc.indiana.edu/vol7/issue3/boyd.html.

37. *Legba's Crossroads: Vodou Services and Supplies*, last accessed 1 December 2009, http://www.legba.biz/.

38. *Legba's Crossroads: Vodou Services and Supplies*, last accessed 1 December 2009, http://www.legbastore.com/aksyon-sevis-quotactionquot-ritual-package-for-rada-lwa.html.

39. "More About Haitian Vodou," *Erzulie's Authentic Vodou*, last accessed 1 December 2009, http://www.erzulies.com/site/articles/view/6.

40. The U.S. Department of State Bureau of Consular Affairs' website, for example, warns "travel in Haiti can be dangerous and all visitors are urged to exercise vigilance and caution"; last accessed 1 December 2009, http://travel.state.gov/travel/cis_pa_tw/cis/cis_1134.html.

41. David Nicholls, *From Dessalines to Duvalier: Race, Color and National Independence in Haiti* (Cambridge: Cambridge University Press, 1979), 36.

42. "Race in Vodou," *Roots Without End Society*, last accessed 1 December 2009, http://www.rootswithoutend.org/race.html.

43. Ibid.

44. Anthony Giddens, *Modernity and Self-Identity: Self and Society in the Late Modern Age* (Stanford: Stanford University Press, 1991), 64.

45. See, for example, "Vodou Initiation," *Roots Without End Society*, last accessed 1 December 2009, http://www.rootswithoutend.org/emporium/kanzo_regis1.html.

46. "Initiation Candidates: Being a Candidate for Vodou Initiation," *Gada Nou Leve Society*, last accessed 1 December 2009, http://www.ezilikonnen.com/vodou/initiation.html.

47. Ibid.

48. In addition to providing aid to Haiti, the organization also provides aid around the world, according to the website; see "Vodou Aid," *Roots Without End Society*, last accessed 1 December 2009, http://www.vodouaid.org/.

49. "Mambo Racine," *MySpace*, last accessed 1 December 2009, http://www.myspace.com/mamboracine.

50. House, in this case, refers to *djevo*, or initiatory room where initiates are kept apart from others during part of the initiation ritual. Heaven's comments were made on the *culture.religion.voodoo* list; see "Djevo Secrets, Courtesy of Ross Heaven," last accessed 1 December 2009, http://osdir.com/ml/culture.religion.voodoo/2005-12/msg00120.html.

51. Review by Kathy Sue Grey, Amazon.com, last accessed 1 December 2009, http://www.amazon.com/gp/pdp/profile/A2F5JUEY6ETZO1/ref=cm_cr_pr_pdp. In other forums Racine has acknowledged she made this comment and has made others like it.

52. "Author Lives Under Voodoo Curse," *The Argus*, 5 January, 2004, last accessed 1 December 2009, http://archive.theargus.co.uk/2004/1/5/119580.html.

53. "Britain Under the Spell: Representations of Voodoo in British TV and Films," *The Zone*, last accessed 1 December 2009, http://www.zone-sf.com/voodoouk.html.

54. "Author Lives Under Voodoo Curse," *The Argus*.

55. *Legba's Crossroads: Vodou Services and Supplies*.

56. "Taking the asson" refers to the highest level of initiation in Haitian Vodou.

57. *Legba's Crossroads: Vodou Services and Supplies*.

TV ST. CLAIRE
Maria José A. de Abreu

I thank Jeremy Stolow for inviting me to take part in the *Deus in Machina* conference. Special thanks go to Thomas Carlson, Reinhilde König, David Morgan, Rafael Sanchez, Samuel Weber, and, again, to Jeremy Stolow, for their valuable comments on earlier versions of this essay. Thanks also to the audience of the conference *Trance Mediums and New Media*, Cologne, 1–2 June 2009. This study has been financed by the Fundação para a Ciência e a Tecnologia (FCT), Portugal (Project Ref. U4038—2011–2012) and dedicated to Candida Isabel Fragoso da Costa, the wise one.

1. I have described and analyzed this story in more detail in Maria José A. de Abreu, "Breath, Media and the Making of Community Canção Nova," in *Aesthetics Formations: Media, Religion and the Senses*, ed. Birgit Meyer (New York: Palgrave Macmillan, 2009), 161–81.

2. As Laércio Ribeiro, one of the pioneers of Canção Nova Community described to me during my visit to the campus on 7 November 2001.

3. I borrow this expression from Manfred Schneider, "Luther with McLuhan," in *Religion and Media*, ed. Hent de Vries and Samuel Weber (Stanford: Stanford University Press, 2001), 198–215.

4. See John Lardas Modern, "Thinking about Melville, Religion, and Machines That Think," in this volume.

5. Jean-Luc Marion is among the most sonant of contemporary authors who define and argue for an intrinsic opposition between technique and

contemplation, alongside the one between idol and icon; see Marion, *The Crossing of the Visible* (Stanford: Stanford University Press, 2003). For an engaging reassessment of these oppositions, see Thomas A. Carlson, *The Indiscrete Image: Infinitude and Creation of the Human* (Chicago: University of Chicago Press, 2008); Jenny Slatman, "Tele-vision: Between Blind Trust and Perceptual Faith," in *Religion and Media*, ed. Weber and de Vries (Stanford: Stanford University Press, 2001), 216–26.

6. See Charles Hirschkind, *The Ethical Soundscape: Cassette Sermons and Islamic Counterpublics* (New York: Columbia University Press, 2006); see also de Abreu, "Goose Bumps All Over: Breath, Media, Tremor," *Social Text* 96 (2008): 59–78.

7. That wall-to wall sound, as Steven Connor expresses about the word *mur-mur*; see Connor, *Building Breathing Space*, last accessed 21 November 2009, http://www.stevenconnor.com/bbs/.

8. The relation of antagonism or convergence between the Catholic Charismatic Renewal and the Liberation Theology movement—as two parallel movements of the Catholic Church that derived from the reforms introduced by the Second Vatican Council in 1964—has been subjected to a variety of theological, sociological, and anthropological interpretations, and it remains a theme that active members within and across both movements much enjoy to discuss. For a sociological and anthropological interpretation of the phenomenon, see Marjo De Theije, "Ceb's and Catholic Charismatics in Brazil," in *Latin American Religion in Motion*, ed. Christian Smith and Joshua Prokopy (New York: Routledge, 1999), 111–24.

9. The expression "demons from the north," very much in vogue during the military years, was subsequently canonized in Délcio M. De Lima, *Os Demónios Descem do Norte*, 3rd ed. (Rio de Janeiro: Alves Editora, 1985).

10. A substantial archive of such alternative media can be found at the ABVP—Associação Brasileira de Video Popular (Brazilian Association of Video Popular Movement)—located in the center of São Paulo. Originally constituted by students, activists, unionists, priests, documentary filmmakers, and renowned academics such as Fernando Santoro, the ABVP went from being a very active center of human rights social activism and video production into little more than a run-down headquarters by the end of the 1990s. While I had planned to study the political aesthetics of video activism within São Paulo, this attempt was abated during my visits to the archive of the ABVP in 2000 and 2001. It was with regret that the one of the two remaining volunteers of the Association expressed during my first visit that television and televangelism had "won the contest" (*ganharam a parada*), as illustrated by the success of TV Canção Nova and likeminded

televangelicals Pentecostal and Catholic Charismatic within the cultural and religious scene of contemporary Brazil. On Pentecostal media production in Brazil, see Patricia Birman, "Future in the Mirror, Media, Evangelicals and Politics in Rio de Janeiro," in *Religion, Media and the Public Sphere*, ed. Birgit Meyer and Annelies Moors (Bloomington: Indiana University Press. 2006), 52–72; Martijn Oosterbaan, "Purity and the Devil: Community, Media and the Body; Pentecostal Adherents in a Favela in Rio de Janeiro," in *Aesthetic Formations: Media, Religion and the Senses*, ed. Meyer (New York: Palgrave Macmillan, 2009), 53–70.

11. Annabelle Sreberny-Mohammed and Ali Mohammadi, *Small Media, Big Revolution: Communication, Culture and the Iranian Revolution* (Minneapolis: University of Minnesota Press, 1994).

12. De Abreu, *In Midair: Breath, Media, Body, Space; A Study of the Catholic Charismatic Renewal Movement in Brazil* (unpublished PhD diss., University of Amsterdam, 2009).

13. See Luce Irigaray, *The Forgetting of the Air in Martin Heidegger* (Austin: University of Texas Press, 1999).

14. See Connor, *Castles in the Air: Transdisciplinarity, Space and Rem Koolhaas*, last accessed 15 October 2008, in http://www.coa.uncc.edu/arch_on_air/.

15. See, for example, Leslie Rossi, *Medieval Art: A Topical Dictionary* (Westport, Conn.: Greenwood 1996).

16. For an illustrative account on colonial encounters with the air of the Pacific, see Bernard Smith, *Imagining the Pacific in the Wake of the Cook Voyages* (New Haven: Yale University Press, 1985); Bernard Smith, *European Vision and the South Pacific* (South Melbourne: Oxford University Press, 1998).

17. Alberto Santos-Dummont (1873–1937), who played a pivotal role in the nationalistic project of "Conquest of the Air" and in the world history of aircraft, eventually committed suicide upon seeing his much beloved machines being used in WWII.

18. See David G. Storck, "Optics and Realism," in *Scientific American* (December 2004): 76–83, last accessed 28 August 2010, http://sirl.stanford.edu/~bob/teaching/pdf/arth202/Stork_SciAm04.pdf.

19. On this topic, see Sudeep Dasgupta, "Multiple Symptoms and the Visible Real: Culture, Media, and the Displacement of Vision," in *Invisible Culture: An Electronic Journal for Visual Culture* 10, no. 10 (2006), http://www.rochester.edu/in_visible_culture/Issue_10/issue10_dasgupta.pdf.

20. See Alena Alexandrova, "Image Instant/Image Plastique in Metamorphoses de L órigine," *La Metamorphose* 64 (May 2009).

21. According to *Webster's Third New International Dictionary* [Unabridged], Merriam-Webster (June 2002), the French term *comtemplari*,

formed by the conjugation of the terms *com* + *templari*, referred to "a space for observation marked out by the augur."

22. Thus Steven Connor refers to Rick Altman's "sound hermeneutic," whereby the sound asks, "where?" and the image responds, "here!"; see Connor, "Sound and the Self," in *Hearing History: A Reader*, ed. Mark M. Smith (Athens: University of Georgia Press, 2004), 61.

23. Gaston Bachelard, *Air and Dreams: An Essay on the Imagination of Movement*, trans. Edith R. Farrel and C. Frederick Farrel (1943; Dallas: Dallas Institute of Humanities and Culture Publications, 1988), 49.

24. Hannah Arendt, "The Vita Activa and the Modern Age," in idem, *The Human Condition* (Chicago: University of Chicago Press, 1958), 290.

25. Walter Benjamin, "The Work of Art in the Age of Mechanical Reproduction," in *Illuminations*, ed. Harry Zohn (1968): 219–53.

26. Ibid.

27. Samuel Weber, *Mass Mediauras: Form, Techniques, Media* (Stanford: Stanford University Press, 1996), 86–87, emphasis added.

28. Ibid, 91; see also Rafael Sanchez, "Channel-Surfing: Media, Mediumship and State Authority in the Maria Lionza Possession Cult (Venezuela)," in *Religion and Media*, ed. Weber and de Vries (Stanford: Stanford University California Press, 2001), 388–434.

29. This transcription of Benjamin's text is not included in Harry Zohn's translation in *Illuminations*, which simply reads, "You experience the aura of these mountains, of this branch"; Benjamin, "Work of Art," 223. For reference to "breathing in the aura," see Weber, *Mass Mediauras*, 85; see also Willem Van Reijen, "Breathing the Aura: The Holy, the Sober Breath," in *Theory, Culture and Society* 18, no. 6 (2001): 31–50

30. Van Reijen, "Breathing the Aura," 33.

31. See de Abreu, "Breathing into the Heart of the Matter: Why Padre Marcelo Needs no Wings," in *Postcripts* 1 (2005): 325–49.

32. It is worth noting that the CCR was only officially recognized by the Brazilian Catholic Church—represented by the national main organ of CNBB (Conference of the National Bishops of Brazil)—in 1994—that is, after twenty-five years of existence in Brazil.

33. The full quote, according to the King James Version, is, "Do you know that your body is a temple of the Holy Spirit, who is in you. . . . You are not your own. You were bought at a price. Therefore, honor God with your body"; 1 Cor. 6:19–20.

34. See WebTVCN, accessed 19 June 2012, http://www.webtvcn.com.br/.

35. St. Claire is also the patron saint of other telecommunications technologies, such as the telegraph and the telephone, in addition to her patronage of embroidery, goldsmithery, and eye diseases.

36. This vacillation produces what Brazilian anthropologist Carlos Alberto Steil calls a "chain of generational influence"; see Steil, "Renovação Carismática Católica: Porta de Entrada ou Saida do Catolicismo; Uma Etnografia do Grupo de São José, Porto Alegre," *Religião e Sociedade* 24, no. 1 (2004): 182–90.

37. Here I am making a parallel with *TV Buddha* (1974), the well-known installation by the pioneering Korean-American video artist Nam June Paik; see *Nam June Paik Studio*, accessed 19 June 2012, http://www.paikstudios.com/gallery/1.html.

38. Weber, *Mass Mediauras*, 86.

CONTRIBUTORS

Maria José de Abreu is a cultural anthropologist and post-doctoral fellow at the University of Lisbon. Her principal areas of research are religion, the body, and its technological extensions. Her latest project deals with theories of indeterminacy in media, religion, and politics, with a particular focus on Portugal and Brazil.

Alexandra Boutros is an assistant professor in communication studies and cultural studies at Wilfrid Laurier University, Canada. Her research is generally concerned with the intersection of media, technology and identity within the context of religious, social and cultural movements.

Wolfgang Ernst holds the Chair of Theories of Media, Institute of Musicology and Media Studies, Humboldt University Berlin, where he teaches media archaeology as a research practice. His current focus is on the temporality and chronopoetics of technical media. His first English-language book is *Digital Memory and the Archive*, edited and with a foreword by Jussi Parikka (2012).

Faye Ginsburg is David B. Kriser Professor of Anthropology at New York University, where she is also director of the Center for Media, Culture and History, co-director of the Center for Religion and Media, and co-director of the NYU Council for the Study of Disabilities. She is author/editor of four books, including, most recently, *Media Worlds: Anthropology on New Terrain* (2002).

Sherine F. Hamdy is an assistant professor of anthropology and Kutayba Alghanim Professor of Social Science at Brown University. Her research involves cross-cultural approaches to medicine, health, and the body. She is the author of *Our Bodies Belong to God: Organ Transplants, Islam, and the Struggle for Human Dignity in Egypt* (2012).

Jason Ananda Josephson is an assistant professor of religion at Williams College. He received his PhD from Stanford University in 2006 and has held visiting positions at Princeton University, École Française d'Extrême-Orient, and Ruhr Universität. He is the author of *The Invention of Religion in Japan* (2012).

JOHN LARDAS MODERN is an associate professor of religious studies at Franklin and Marshall College. He practices history as a trade. He is the author of *The Bop Apocalypse: The Religious Visions of Kerouac, Ginsberg, and Burroughs* (2001) and *Secularism in Antebellum America* (2011).

PETER PELS is Professor of the Anthropology of Africa at the Institute of Cultural Anthropology and Development Sociology of the University of Leiden. He specializes in the study of how people classify each other as different in religion, politics, and consumerist popular culture. He currently conducts research into global images of the future and the temporality of heritage and material culture.

JOHN DURHAM PETERS is the A. Craig Baird Professor of Communication Studies at the University of Iowa. A media historian and social theorist, he is the author, among many other works, of *Speaking into the Air: A History of the Idea of Communication* (1999).

JEREMY STOLOW is an associate professor of communication studies at Concordia University, Montreal, where he studies and teaches media history. Among various publications about religion and media is his book *Orthodox by Design: Judaism, Print Politics, and the ArtScroll Revolution* (2010).

MARLEEN DE WITTE is a cultural anthropologist affiliated with the Vrije Universiteit, Amsterdam. Her main research foci are media and religion, popular culture, and urban Africa.

www.ingramcontent.com/pod-product-compliance
Lightning Source LLC
Chambersburg PA
CBHW031231290426
44109CB00012B/243